Skills for Communicating with Patients

Third Edition

Jonathan Silverman

Associate Clinical Dean and Director of Communication Studies
School of Clinical Medicine, University of Cambridge, UK
President-elect, European Association for Communication in Healthcare

Suzanne Kurtz

Professor Emerita
University of Calgary, Alberta, Canada
Clinical Professor and Director of the Clinical Communication Program
College of Veterinary Medicine, Washington State University, US

and

Juliet Draper

Retired General Practitioner
Past Director, Eastern Deanery Cascade Communication Skills Teaching Project, UK

Forewords by

Professor Myriam Deveugele
Professor in Communication in Health Care
Department of Family Medicine and Primary Health Care, Ghent University, Belgium
President, European Association for Communication in Healthcare

and

Anthony L Suchman MD, MA
Organisational Consultant, McArdle Ramerman Center
Clinical Professor of Medicine,
University of Rochester School of Medicine and Dentistry,
Rochester, NY, US

Radcliffe Publishing
London • New York

Radcliffe Publishing Ltd
33–41 Dallington Street
London
EC1V 0BB
United Kingdom

www.radcliffehealth.com

British Library Cataloguing in Publication Data

A catalogue record for this book is available from the British Library.

ISBN-13: 978 184619 365 1

Typeset by Darkriver Design, Auckland, New Zealand
Printed and bound by Cadmus Communications, USA

Contents

Foreword by Myriam Deveugele

There used to be a time when medical professionals were at the centre of care. The professionals, mostly doctors, undertook the history taking and investigation from their own point of view, in order to make a diagnosis. They told the patient what to do, how and when. Healthcare providers hoped or believed that the patient would follow their instructions. And if the patient was not relieved of the symptoms or if the disease could not be cured, it was thought to be due to the patient's poor compliance. Is this a caricature or an old-fashioned view? Of course it is. Even in ancient times medical professionals tried to do the best they could to help the patient.

Nevertheless times have changed. Research on provider–patient communication reveals that the patient is an important co-player in the medical consultation. He or she is the 'expert' and best placed to tell about his or her body functioning, about the complaint, about the reason for looking for help. Therefore terms such as 'patient/person/people-centred care' are adopted, even by important bodies such as the WHO. We know that effective communication has important benefits for both patient and caregivers. You can find a research overview on this topic in the first chapter.

Moreover, people live longer and as a consequence have more co-morbidity and suffer more from diseases that often cannot be cured. Quality of life becomes more and more a core issue in health sciences. If a serious condition cannot be ameliorated, the patient is the only one who can give an idea of his or her most important wishes for the remaining time. If a medical professional has to deal with a patient who has two or more health issues for which the ordinary treatments are contradictory, the only person able to help is the patient. At that moment the best way to handle this problem is to listen to the patient, to his or her wishes, to make decisions on what and how to treat together with the patient.

These new insights need a changing attitude from all players in the medical field, patients and healthcare professionals. The patients have more responsibility, have to be more prepared before entering the consultation and have to be willing to engage in the conversation. The caregiver needs to establish a good relationship, to be able to listen, to discover the reason(s) for the encounter, to give information and to discuss and share the decision making with both patients and other healthcare providers, in combination with good medical reasoning and medical technical skills.

Since healthcare professionals have always demonstrated their compassion and care for the patient, one could argue that these insights, attitudes and behaviours will easily be achieved. As a consequence, a book on 'skills for communicating with patients' would then be unnecessary. We all know that this premise is incorrect – attitude and behaviour change do not follow automatically out of knowledge. Change needs training. Communication is more than being nice, communication deals with core skills that need to be learned.

Therefore, I am happy that Jonathan Silverman, Suzanne Kurtz and Julie

Draper have made the effort to publish a third edition of their very important book on communication skills. Although the Calgary–Cambridge Guides and the two companion books describing their approach (this book and *Teaching and Learning Communication Skills in Medicine*) were already established as standard texts in many medical curricula and were referred to as 'the first entirely evidence-based textbook on medical interviewing', this third edition incorporates the latest research on medical communication. This resulted in, on the one hand, added evidence and on the other some changes to the application of skills themselves, especially shared decision making, risk communication and health literacy, all topics gaining in importance and receiving more attention.

The importance of this skills-based consultation model cannot be overstressed. The Calgary–Cambridge Guides describe the core skills useful for all learners and teachers in medical sciences, for all levels of education, for specialists as well as for family doctors. These skills are useful in all conditions. Core skills pertain in difficult and challenging circumstances although it might be necessary to use them with greater intensity and awareness.

The book you have in your hands gives an answer to the challenge healthcare providers encounter when conducting accurate, effective and efficient medical consultations.

I wish you as much pleasure in reading this important work as I had myself.

Myriam Deveugele
Professor in Communication in Health Care
Department of Family Medicine and Primary Health Care,
Ghent University, Belgium
President, European Association for Communication in Healthcare
July 2013

Foreword by Anthony L Suchman

Nothing in healthcare is more important than good communication.

Healthcare is by definition interpersonal – one person seeking care from another. Without good communication, healthcare is at best wasteful and at worst dangerous. Everything depends upon the degree to which the patient and clinician understand each other accurately, develop a shared understanding of the patient's illness and commit to work together on a course of treatment.

We're not talking about good bedside manner here, a quaint term that connotes a nice but optional flourish. We're talking about clinical outcomes. Every bit of biomedical technology (the hard stuff) must be deployed within a social context of effective communication and relationships (the soft stuff) if it is to be safe and successful. There are no exceptions. The time of disdaining communication skills as 'touchy feely' is over. Communication competence is a critical component of clinical competence, and the commitment to assess and improve one's communication competence is a core element of professionalism.

Skills for Communicating with Patients is an outstanding resource in which clinicians in any health profession and at any level of experience can find insights to help them advance their communication competence. It offers very specific, practical descriptions of communication techniques and the evidence base in which they are grounded.

The methods described here will make you a better practitioner. They will also add to the quality and satisfaction of your professional life. For example, to cite one of my own personal favorites, a technique called screening, described on p. 52 ff, helps me elicit the patient's full agenda early in the visit, before I've committed all our time to the very first issue mentioned, which often is not the most important one. This is the single most powerful tool I possess for staying on schedule and avoiding the stress of running late. Another of my favorites is the approach to breaking bad news. Before I had any skills, I feared such situations, felt incompetent, rushed through them and undoubtedly added to my patients' suffering. But now, equipped with the principles and skills described on p. 224 ff, I know what to do, so I can be calmly present to my patients during a time of great need. I can be of much greater service and a previously dreaded situation is now a source of great meaning.

While *Skills for Communicating with Patients* focuses on dyadic interactions between patients and clinicians the communication skills it describes apply equally well to any kind of collaboration: conducting rounds, exploring a disagreement with a colleague, or developing a process improvement plan. Attending to content and process, to task and relationship are essential skills for success in this age of system-based care. Individuals, teams and even organizations must manage their interdependence better than they ever have before if they are to implement new models of care, interprofessional education and translational science. It's all about relationships.

For the clarity, timeliness and intellectual rigor of this book, the authors, Jonathan Silverman, Suzanne Kurtz and Julie Draper, deserve our deep appreciation. The appearance of the third edition – a spectacular sign of success – is an opportunity to celebrate their achievement, their ongoing dedication and their enormous contribution to the field of healthcare communication.

Anthony L Suchman MD, MA
Organisational Consultant,
McArdle Ramerman Center
Clinical Professor of Medicine,
University of Rochester School of Medicine and Dentistry,
Rochester, NY, US
July 2013

Preface to the third edition

Skills for Communicating with Patients is one of a set of two companion books on improving communication in medicine that together provide a comprehensive approach to teaching and learning communication throughout all three levels of medical education (undergraduate, residency and continuing medical education) and in both specialist and family medicine. Since their first publication in 1998, this book and its companion, *Teaching and Learning Communication Skills in Medicine*, have become established as standard texts in communication skills teaching throughout the world, 'the first entirely evidence-based textbook on medical interviewing' (Suchman 2003). For notification of digital developments relating to both books, please refer to www.radcliffehealth.com.

Since we wrote the second edition in 2005, there has been a considerable and sustained increase in research on healthcare communication, with approximately 400 papers per year listed on Medline on physician–patient relations and communication. In this edition, we have attempted to fully update our text to incorporate the research evidence that has accumulated during the last eight years. Updating the literature has added considerable evidence in support of the skills of the Calgary–Cambridge Guides but has resulted in very few changes to the skills themselves. The guides, which hold a central position in both books, continue to offer a comprehensive and now even more evidence-based delineation of the skills that make a difference in communicating with patients. We have not redesigned the structure of the book, which remains very similar to the second edition and is described in detail in our earlier Preface.

Much of the research evidence over the last few years has related to the burgeoning fields of shared decision making, explanation of risk and health literacy. This is reflected in Chapter 6 ('Explanation and planning') having the most new references added. However, we have incorporated new research into all chapters in this book and we hope this will enable learners and teachers to fully understand the evidence base behind contemporary medical interviewing and health communication.

Jonathan Silverman
Suzanne Kurtz
Juliet Draper
July 2013

Preface to the second edition

In producing the second editions of both evidence-based books, we seek to reflect developments and changes since the 1998 editions were published regarding:

- research on communication in healthcare
- theoretical and conceptual approaches to communication in healthcare
- medical and educational practices
- healthcare systems and other contexts where health communication occurs.

There have been enormous advances in the field of communication skills teaching in the last six years. Communication programmes have become a part of mainstream education at all levels of medical training and in many countries. Certifying summative assessment of communication skills has become an established component of many undergraduate curricula and residency training programmes, both locally and nationally. There has been increasing development of courses for faculty in communication skills teaching. And there continues to be an explosion of research in this arena, with over 2000 papers listed on Medline on physician–patient relations and medical education with respect to communication over the last six years.

The second editions of these two books reflect all of these developments. We have updated both books in relation to the current burgeoning research evidence and to changes in teaching and assessment practices. We have of course also been developing our own teaching over the last six years and have included many ideas that have been borne of that experience.

This labour of love has had many benefits for the authors of these books. We have learned much from professional colleagues, both in writing and in person, and we have benefited greatly from suggestions and ideas from our readers. We have enjoyed immensely the opportunity to reflect on our teaching approaches and consider the evidential base again. We have valued the chance to consider, conceptualise and formalise our varying experiences over the last few years. We hope that our readers enjoy the final product as much as we have constructing it.

Here, we would like to explain the rationale for the two books and briefly outline the changes we have made to the second editions. In the first edition of our companion book, *Teaching and Learning Communication Skills in Medicine*, we examined how to construct a communication skills curriculum, documented the individual skills that form the core content of communication skills teaching programmes and explored in depth the specific teaching and learning methods employed in this unique field of medical education. Our first book presented:

- an overall rationale for communication skills teaching – the 'why', the 'what' and the 'how' of teaching and learning communication skills in medicine
- the individual skills that constitute effective doctor–patient communication
- a systematic approach for presenting, learning and using these skills in practice

- a detailed description of appropriate teaching and learning methods, including:
  - innovative approaches to analysis and feedback in experiential teaching sessions
  - key facilitation skills that maximise participation and learning
- principles, concepts and research evidence that substantiate the specific teaching methods used in communication skills programmes
- strategies for constructing a communication skills curriculum in practice.

In the second edition of our companion book, we have:

- fully updated the research evidence throughout the book
- rewritten Chapter 2 to incorporate a new enhanced version of the Calgary–Cambridge Guides that was introduced in 2003 (Kurtz *et al.* 2003) (these new guides form the centrepiece of both of our second editions; the original Calgary–Cambridge Guides were developed to delineate effective physician–patient communication skills and provide an evidence-based structure for the analysis and teaching of these skills in the medical interview; the enhanced versions more explicitly delineate the content and process of medical communication, promoting a comprehensive clinical method that explicitly integrates traditional clinical method with effective communication skills)
- considerably expanded our discussion of the value and use of simulated patients in Chapter 4
- redesigned Chapters 5 and 6 to enable a more comprehensive discussion of the analysis and feedback of communication skills and the strategies for facilitating experiential teaching sessions in different learning contexts
- amplified our discussion of curriculum and programme development across all levels of medical education, first describing common elements that run across curricula in Chapter 9, and then offering specific strategies for communication teaching and learning at the different levels of medical education in Chapter 10; given the wide-ranging and burgeoning changes regarding communication teaching at the residency level, we have specifically included a number of curriculum and programme suggestions that have been implemented in specialist and primary care residency programmes
- provided a new expanded chapter on the increasingly important field of assessment of communication skills (Chapter 11)
- included a new chapter on facilitator training and faculty development which expands our discussion of this important topic (Chapter 12)
- expanded our vision of where communication training is headed next (Chapter 13).

The first edition of our second book, *Skills for Communicating with Patients*, undertook a more detailed exploration of the specific skills of doctor–patient communication. We not only examined how to use these skills in the medical interview, but also provided comprehensive evidence of the improvements that communication skills can make both to everyday clinical practice and to ensuing health outcomes. The first edition presented:

- the individual skills that form the core content of communication skills teaching programmes

- an overall structure to the consultation which helps to organise the skills and our teaching and learning about them
- a detailed description of and rationale for the use of each of these core skills in the medical interview
- principles, concepts and research evidence that validate the importance of the skills and document the potential gains for doctors and patients alike
- suggestions on how to use each skill in practice
- a discussion of the major role that these core communication skills play in tackling specific communication issues and challenges.

In the second edition of this book, we have:

- fully updated the research evidence throughout the book
- redesigned the structure of the book and each individual chapter to incorporate an enhanced version of the Calgary–Cambridge Guides that was introduced in 2003 (Kurtz *et al.* 2003), described in detail in Chapter 1
- ensured that the entire book now describes a comprehensive clinical method, explicitly integrating traditional clinical method with effective communication skills
- expanded Chapter 3 ('Gathering Information') to consider both the content and the process skills of information gathering, the complete vs. the focused history and the effect of clinical reasoning on communication process skills
- separated the material on structuring the interview into a separate chapter (Chapter 4), rather than a subsection of information gathering, and conceptualised it as a continuous thread running throughout the interview just like relationship building
- added to our consideration of relationship building in Chapter 5 the need to enhance relationships and co-ordination within healthcare organisations and with communities, as well as between patients and clinicians
- deepened the exploration in Chapter 6 ('Explanation and Planning') of the increasingly important and linked issues of shared decision making, concordance and explanation of risk
- explored in more detail in Chapter 8 how to approach specific communication issues in the medical interview and their relationship to the core process skills of the Calgary–Cambridge Guides.

We encourage our readers to study both volumes. While at first glance, it would appear that this volume might be exclusively for learners, and our companion volume exclusively for teachers, this is far from our intention.

- Facilitators need as much help with 'what' to teach as with 'how' to teach. We demonstrate how in-depth knowledge of the use of communication skills and of the accompanying research evidence is essential if facilitators wish to maximise learning in their experiential teaching sessions.
- Learners need to understand 'how' to learn as well as 'what' to learn. Understanding the principles of communication skills teaching will enable learners to maximise their own learning throughout the communication curriculum, improve their own participation in that learning, understand the value

of observation and rehearsal, provide constructive feedback and contribute to the formation of a supportive climate.

In communication skills teaching there is a fine line between teachers and learners. Teachers will continue to make discoveries about communication throughout their professional lives and to learn from their students. Learners not only teach their peers but also soon become the communication skills teachers of the next generation of doctors, whether formally, informally or as role models. No doctor can escape this responsibility.

Jonathan Silverman
Suzanne Kurtz
Juliet Draper
September 2004

About this book

This book and its companion volume, *Teaching and Learning Communication in Medicine*, are the result of a happy and fruitful collaboration between the three authors. It began with Dr Silverman taking a sabbatical with Professor Kurtz at the Faculty of Medicine, University of Calgary, Canada, in 1993. Professor Kurtz and her colleagues had been developing and extending communication curricula in medicine as well as methods for improving communication in other areas of healthcare since the mid-1970s. Dr Silverman and Dr Draper had been working together to run communication skills teaching in postgraduate general practice in East Anglia since 1989. Over a period of 20 years, the collaboration between the three authors has led to cross-fertilisation of ideas and methods and has resulted in the writing of three editions of this book and two editions of its companion volume.

About the authors

Dr Jonathan Silverman FRCGP is Associate Clinical Dean and Director of Communication Studies at the School of Clinical Medicine, University of Cambridge, and a retired general practitioner. He has been actively involved in teaching communication skills since 1988 and in 1993 he undertook a sabbatical with Professor Suzanne Kurtz, teaching and researching communication skills at the Faculty of Medicine, University of Calgary. In 1999, he became Director of Communication Studies for the undergraduate curriculum in Cambridge, which now involves over 650 half-day small group sessions per year. He has conducted communication skills teaching seminars throughout the UK, Europe and North America. In 2005, he founded the UK Council for Communication Skills Teaching in Undergraduate Medical Education for all 33 UK medical schools and served as chair until 2012. From 2008 to 2013 he was chair of the teaching committee of the European Association for Communication in Healthcare and is currently President-elect.

Dr Suzanne M Kurtz PhD is Professor Emerita, University of Calgary, Canada, where she served the faculties of education and medicine from 1976 to 2005 and directed the Faculty of Medicine's communication programme. Since 2006, she has been Clinical Professor and founding Director of the Clinical Communication Program, College of Veterinary Medicine, Washington State University. Focusing her career on improving communication and educational practices in the professions and in the community, development of communication curricula, and clinical skills evaluation, she has worked with students, residents, practising physicians and veterinarians across the specialties, nurses and allied health professionals, patient groups, teachers, administrators, industry partners, lawyers, and government and professional organisations. Contributing across diverse cultural and disciplinary lines, she continues to consult nationally and internationally at all levels of medical and veterinary practice and education and has collaborated on several health-related international development projects in Nepal, South East Asia and South Africa. Her publications include many articles and chapters, as well as an earlier book co-authored with VM Riccardi, entitled *Communication and Counseling in Health Care* (published by Charles C Thomas in 1983).

Dr Juliet Draper FRCGP, MD is a past director of the UK Eastern Deanery cascade communication skills teaching project. She has now retired from clinical work in general practice and has recently hung up her teaching boots too. For the last 10 years she has worked in the Middle East, North Africa, India and countries previously behind the Iron Curtain, helping them to set up communication curricula. This has proved to be an enormous delight and privilege. She is now a patient, among many other things, and she continues to be interested in the patient and the doctor point of view, and psychological therapies in particular.

Acknowledgements

This book would not have been written without the help of patients, learners and research and teaching colleagues from all over the world. They have taught us so much and we owe them a great debt.

Many people have helped us directly and indirectly with their ideas, support and time, in particular our families and the people we work with regularly – the facilitators, coaches and trainers in our courses and the administrative assistants, simulated patients and clients, and audiovisual technicians who assist us.

We are especially grateful to Dr Vincent M Riccardi for his foresight and seminal efforts regarding communication in medicine and patient advocacy, his early support and foundational contributions to our work, and his perceptive questions and comments.

We also especially want to acknowledge Dr Catherine J Heaton for her creative work and continual support over a period of 15 years as co-director and co-author of the undergraduate communication curriculum in Calgary. Her substantive professional contributions to the teaching and evaluation programmes and her work with learners and patients during all of that time have influenced our work and our two books greatly. We are also grateful to Meredith Simon for her insight, contributions, and support over many, many years as a veteran preceptor and, from 1999 to 2003, as co-director of Calgary's communication course.

We are particularly grateful to Bob Berrington and Arthur Hibble for providing protected time for us to write a manual for general practitioner facilitators in East Anglia in 1996. This protected time provided considerable impetus for the writing of the first edition of this book. We also thank Chris Allen, Paul Siklos and Diana Wood for their continuing and enthusiastic support of communication training at the School of Clinical Medicine, University of Cambridge. Special thanks go to John Benson for his creative vision in promoting communication skills teaching in Cambridge, for his unceasing support within the Clinical School and for co-writing the enhanced version of the Calgary–Cambridge Guides. We would like to thank Sally Quilligan, Mandy Williams, Steve Attmore (School of Clinical Medicine) and all members of the cascade programme in East Anglia for their constructive ideas and dialogue over many years.

We are similarly grateful to Annette La Grange and Bruce Clark (Faculty of Education) and Penny Jennett, Wally Temple, John Baumber, Allan Jones, Jill Nation, John Toews and the members of the Medical Skills Program Committee (Faculty of Medicine) for their ongoing and substantial administrative support of communication programmes at the University of Calgary. Special thanks also to Julie Cary, Rick DeBowes, Bryan Slinker, Warwick Bayly, Karen Hornfelt, Rachel Jensen and Daniel Haley (College of Veterinary Medicine, Washington State University) for their invaluable support and insights.

For their advice, help and encouragement we also sincerely thank Arthur Clark, Kathy Frankhouser, Brian Gromoff, Renee Martin, Roberta Walker, Cindy Adams,

Sherry George, Marcy Rosenbaum, John Spencer, Annie Cushing and Rachel Howells.

And finally, we would like to acknowledge Gillian Nineham and all the team at Radcliffe Publishing and Undercover Project Management for their continuing faith in our work and all of their suggestions and efforts on behalf of the books.

We dedicate these two books to our families, who have supported us through the long haul and who have taught us so much about communication and relationships and love.

To my father and mother, Earl and Esther Kurtz, in loving memory, Kathy (Kurtz) and Sam Frankhouser, John Kurtz and Ellen Manobla, Doug and Cat, John and Debbie, David, Kristin, Steven, Peter, Max and Dylan.

Suzanne Kurtz

To my parents, Alma and Sydney Silverman; my wife, Barbara; our children, David, Cathy and Ellie; and our grandson Max.

Jonathan Silverman

To my large extended family who perhaps knowingly and unknowingly have taught me so much, but especially to my husband, Peter; our children, Chloe, Susie and Tim; and our five grandchildren.

Julie Draper

Introduction

An evidence-based approach

The authors of this book believe passionately in the importance of communication skills in medicine – our overriding objective in writing this book and its companion has been to help improve the standard of doctor–patient communication. However, belief and passion are not enough to produce changes in medical education or clinical practice. Without evidence to back our claims that improving doctors' communication skills results in better outcomes for patients and doctors, we cannot expect a relatively new discipline such as communication skills to make substantial inroads into an already crowded curriculum of learning, whether in undergraduate, residency or continuing medical education.

So our aim for this book is to provide an evidence-based approach to communication skills in medicine. We wish not only to demonstrate how to use communication skills in the medical interview, but also to provide the research evidence that validates the importance of communication skills and which documents the potential gains to both doctors and patients alike. There is now comprehensive theoretical and research evidence to guide the choice of communication skills to include in the communication curriculum – we know which skills can actually make a difference to clinical practice. These research findings should now inform the educational process and drive the communication skills curriculum forward (Stewart and Roter 1989; Makoul 2003; Suchman 2003; Street *et al.* 2009). We provide this evidence throughout the following chapters to help learners at all levels of medical education and practice to fully understand the theoretical and research basis of the subject.

This book strives to:

- enhance the communication skills of *students, residents and established practitioners of medicine*
- provide *learners, facilitators and programme directors* with the research evidence and knowledge to understand and teach this vital subject
- convince *medical educators* of the importance of developing extensive and excellent communication skills teaching within their institutions.

In our companion book *Teaching and Learning Communication Skills in Medicine*, we explore how to actively use the evidence described here in communication skills teaching. We describe teaching and learning methods that enable the evidence not only to be used in formal presentations but also, and more important, to be introduced opportunistically to help to illuminate and deepen experiential small group or one-to-one learning.

A skills-based approach

In our companion book, we identify three areas that communication skills programmes need to address: skills, attitudes and issues. We emphasise the importance of a skills-based approach and how it should be seen as the final common pathway for all communication learning. This book therefore focuses primarily on skills rather than on attitudes or issues. We define a curriculum of core communication skills, document how to use these skills in the medical consultation and describe the theoretical and research evidence that substantiates their value.

Core skills are of fundamental importance. Once they have been mastered, more specific communication issues and challenges, such as anger, addiction, breaking bad news or cultural issues, are much more readily tackled. Many previously published texts quickly move on to these specific issues after only a brief description of core skills. Our aim is to redress this balance. We wish to provide a secure platform of core skills that will serve as the primary resource for dealing with all communication challenges. There is no need to invent a new set of skills for each issue. Instead, we need to be aware that although most of the core skills are still likely to pertain, some of them will need to be used with greater intention, intensity and awareness. We need to deepen our understanding of these core skills and the level of mastery with which we apply them. The core skills that we describe represent the foundations for effective doctor–patient communication in all circumstances.

A unified approach throughout undergraduate, residency and continuing medical education

We are especially keen to tie together the teaching of communication skills in undergraduate, residency and continuing medical education. In our own work, we use the same principles of learning and teach the same core skills in all three settings. We wish to demonstrate the need for a continuing coherent programme of communication skills teaching that extends throughout all three levels of medical education (Laidlaw *et al.* 2002), the need to both review and to reiterate previous learning and the importance of moving on to more complex situations and challenges as learners move from one level to the next. The curriculum of core skills that we offer provides a common foundation for communication programmes throughout undergraduate, residency and continuing medical education.

A unified approach to communication skills teaching in specialist and family medicine

Some commentators have suggested that it is not possible for a text on communication skills teaching to be appropriate to both general practice and the wide range of settings found in specialist medicine, as these different contexts require very different skills. We disagree with this view and feel strongly that these arguments have in the past been responsible for holding back the expansion of communication training. As many of the concepts and research efforts concerning communication skills were initially forged in general practice or psychiatry, it has been easy for specialists to say that the findings are irrelevant to the special needs of their work and that the lessons from one discipline cannot be transferred to another. The authors have considerable experience in teaching communication across a wide range of specialties and we have observed doctors' and medical students' communication skills in a wide variety of settings. Although different contexts may require a subtle shift in emphasis, our overwhelming common experience is that the similarities far outweigh the differences and that the underlying principles and core communication skills remain the same – the barriers between specialties are more in subject matter than in communication skills. In this book, we present evidence from a variety of diverse specialist settings that lends support to this approach. Our experience of facilitating the introduction of communication skills teaching into veterinary medicine, developing clinical communication programmes at all levels of veterinary education and working with veterinarians across the specialties in the UK, Australia and North America reinforces our belief that in a wide range of healthcare situations it is the same set of core communication skills that pertains.

A unified approach to communication skills teaching on both sides of the Atlantic and beyond

It has also been said that there are such important differences in culture, patient expectations, medical training, clinical management and healthcare systems between the UK, North America and other countries that it is very difficult to write a book on communication skills that appeals to such a wide audience. Again we disagree. The authors use the same principles of learning and teach the same basic skills both in England and in Canada. Professor Kurtz in particular has observed medical consultations in many countries and cultures, and the similarities are far greater than the differences. Indeed, the first two editions of both our books have been taken up in many countries and both the books and the guides that delineate the core skills (a centrepiece of both books) have now been translated into several languages.* Strangely, research and theory have not always travelled well across the oceans in any direction and teaching programmes tend not to take account of the progress made elsewhere. Consensus statements (Simpson *et al.* 1991; Makoul and Schofield 1999; Participants in the Bayer-Fetzer Conference on Physician–Patient Communication in Medical Education 2001; Von Fragstein *et al.* 2008; Bachmann *et al.* 2012), the major international conferences on communication in healthcare that have been held since 1996 and which now occur annually, and international organisations such as the American Academy on Communication in Healthcare (AACH) and the European Association for Communication in Healthcare (EACH) have begun to break down these international barriers, as did the first two editions

---

* The books have been translated into Dutch, French, Arabic and Korean and are currently being translated into Spanish and Portugese. Translated versions of the Calgary–Cambridge Guides are available in Arabic, Dutch, French, Korean, Norwegian, Spanish and several other languages.

of our books. We would like to continue the process with the third edition of this book.

Who is the intended audience for this book?

Learners at all levels of medical education

This book is intended as core material for learners in communication skills programmes whether at undergraduate, residency or continuing medical education levels. We are keen for learners to read this book to complement their experiential training. However, we emphasise that reading alone cannot replace experiential learning. As we discuss in our companion book on teaching, learning and curriculum building, cognitive knowledge by itself does not change learners' behaviour in the consultation – experiential methods are required to cement learning from knowledge-based methods into place. However, knowledge does allow learners to understand more fully just what each skill involves, the evidence for each skill leading to improved outcomes in the consultation and the issues behind communication skills training. Intellectual understanding can greatly augment and guide our use of skills and aid our exploration of attitudes.

Facilitators and programme directors

Another major audience for our book consists of the facilitators and programme directors who wish to teach, plan and develop communication skills training programmes, whether in undergraduate, residency or continuing medical education. As we discuss in our companion book, facilitators and programme directors need help with both the 'what' and the 'how' of communication skills teaching. Although the situation is beginning to change, most medically trained facilitators and programme directors were themselves educated in an era when communication skills were hardly taught at all. Too often it has been assumed that facilitators through their very practice of medicine will have gained sufficient knowledge of the specific skills involved in medical communication – the 'what' of communication skills teaching – and that all they need to learn is 'how' to teach this subject. We place equal emphasis on training facilitators and programme directors in both the 'what' and the 'how'. Both are vitally important. Our companion book tackles 'how' to teach. In this book, we help facilitators and programme directors to increase their knowledge of 'what' to teach and to understand the research basis of communication in medicine.

We recognise that facilitators and programme directors are not a uniform group. Some will have little if any communication training while others will have extensive training. Some will have just started to develop an interest in communication in healthcare while others will have already made a commitment to it that they want to strengthen and build upon. Both groups will find confirmation as well as challenge in these books.

Facilitators and directors may also come from the following very diverse backgrounds:

- *medical*:
  - community, hospital or academic-based doctors

- general practice and family practice physicians
- psychiatrists
- specialists
- nurses
- allied health professionals
● *non-medical*:
  - communication specialists
  - psychology or counselling backgrounds.

Newer additional audiences consist of learners, practitioners, educators and research-ers in pharmacy and veterinary medicine, who are using the lessons from research and experience concerning communication skills in human medicine as a foundation for their increasing efforts to enhance clinical communication in those disciplines.

This diversity has caused some stylistic difficulties in writing this book. We have often chosen to refer to facilitators in this book as if they were all doctors – we might quote the facilitator as saying to a learner group, '*we* all have similar prob-lems with patients', even though our readers, like the three authors of this book, are not all medical practitioners. We use this device because we feel that it is pref-erable to saying, 'what you doctors all do is …': it is helpful to include ourselves in such descriptions even if we are not all doctors, so as to align ourselves with the medical profession rather than seem to be 'doctor bashing'. Those of us who are not doctors have interactions with our learners that are similar to those interac-tions that doctors have with their patients, and the lessons to be learned are very similar for us all. The interdisciplinary nature of communication in medicine has strengthened and enriched the field. We hope that non-medical facilitators will understand we are not implying that all facilitators are or should be doctors.

Medical education administrators, funding agencies and medical politicians

It is vital that the importance of communication skills teaching is understood by those in positions of authority and power, including deans of medical institutions, administrators of health management organisations, hospitals and health authori-ties, medical societies, royal colleges, medical associations, funding agencies and medical politicians. It is also vital that this audience appreciates the complexity of the communication curriculum and the scholarship that underpins and validates this subject.

How have we addressed style issues in a book intended for the European, North American and wider international market?

A particular problem has been how to write this book for a diverse audience. So many words and phrases have subtly different meanings that we have had to tread carefully to avoid unnecessary confusion. Throughout the book, we have decided to use certain words consistently – we apologise for this shorthand and hope that readers will be able to translate our convention to fit their own context. For instance, we have tried to use the following terms:

specialist rather than *consultant*
resident rather than *registrar* or *trainee*
programme director rather than *course organiser*
facilitator rather than *preceptor* or *trainer*
learner rather than *student*
office or *clinic* rather than *surgery*
follow-up visit rather than *review*.

Some areas have proved to be more difficult. We use the terms *medical interview* and *consultation* interchangeably. We also use the British term *general practice* and the North American term *family medicine* to mean the same thing, despite their different meanings in North America.

Chapter 1

Defining what to teach and learn: an overview of the communication skills curriculum

Introduction

In our companion book, *Teaching and Learning Communication Skills in Medicine*, we presented a detailed rationale for communication skills training that showed the following:

- doctor–patient communication is central to clinical practice
  - doctors perform 200 000 consultations in a professional lifetime, so it is worth struggling to get it right
  - there are major problems in communication between doctors and patients
  - effective communication is essential to high-quality medicine; it improves patient satisfaction, recall, understanding, adherence and outcomes of care
- communication is a core clinical skill, an essential component of clinical competence
  - knowledge base, communication skills, physical examination and problem-solving ability are the four essential components of clinical competence, the very essence of good clinical practice
  - communication skills are not an optional add-on extra; without appropriate communication skills, our knowledge and intellectual efforts are easily wasted
  - communication turns theory into practice; how we communicate is just as important as what we say
- communication skills need to be taught and learned
  - communication is a series of skills that can be both learned and retained; it is not just a personality trait
  - experience alone can be a poor teacher
  - communication needs to be taught with the same rigour as other core skills, such as the physical examination
  - shifts in the nature of healthcare and medical practice amplify the need for even experienced doctors to continually enhance their communication skills and knowledge
- specific teaching and learning methods are required in communication skills training
  - a skills-based approach is essential to achieve change in learners' behaviour
  - experiential learning methods incorporating observation, feedback and rehearsal are required
  - a problem-based approach to communication skills learning is necessary
  - cognitive and attitudinal learning and ongoing development of capacities

such as compassion, integrity and mindfulness complement a skills-based approach, and vice versa.

We hope that we have convinced our readers not only that teaching and learning communication skills is of the utmost importance but also that appropriate teaching methods can produce effective and long-lasting change in learners' communication skills.

In this book, we develop a theme that we have already outlined in our companion volume: by undertaking communication skills training we can improve our clinical practice (*see* Box 1.1).

Box 1.1   The prize on offer from communication skills training is improved clinical performance

- Communication is not just 'being nice'; it produces a more effective consultation for both patient and doctor.
- Effective communication significantly improves:
  - accuracy, efficiency and supportiveness
  - health outcomes for patients
  - satisfaction for both patient and doctor
  - the therapeutic relationship.
- Communication bridges the gap between evidence-based medicine and working with individual patients.

More effective consultations

Throughout this book, we return to the concepts outlined in Box 1.1 and examine how the communication skills that we discuss can produce more *effective* consultations for both doctor and patient. We show how communication skills can make history taking and problem solving more *accurate* and we explore how attention to communication skills helps us to be more *supportive* to patients.

In particular, we stress how the appropriate use of communication skills enables us to be more *efficient* in day-to-day practice. We are not interested in promoting skills that are inappropriate given the time constraints within which we have to practise medicine in the real world. We argue throughout this book that using the communication skills that we suggest will enhance efficiency and we take pains to provide evidence to validate our assertions.

Improved health outcomes

We will also see how communication can significantly improve *health outcomes* for patients. Throughout this book, we relate the use of individual skills to improvements in the following parameters of care: patient satisfaction, adherence, symptom relief and physiological outcome.

To substantiate these claims for improvements in patient care, this book takes *an evidence-based approach* to communication skills that not only describes the skills and demonstrates their use in the medical interview but also provides the research and theoretical evidence that validate their importance and document the potential gains for doctor and patient alike.

Communication can also improve *outcomes for doctors*. We shall see how the use of appropriate communication skills can not only increase patients' satisfaction with their doctors but also help doctors to feel less frustrated and more satisfied in their work. Not least, effective communication can prevent patient complaints (Adamson *et al.* 2000; Kinnersley and Edwards 2008). In a very important study, Tamblyn *et al.* (2007) have demonstrated that scores achieved in patient–physician communication in the Canadian national licensing examination significantly predict complaints to medical regulatory authorities, with a linear relationship over a 12-year follow-up period.

A collaborative partnership

Together the skills that we identify support both *patient-* and *relationship-centred approaches* that promote *collaborative partnership* between the patient and the health professional. This is not because of our own subjective opinion or personal beliefs – we take this approach because the skills that enable these theoretical views of the doctor–patient relationship to be achieved have been shown both in practice and in research to produce better outcomes for both patients and doctors.

The concept of a collaborative partnership implies a more equal relationship between patient and doctor, and a shift in the balance of power away from medical paternalism towards mutuality (Roter and Hall 1992; Coulter 2002). This book explores the communication skills that doctors can employ to enhance their patients' ability to become more involved in the consultation and to take part in a more balanced relationship.

We do not mean to imply that directive or doctor-centred communication is never useful – a life-or-death emergency, for example, often requires a directive approach. The question is not which paradigm is best – doctor-, patient- or relationship-centred care – but rather which is most appropriate at any given moment. As Lussier and Richard (2008) point out, the answer to the latter question depends on the specific context and nature of the problem at that moment, as well as the needs and preferences of both the patient and the clinician at that point in time.

There is a further dimension of equal importance that is beyond the scope of this book; namely, what patients can do in the interview to influence communication and their own healthcare. Far from being passive recipients of changes that doctors adopt, patients have a major part to play in the process of the consultation. How individual patients can participate differently in the consultation, how they can take responsibility themselves to alter the doctor–patient relationship and how they can adopt a more active role in the interview are questions that equally deserve attention and investigation. Although this book touches on research that demonstrates the value of providing patients with skills to enable them to adopt a more active role in the medical interview, here we concentrate on what doctors can do in the interview to facilitate their patients' involvement.

Plan of chapter

The next six chapters of this book follow through the sequence of the medical interview and examine each individual skill in depth. They provide learners and teachers with a detailed understanding of the skills of clinical communication. First, however, to make the skills easier to understand and use, we provide an overview of what to teach and learn in the communication skills curriculum – this foundational material also appears in our companion book, *Teaching and Learning Communication Skills in Medicine*, along with additional detail. In this chapter we explore the following key questions.

- **What are the skills?**

Is it possible to break down such a complex, worthy and important task as the medical interview into its individual components? Can we identify and define the individual skills that together constitute clinical communication and that we wish to include in the communication curriculum?

- **How do the skills fit together?**

Can we present the skills within an overall conceptual framework that enables learners and teachers to make sense of the skills themselves and how they relate to the consultation as a whole?

- **Is there evidence that these skills make a difference to doctor–patient communication?**

What is the theoretical and research basis that justifies the inclusion of the skills in our communication programmes? Is there good evidence for the efficacy of these skills or is it all subjective opinion?

Types of communication skills and how they interrelate

Three broad types of skills need to be addressed in communication skills training.

1. **Content skills** – *what healthcare professionals communicate* – the substance of their questions and responses, the information they gather and give, the treatments they discuss.
2. **Process skills** – *how they do it* – the ways they communicate with patients, how they go about discovering the history or providing information, the verbal and non-verbal skills that they use, how they develop the relationship with the patient, the way in which they organise and structure communication.
3. **Perceptual skills** – *what they are thinking and feeling* – their internal decision-making, clinical-reasoning and problem-solving skills; their attitudes; their personal capacities* for compassion, mindfulness, integrity, respect and flexibility; their awareness of feelings and thoughts about the patient, about the

---

* We credit David Sluyter (2004, personal communication), a past officer of the Fetzer Institute and editor of a book on emotional intelligence, for contributing the notion of personal capacities. As he suggests, 'it is really necessary to have both the capacity ... and the skills to communicate that capacity to others.'

illness and about other issues that may be concerning them; awareness of their own self-concept and confidence, of their own biases and distractions.

It is important to emphasise that content, process and perceptual skills are inextricably linked and cannot be considered in isolation. We must give attention to all three types of skills when studying the medical interview (Riccardi and Kurtz 1983; Beckman and Frankel 1994; Kurtz *et al.* 2003; Windish *et al.* 2005; Silverman 2009). Although particular content skills, such as the questions that constitute the review of systems or that need to be asked to investigate a specific problem, are vitally important; these aspects of content are well described in many textbooks and so we devote little space to them here. The same can be said of the clinical reasoning and medical problem-solving aspects of perceptual skills. On the other hand, communication process skills and the ways in which the three types of skills interact receive considerably less attention in medical curricula. Therefore, this book and its companion focus primarily on process skills, devote attention to significant aspects of content and perceptual skills that are relevant to communication in healthcare, and look carefully at how all three types of skills influence and are influenced by one another.

Here are some examples that demonstrate the interdependence between process, content and perceptual skills.

EXAMPLE I

Say you ask a series of closed questions (process) early on in the consultation about one specific area (content). This apparently efficient way of obtaining answers to your own questions can lead to problems in effective diagnosis by preventing you from considering the wider picture. Questioning skills used inappropriately (process) can lead directly to poor hypothesis generation (perceptual).

Compare

Patient:	*'I've been having to get up in the night to pass water lately'*
Doctor:	*'OK.*
	How many times each night?
	Is there a poor stream?
	Is it difficult to start the flow?
	Do you dribble afterwards?' etc.

with

Patient:	*'I've been having to get up in the night to pass water lately.'*
Doctor:	*'Yes …'*
Patient:	*'And I've been drinking a lot.'*
Doctor:	*'Ah ha.'*
Patient:	*'My mother's diabetic. Do you think I could be?'*

EXAMPLE 2

It is fascinating to examine the link between inner thoughts and feelings and outward communication. Thoughts and feelings about a patient (perceptual) can interfere with our normal behaviour and block our communication. For instance:

- irritation with a patient's personality (perceptual) can interfere with listening and lead us to miss important cues (process)
- physical attraction to a patient (perceptual) can prevent us from asking questions about sexual matters (content) that are vital to making a correct diagnosis.

EXAMPLE 3

Unchecked erroneous assumptions (perceptual) can block effective information gathering (process) and lead us into the wrong area for discussion (content). For instance:

- assuming that a patient has come back for a routine check of an ongoing problem can prevent us from finding out until late in the proceedings that the patient has a more important problem or a new symptom to discuss.

The problem of separating content and process skills in teaching and learning about the medical interview*

Clearly, content, process and perceptual skills must be integrated in our teaching – all are essential clinical skills. Yet too often these three types of skills have been artificially divided in medical education to the detriment of learners. Separating content and process skills in the teaching of the medical interview has proven to be particularly problematic. One unfortunate result is that learners have been confronted with two apparently conflicting models of the medical interview, whether as medical students, residents or practising physicians. The first is the 'traditional medical history' (*see* Box 1.2), which details a framework for the information that clinicians are generally expected to obtain when taking a clinical history and to consider when formulating a diagnosis. This is the *content* of the medical interview.

Box 1.2   Traditional medical history

- Chief complaint
- History of the present complaint
- Past medical history
- Family history
- Personal and social history
- Drug and allergy history
- Functional enquiry/systems review

---

* Material in this section was originally published in Kurtz, Silverman, Benson and Draper (2003).

The second type of model that learners face is commonly referred to as a 'communication model'. Models such as these provide an alternative framework and list of skills that detail the means by which doctors conduct the medical interview, develop rapport, obtain the required information described in the traditional medical history and then discuss their findings and management alternatives with patients. This is in fact the *process* of the medical interview.

Confusion over process

When confronted with these two models (i.e. traditional history describing content and communication skills describing process), it is all too easy for learners to think of them as alternatives and to confuse the models' respective roles. Too often, students disregard their communication process skills learning and use the traditional medical history model as a guide not just to the content but also to the process of the medical interview. Unfortunately, this leads learners to use the framework of the traditional medical history as their process guide, reverting to closed questioning and a tight structure to the interview dictated by the search for biomedical information.

Confusion over content

Another source of confusion concerns content. Although communication models are commonly perceived to focus solely on process skills, many have introduced a new area of content to history taking – namely, the patient's perspective of their illness (McWhinney 1989). As we describe in detail in Chapter 3 of this book, the traditional medical history concentrates on pathological disease at the expense of understanding the highly individual needs and perspectives of each patient. As a consequence, much of the information required to understand and deal with patients' problems is never elicited. Studies of patient satisfaction, adherence, recall and physiological outcome validate the need for a broader view of history taking that encompasses the patient's life-world as well as the doctor's more limited biological perspective (Stewart *et al.* 1995).

The fact that patients' ideas, concerns and expectations are not a component of the traditional medical history has all too often resulted in their omission from everyday clinical practice (Tuckett *et al.* 1985) and has led communication process guides to include this area of content as a counterbalance. However, if different areas of content appear in traditional history-taking guides and communication skills guides, learners may think they need either to discover patients' ideas and concerns *or* to take a full and accurate biomedical history, when in fact they need to do both.

Marrying content and process

Later in this chapter, we discuss an approach that we have developed to solve the dilemmas mentioned here. We demonstrate a unified model of the medical interview that highlights both process and content components of the medical interview and combines the 'old' content of the biomedical history with the 'new' content of the patient's perspective.

An overall curriculum of doctor–patient communication skills

The process, content and perceptual skills described in the preceding section provide a broad frame of reference to work from. But what exactly are the specific skills of doctor–patient communication? How can we define the individual skills that we wish to include in the curriculum? How do we make them more readily accessible to facilitators and learners so that they can understand the extent of the overall curriculum? And how can we present them so that learners can remember the individual skills and understand how they relate to each other and the consultation as a whole?

We present our overview of what to teach and learn in the form of the Calgary–Cambridge Guides, the centrepiece of our whole approach to communication skills teaching and a major feature of both this book and its companion volume, *Teaching and Learning Communication Skills in Medicine*. The guides provide a concise and accessible summary of the communication skills curriculum. They establish the structure that we follow throughout this book and serve as an aide-memoire of the individual skills that we discuss.

We would like to stress that the guides do not just summarise the 'what' of the communication curriculum; they are also an important part of the 'how' of communication skills teaching and learning. In our companion volume, we provide a more detailed presentation of how to use the guides as a teaching and learning tool. Here, we repeat the rationale for the guides' derivation and approach.

The Calgary–Cambridge Guide (as presented in the 1998 editions of our companion books)

The Calgary–Cambridge Guide (Kurtz and Silverman 1996; Kurtz *et al.* 1998; Silverman *et al.* 1998) was designed to answer the aforementioned questions in a concrete, concise and accessible format. That guide was the centrepiece of the first edition of this book and its companion volume. The guide defined a skills-based curriculum built upon four main elements that influence 'what to teach and learn' in skills-based communication programmes.

1. **Structure** – how do we organise communication skills?
2. **Skills** – what are the skills that we are trying to promote?
3. **Validity** – what evidence is there that these skills make a difference in doctor–patient communication?
4. **Breadth** – what is the scope of the communication curriculum?

The guide had two broad aims:

1. to help facilitators and learners conceptualise and structure their teaching and learning
2. to assist communication programme directors, whether working in undergraduate, residency or continuing medical education, in their efforts to establish training programmes for both learners and facilitators.

Although only a few pages in length, the guide:

- proposed a framework for organising the skills of medical communication that corresponds directly to the way we structure the consultation, and therefore aids teaching, learning and medical practice
- delineated and described the individual skills that make up effective doctor–patient communication
- summarised and made more accessible the literature regarding doctor–patient communication skills
- formed the foundation of a comprehensive curriculum (Kurtz 1989; Riccardi and Kurtz 1983), providing students, facilitators and programme directors alike with a clear idea of the curriculum's learning objectives
- provided a concise summary of the skills for both facilitators and learners that they can use on an everyday basis during teaching sessions as an accessible aide-memoire and a way to structure observation, feedback and self-evaluation
- provided a common language for labelling and referring to specific behaviours
- provided a sound basis for the content of facilitator training programmes, creating coherence and consistency in the teaching of the large number of facilitators required in a communication programme
- provided a common foundation for communication programmes at all levels of training – undergraduate, residency and continuing medical education – by specifying a comprehensive set of core patient–doctor communication skills equally valid and applicable in all three contexts.

Although many people have clarified what to teach in the past and numerous guides and checklists had been available, including our own previous versions (Stillman *et al.* 1976; Cassata 1978; Sanson-Fisher 1981; Riccardi and Kurtz 1983; Cohen-Cole 1991; van Theil *et al.* 1991; van Thiel and van Dalen 1995; Novack *et al.* 1992), the Calgary–Cambridge Guide as presented in the 1998 editions of our books made significant advances by:

- providing a comprehensive repertoire of skills that is validated by research and theoretical evidence
- referencing the skills to the then current evidence
- taking into account the move to a more patient-centred and collaborative style
- increasing the emphasis on the highly important area of explanation and planning (Carroll and Monroe 1979; Riccardi and Kurtz 1983; Maguire *et al.* 1986b; Tuckett *et al.* 1985; Sanson-Fisher *et al.* 1991); more recent literature underscores the need for greater emphasis here (Towle and Godolphin 1999; Edwards and Elwyn 2001a)
- providing guidance on skills that make a difference in medical communication while allowing considerable latitude for individual style and personality.

Equally suited to both small group and one-to-one teaching, the guide has been carefully developed and refined over many years and in many different medical contexts. We are particularly indebted to Dr Rob Sanson-Fisher (Australia) for his contributions to the structure and skills of parts of the guide and to Drs Vincent Riccardi (United States) and Catherine Heaton (Canada) who were joint authors of earlier versions. This evolving guide has been used as a central feature of the undergraduate communication curriculum in the University of Calgary Faculty of Medicine in Canada for the last 25 years (Riccardi and Kurtz 1983, Kurtz 1989) and more recently in a variety of Calgary's residency and continuing medical education programmes. We are grateful to Dr Meredith Simon, who has recently helped to develop the guide further in Calgary.

It has also been introduced into the teaching of British general practice regis-trars and their facilitators in the East Anglian region and has been refined there through a process of experimentation in workshops with practising physicians and facilitators. With the help of Dr John Benson, the guide has become the central component of an extensive medical interviewing course in the undergraduate cur-riculum in the School of Clinical Medicine at the University of Cambridge.

Since their publication in 1998 and the development of the enhanced guides that we describe shortly, a number of other organisations at all levels of medical education and across a wide range of specialties have adopted the guides as the underpinning to their communication skills programmes. Institutions in Australia, New Zealand, South Africa, South America (Argentina, Brazil, Chile), the Middle East, Scandinavia, Western Europe (Italy, Germany, France, the Netherlands, Portugal, Spain), eastern Europe, Russia, Southeast Asia, Taiwan, Nepal, the UK, Canada and the United States and elsewhere have used the guide as a primary teaching resource, an assessment tool or a research instrument. The guide has also been used with only slight modification in other health professions, includ-ing pharmacy, nursing and veterinary medicine (Adams and Ladner 2004; Adams and Kurtz 2006; Radford *et al.* 2006; Greenhill *et al.* 2011; Hecker *et al.* 2012). In our companion book, we explore the use of the guide as a teaching and assess-ment tool and discuss the guide's validity, reliability and educational impact in the context of the larger issues related to curriculum development and the assessment of communication skills.

The enhanced Calgary–Cambridge Guides*

Several important issues surfaced as the 1998 version of the guide became more widely used in both our own and others' institutions. The first issue was how to enable learners to perceive the value and helpfulness of the guide without being discouraged initially by the guide's 70 individual communication process skills. We appreciate that this number of skills can seem daunting at first sight. Yet at the same time we want to be careful not to oversimplify clinical communication – it is a complex and challenging field and we would not do justice to it if we reduced the guide to only a few skills.

The second issue was how to integrate more explicitly the content and process of communication within the Calgary–Cambridge Guide.

Closely related to the first two, a third issue was how to ensure that clinical faculty and learners integrate, teach and learn communication beyond the under-graduate communication course and extend communication teaching and learning coherently into clerkship and residency programmes.

In response to these dilemmas and as a result of the experience gained since

---

* The following discussion and diagrams of the enhanced Calgary–Cambridge Guides were originally published in Kurtz *et al.* (2003).

1998, we developed an enhanced version of the Calgary–Cambridge Guides (Kurtz *et al.* 2003). Our enhancements included:

- developing a framework of three diagrams that visually and conceptually improve the way we introduce communication skills teaching and place communication process skills within a comprehensive clinical method
- devising a new content guide for medical interviewing that is more closely aligned with the structure and process skills of communication skills training
- incorporating the patient's perspective into both process and content aspects of the medical interview.

These enhancements continue to enable us to introduce the guides in three distinct stages. First, we provide a set of three diagrams that outline the framework of a communication curriculum and place it in the context of a comprehensive clinical method. The three diagrams depict this framework graphically in increasing detail and provide a logical organisational schema for both physician–patient interactions and communication skills education.

Second, we provide a comprehensive list of some 70 communication process skills that fit explicitly into this framework. By following this sequence, learners can be introduced initially to the 'essential elements' as depicted in the basic conceptual model and can then progress gradually to the comprehensive list of specific process skills relevant to each broad area. Readers familiar with the 1998 version will also notice modifications and improvements regarding some of the specific skills that comprise the process guides themselves.

As a third and final stage, we provide a guide to the content of the medical interview that offers an enhanced method for conceptualising and recording information during the consultation and in the medical record.

This content guide is more closely aligned with patient- and relationship-centred care and the specific communication skills of the Calgary–Cambridge process guide. Because of this 'fit', the two guides reinforce each other and encourage integration of content with process skills. This arrangement marries the content and process elements of the medical interview within a single model for the practice of a truly comprehensive clinical method. It also makes more apparent the relationship between clinical reasoning, content, and process skills. The enhanced Calgary–Cambridge Guides, like their predecessor in 1998, once again serve as the centrepiece for both our books.

Three diagrams: the framework of the enhanced Calgary–Cambridge Guides

The three diagrams depicting the enhanced Calgary–Cambridge Guides make it easier for learners and physicians who teach them to conceptualise:

- what is happening in a medical interview
- how the skills of communication and physical examination work together in an integrated way.

The three diagrams introduce the skills of communication and place them within a comprehensive clinical method.

The basic framework

Figure 1.1 is a graphic representation of the medical interview. Including both communication tasks and physical examination, this 'bare bones' map depicts the flow of these tasks in real-life clinical practice:

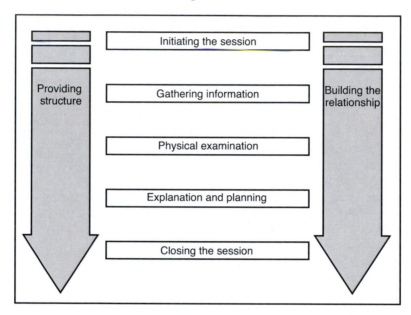

Figure 1.1   Basic framework.

In previous incarnations of the guide, we organised the skills around five basic tasks that physicians and patients routinely attempt to accomplish in everyday clinical practice: (1) initiating the session, (2) gathering information, (3) building relationship, (4) explanation and planning and (5) closing the session. The tasks made intuitive sense and provided a logical organisational schema for both physician–patient interactions and communication skill education. This structure was first proposed by Riccardi and Kurtz in 1983 and it is similar to that adopted by Cohen-Cole in 1991.

Figure 1.1 introduces two changes in the enhanced Calgary–Cambridge Guides. Instead of mapping communication only, the guides now include physical examination as one of five key tasks that physicians tend to carry out in temporal sequence during a full medical interview. Depicting physical examination in its appropriate place in the sequence reflects what happens in real-life interviews and enables learners to see the fit between physical examination and the other communication tasks more readily.

The second change sharpens the distinction between the five tasks that are performed more or less in sequence in medical interviews and the two that occur as continuous threads throughout the interview – namely, building the relationship and structuring the interview. Previously, structuring the interview was represented as a subset of gathering information, but we now realise that structuring the interview, like relationship building, is a task that occurs throughout the interview rather than sequentially. Both continuous tasks are essential for the five sequential tasks to be achieved effectively.

These changes help learners conceptualise more accurately the communication process itself as well as the relationships between the various tasks that comprise it.

The expanded framework

Figure 1.2 expands the basic framework by identifying the objectives to be achieved within each of its six communication tasks. This expanded framework of tasks and objectives provides an overview that helps the learner organise and apply the numerous communication process skills that are delineated in the more complex Calgary–Cambridge Guides. The guides then spell out the specific, evidence-based skills needed to accomplish each objective.

The complete guides include an additional 'options' section under explanation and planning that is not depicted in Figure 1.2. It contains both content and process skills related to three of the most common focuses of explanation and planning: (1) discussing the doctor's opinion and significance of problems, (2) negotiating a mutual plan of action and (3) discussing investigations and procedures. The communication skills associated with ensuring respectful conduct and keeping the patient appropriately informed during the physical examination are incorporated under relationship building, structuring, and explanation and planning.

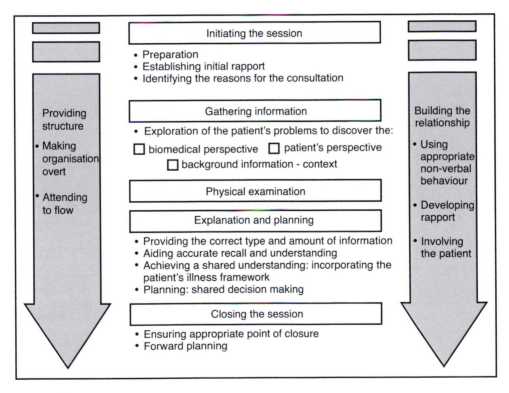

Figure 1.2   Expanded framework.

An example of the interrelationship between content and process

Figure 1.3, the third diagram, takes one task – gathering information – as an example and shows an expanded view of how content and process specifically interrelate in the medical interview.

Gathering information

Process skills for exploration of the patient's problems
- Patient's narrative
- Question style: open-to-closed cone
- Attentive listening
- Facilitative response
- Picking up cues
- Clarification
- Time-framing
- Internal summary
- Appropriate use of language
- Additional skills for understanding the patient's perspective

Content to be discovered

THE BIOMEDICAL PERSPECTIVE - DISEASE

    Sequence of events
    Symptom analysis
    Relevant systems review

THE PATIENT'S PERSPECTIVE - ILLNESS

    Ideas and beliefs
    Concerns
    Expectations
    Effects on life
    Feelings

BACKGROUND INFORMATION - CONTEXT

    Past medical history
    Drug and allergy history
    Family history
    Personal and social history
    Review of systems

Figure 1.3 An example of the interrelationship between content and process.

Together, the three diagrams in Figures 1.1–1.3 form a framework for conceptualising the tasks of a physician–patient encounter and the way that they flow in real time. This framework helps learners (and those faculty who are less familiar with communication teaching) visualise and understand the relationships between the discrete elements of communication content and process.

Increasingly, communication programmes are attempting to extend communication training beyond formal communication courses and integrate it into clerkships, residency programmes, and other bedside or clinic teaching settings. In these contexts, clinical faculty vary in their own training and knowledge base regarding communication as well as in their expertise and comfort with teaching communication skills. The three diagrams offer ways to conceptualise communication skills in the medical interview that clinical teachers and role models outside the formal communication course can relate to and use more easily.

More detailed process and content guides are then needed to move learners from merely thinking effectively about the objectives of physician–patient interaction to actually identifying the communication process skills involved and using them to discover and communicate the appropriate content of the medical interview.

Calgary–Cambridge Guides: communication process skills

With regard to communication process skills, the Calgary–Cambridge process skills guide provides that detail. This guide delineates and briefly defines 73 core, evidence-based communication process skills that fit into the framework of tasks and objectives shown in Figure 1.2. In our experience, learners and clinical faculty who understand the framework in Figures 1.1–1.3 first are better able to accept and assimilate the true complexity of doctor–patient communication as detailed in the many individual skills of the Calgary–Cambridge guides. The guides present a comprehensive repertoire of skills to be used as required, not a list to be slavishly followed. While the enhanced Calgary–Cambridge process guides are very similar to those published in 1998, readers familiar with the 1998 version will notice modifications and improvements to some of the skills. For the most part, in the second edition (2005) we made changes primarily to describe existing skills items more clearly or to make it easier to use the guides in teaching and evaluations. The most obvious changes were in the shared decision-making section, where we reconfigured items 48 to 52. In 2005, we did not add new skills or make major changes in interpretation. In this third edition, we have made only one significant change to the guides themselves and that is the addition of 'preparation' in the section on 'Initiating the session'. Significantly, the literature published since 2005 once again deepens the evidence base for the skills that are already on the guides, thus reinforcing those skills, rather than suggesting changes in interpretation or new skills to add.

CALGARY–CAMBRIDGE GUIDES COMMUNICATION PROCESS SKILLS

Initiating the session

Preparation

1. **Puts aside last task**, attends to self-comfort
2. **Focuses attention** and prepares for this consultation

Establishing initial rapport

3. **Greets** patient and obtains patient's name
4. **Introduces** self, role and nature of interview; obtains consent if necessary
5. **Demonstrates respect** and interest; attends to patient's physical comfort

Identifying the reason(s) for the consultation

6. **Identifies** the patient's problems or the issues that the patient wishes to address with appropriate **opening question** (e.g. *'What problems brought you to the hospital?'* or *'What would you like to discuss today?'* or *'What questions did you hope to get answered today?'*)
7. **Listens** attentively to the patient's opening statement, without interrupting or directing patient's response
8. **Confirms list and screens** for further problems (e.g. *'so that's headaches and tiredness, anything else?'* or *'do you have some other concerns you would like to discuss today?'*)
9. **Negotiates agenda** taking both patient's and physician's needs into account

Gathering information

Exploration of patient's problems

10. **Encourages patient to tell the story** of the problem(s) from when first started to the present, in own words (clarifying reason for presenting now)
11. **Uses open and closed questioning techniques**, appropriately moving from open to closed
12. **Listens** attentively, allowing patient to complete statements without interruption and leaving space for patient to think before answering or go on after pausing
13. **Facilitates** patient's responses, verbally and non-verbally, e.g. by use of encouragement, silence, repetition, paraphrasing, interpretation
14. **Picks up** verbal and non-verbal **cues** (body language, speech, facial expression); **checks out and acknowledges** as appropriate
15. **Clarifies** patient's statements that are unclear or need amplification (e.g. *'Could you explain what you mean by light-headed?'*)

16. Periodically **summarises** to verify own understanding of what the patient has said; invites patient to correct interpretation or provide further information
17. Uses **concise, easily understood questions and comments**; avoids or adequately explains jargon
18. **Establishes dates and sequence of events**

Additional skills for understanding the patient's perspective

19. **Actively determines and appropriately explores:**
    - patient's **ideas** (i.e. beliefs regarding cause)
    - patient's **concerns** (i.e. worries) regarding each problem
    - patient's **expectations** (i.e. goals, what help the patient had expected for each problem)
    - **effects** – how each problem affects the patient's life
20. **Encourages patient to express feelings**

Providing structure to the consultation

Making organisation overt

21. **Summarises** at the end of a specific line of inquiry to confirm understanding before moving on to the next section
22. Progresses from one section to another using **signposting, transitional statements**; includes rationale for next section

Attending to flow

23. Structures interview in logical **sequence**
24. Attends to **timing** and keeping interview on task

Building relationship

Using appropriate non-verbal behaviour

25. **Demonstrates appropriate non-verbal behaviour:**
    - eye contact, facial expression
    - posture, position, movement
    - vocal cues, e.g. rate, volume, intonation
26. If reads, writes **notes** or uses computer, does so in a **manner that does not interfere with dialogue or rapport**
27. **Demonstrates** appropriate **confidence**

Developing rapport

28. **Accepts** legitimacy of patient's views and feelings; **is not judgemental**
29. Uses **empathy** to communicate understanding and appreciation of the patient's feelings or predicament; overtly **acknowledges patient's views and feelings**

30. **Provides support**: expresses concern, understanding, willingness to help; acknowledges coping efforts and appropriate self-care; offers partnership
31. **Deals sensitively** with embarrassing and disturbing topics and physical pain, including when associated with physical examination

Involving the patient

32. **Shares thinking** with patient to encourage patient's involvement (e.g. *'What I'm thinking now is …'*)
33. **Explains rationale** for questions or parts of physical examination that could appear to be non sequiturs
34. During **physical examination**, explains process, asks permission

Explanation and planning

Providing the correct amount and type of information

Aims: to give comprehensive and appropriate information
to assess each individual patient's information needs
to neither restrict nor overload

35. **Chunks and checks**: gives information in assimilable chunks; checks for understanding; uses patient's response as a guide to how to proceed
36. **Assesses patient's starting point**: asks for patient's prior knowledge early on when giving information; discovers extent of patient's wish for information
37. **Asks patient what other information would be helpful**, e.g. aetiology, prognosis
38. **Gives explanation at appropriate times**: avoids giving advice, information or reassurance prematurely

Aiding accurate recall and understanding

Aims: to make information easier for the patient to remember and understand

39. **Organises explanation**: divides into discrete sections; develops a logical sequence
40. **Uses explicit categorisation or signposting** (e.g. *'There are three important things that I would like to discuss. First …'*; *'Now, shall we move on to …?'*)
41. **Uses repetition and summarising** to reinforce information
42. **Uses concise, easily understood language**; avoids or explains jargon
43. **Uses visual methods of conveying information**: diagrams, models, written information and instructions
44. **Checks patient's understanding** of information given (or plans made), e.g. by asking patient to restate in own words; clarifies as necessary

Achieving a shared understanding: incorporating the patient's perspective

Aims: to provide explanations and plans that relate to the patient's perspective
to discover the patient's thoughts and feelings about the information given
to encourage an interaction rather than one-way transmission

45. **Relates explanations to patient's perspective**: to previously elicited ideas, concerns and expectations
46. **Provides opportunities and encourages patient to contribute**: to ask questions, seek clarification or express doubts; responds appropriately
47. **Picks up and responds to verbal and non-verbal cues**, e.g. patient's need to contribute information or ask questions, information overload, distress
48. **Elicits patient's beliefs, reactions and feelings** regarding information given, terms used; acknowledges and addresses where necessary

Planning: shared decision making

Aims: to allow patients to understand the decision-making process
        to involve patients in decision making to the level they wish
        to increase patient's commitment to plans made

49. **Shares own thinking as appropriate**: ideas, thought processes and dilemmas
50. **Involves patient**:
    - offers suggestions and choices rather than directives
    - encourages patient to contribute their own ideas, suggestions
51. **Explores management options**
52. **Ascertains level of involvement patient wishes** in making the decision at hand
53. **Negotiates a mutually acceptable plan**:
    - signposts own position of equipoise or preference regarding available options
    - determines patient's preferences
54. **Checks with patient**:
    - if accepts plan
    - if concerns have been addressed

Closing the session

Forward planning

55. **Contracts** with patient regarding next steps for patient and physician
56. **Safety nets**, explaining possible unexpected outcomes, what to do if plan is not working, when and how to seek help

Ensuring appropriate point of closure

57. **Summarises** session briefly and clarifies plan of care
58. **Final check** that patient agrees and is comfortable with plan and asks if any corrections, questions or other issues

Options in explanation and planning (includes content and process skills)

If discussing opinion and significance of problem

59. Offers opinion of what is going on and names if possible
60. Reveals rationale for opinion
61. Explains causation, seriousness, expected outcome, short- and long-term consequences
62. Elicits patient's beliefs, reactions, concerns regarding opinion

If negotiating mutual plan of action

63. Discusses options, e.g. no action, investigation, medication or surgery, non-drug treatments (physiotherapy, walking aids, fluids, counselling), preventive measures
64. Provides information on action or treatment offered: name, steps involved (how it works), benefits and advantages, possible side effects
65. Obtains patient's view of need for action, perceived benefits, barriers, motivation
66. Accepts patient's views; advocates alternative viewpoint as necessary
67. Elicits patient's reactions and concerns about plans and treatments, including acceptability
68. Takes patient's lifestyle, beliefs, cultural background and abilities into consideration
69. Encourages patient to be involved in implementing plans, to take responsibility and be self-reliant
70. Asks about patient support systems; discusses other support available

If discussing investigations and procedures

71. Provides clear information on procedures, e.g. what patient might experience, how patient will be informed of results
72. Relates procedures to treatment plan: value, purpose
73. Encourages questions about and discussion of potential anxieties or negative outcomes

Calgary–Cambridge Guides: communication content

The revised content aspect of the guides offers an alternative method of *conceptualising* and *recording* information during the consultation and in the medical record. The traditional ways of recording medical information (*see* Box 1.2) are retained, but they are enhanced by explicitly including:

- a list of the problems that the patient wishes to address (not one 'complaint')
- progression of events
- the 'new' content regarding the patient's perspective
- possible treatment alternatives considered by the physician
- a record of what the patient has been told
- the plan of action that has been negotiated.

With these additions, the content guide (*see* Figure 1.4) parallels current medical practice more closely than the traditional approach.

By making it easier for learners to routinely include both 'old' and 'new' content in real-life practice, these additions result in improvements to both teaching and practice regarding the medical record. (For use in practice, each item in the content guide would be followed by a space where learners can write the appropriate information as they make notes during the interview and later write up their notes in the medical record.)

The headings on the content guide and the sequential tasks of medical interviewing correspond closely:

- the patient's problem list corresponds to initiation
- exploration of the patient's problems corresponds to gathering information
- physical examination is the same in both frameworks
- the rest of the content guide's headings correspond to explanation and planning.

Thus the improved content guide is also more closely aligned with the specific communication skills of the Calgary–Cambridge process guide. As a result, the two guides reinforce each other and encourage integration of content with process skills.

The need for a clear overall structure

An important element of the skills-based curriculum that we have described here is the provision of a clear overall structure within which the individual communication skills are organised. In both this and our companion book, we refer repeatedly to the importance of the structure so explicitly provided by the framework of the Calgary–Cambridge Guides (Figures 1.1 and 1.2). Why do we place such value on defining such an overt structure?

An understanding of the structure has benefits to practitioners, learners and facilitators alike.

- **For practitioners,** an awareness of the structure prevents the consultation from wandering aimlessly and important points from being missed. Communication skills are not used randomly – different skills need to be deployed purposefully

REVISED CONTENT GUIDE TO THE MEDICAL INTERVIEW

Patient's problem list

Exploration of the patient's problems

Biomedical perspective - disease	*Patient's perspective - illness*
Sequence of events	Ideas and beliefs
Symptom analysis	Concerns
Relevant systems review	Expectations
	Effects on life
	Feelings

Background information - context
Past medical history
Drug and allergy history
Family history
Personal and social history
Review of systems

Physical examination

Differential diagnosis - hypotheses
Including both disease and illness issues

Physician's plan of management
Investigations
Treatment alternatives

Explanation and planning with patient
What the patient has been told
Plan of action negotiated

Figure 1.4 Revised content guide.

and intentionally at different points in the consultation. We therefore need to keep the structure in mind so that we can remain aware of the distinct phases of the interview as we proceed. For instance, if the doctor does not recognise that the gathering information phase of the interview involves developing an understanding of the patient's individual reaction to their illness as well as the clinical aspects of their disease, the doctor may enter the explanation and planning phase of the interview prematurely and fail to address the patient's real concerns. Of course, an awareness of structure in the consultation has to be combined with flexibility – consultations do not have a fixed path that can be dictated by the doctor without reference to the patient. But without structure, it is all too easy for communication to be unsystematic and unproductive.

• **For learners**, a list of the individual communication skills alone is not sufficient. There are too many skills to remember if they are simply listed without categorisation. Learners need an overall conceptual model to help to organise the evidence-based skills into a memorable and useful whole. In Chapter 3 of our companion book, we discuss the importance of experiential methods in producing change in learners' communication skills. However, experiential learning is intrinsically random and opportunistic – the feedback and suggestions can be difficult to pull together. Providing a structure into which skills can be placed as they arise helps learners to order the skills that they discover opportunistically in experiential work and to see how the individual pieces fit together into the consultation as a whole.

- **Facilitators** may also lack a clear idea of how to pull together the individual skills or skill sets that they recognise as important learning areas. Without an overall conceptual model, the numerous skills of the medical interview can appear to be a disorganised bag of tricks. Facilitators can find it difficult to link the different skills together in their teaching. Providing them with a clear and overt structure can help overcome this problem. Structure has the added advantage of enabling facilitators to take an outcome-based approach in their communication skills teaching (*see* Chapter 4). Structure establishes an overview enabling facilitators to ask two central questions of learners: 'Where are you in the interview?' and 'What are you trying to achieve?' Having established a direction, the individual skills then help with the next question: 'How might you get there?' The facilitator can also use the structure to ask similar questions with respect to the patient: 'Where is the patient in the interview?' 'What is the patient trying to achieve at that given moment?' 'How might you discover this information and then use communication skills to respond?'

We use the conceptual model to structure our communication learning and effort in much the same way that experienced clinicians use schema in clinical reasoning: to access and apply knowledge or skills systematically, to aid memory, to impose coherence and order on what would otherwise be unusable and random pieces of information.

Choosing the process skills to include in the communication curriculum

At this point we can almost hear readers saying, 'You must be joking – 73 process skills to learn, assimilate and master: that's impossible!' Does it really need to be that complicated? Couldn't we reduce the numbers or amalgamate a few items? Is it really necessary to try to incorporate all of these skills into each consultation? (Silverman 2007).

Our unapologetic answer to this is that the medical interview is indeed very complex and cannot be summed up in a few broad generalisations. We have already seen that communication is a series of learned skills and that it is both possible and essential to break the consultation down into these individual skills if we wish to identify, practise and assimilate new behaviours into our practice of medicine. All of the skills listed in the guides can be of great value to the process of the interview; all, as we shall see shortly, have been validated by theory or research; and all will repay our attention.

Does all this mean that you have to use all 73 process skills in every encounter? The answer, of course, is no. We are not suggesting that every skill needs to be employed on every occasion. The particular skills you need will depend on the situation and the specific outcomes that you and the patient want to achieve. By making this quite clear to learners from the very outset, we can help defuse the anxiety associated with such a long list. For instance, although most of the skills in the gathering information phase of the interview are appropriate to every consultation, the use of many of the items in the explanation and planning phase needs to be tailored to the individual circumstances of the interview – the total repertoire of skills in explanation and planning will not be used in every consultation. Nonetheless, familiarity with all of the skills will undoubtedly benefit learners. At the very least, the skills can then be used intentionally and with appropriate intensity whenever the going gets tough!

Learners can use the guides to develop their learning agenda for a given interview by selecting specific skills from the comprehensive list. When the guides are used as the basis for feedback in small group teaching, facilitators can assign individual observers to focus their attention and feedback on different sections or subsection of the guides.

So, what is the basis for the inclusion of each of the 73 listed skills in the Calgary–Cambridge curriculum? Are we able to validate the importance of each of these skills in any way or is it purely subjective opinion? Where does the justification for these skills come from?

The research and theoretical basis that validates the inclusion of each individual skill

It is no longer appropriate to consider communication skills teaching as simply raising awareness of the importance of communication in the consultation. Nor is it just a matter of sharing various approaches, of increasing the range of possibilities available, of treating all suggestions as equally valid. Certain skills and methods have now been shown to make a substantial difference to doctor–patient communication and to ensuing health outcomes.

We are fortunate that over the last 40 years an extensive cannon of theoretical and research evidence has accumulated that enables us to define the skills that enhance communication between patient and physician. Research clearly demonstrates how the use of specific skills can lead to improvements in patient satisfaction, adherence, symptom relief and physiological outcome. We can now promote these skills as worth teaching in a communication teaching programme and using with intention in clinical practice. We are able to confidently answer the question 'Where's the validity?' and effectively counter the suggestion that communication skills are purely subjective.

The curriculum of skills is not and should not be static. Research will continue to accumulate to challenge our preconceptions and move the goalposts of communication skills teaching (Griffin *et al.* 2004; de Haes and Bensing 2009; Street *et al.* 2009; von Fragstein *et al.* 2008). For instance, in recent years, research findings have enabled the curriculum to shift in two important directions. First, there has been increasing emphasis on the important but often previously neglected field of explanation and planning (information giving). Second, there has been a gradual move towards a more patient-centred, relationship-centred, and collaborative approach.

In this chapter, we have simply delineated a curriculum for communication skills programmes by listing and briefly defining each skill. In the following six chapters, we describe the skills more fully and examine in depth the concepts, principles and research evidence that validate each skill.

Underlying goals and principles of communication that helped in choosing the skills

As well as the research evidence, a straightforward set of *goals* and *principles* of communication also influenced the choice of items to include in the guide. Together, they provide a simple and coherent theoretical foundation for the guide and for the development of communication curricula that result in improved communication in healthcare.

The *goals* that physicians and patients attempt to achieve whenever they communicate with each other are shown in Box 1.3. These are the outcomes we hope to have an impact on by enhancing the communication skills of healthcare providers.

Box 1.3 Goals of communication in healthcare

Increasing:
- accuracy
- efficiency
- supportiveness

Enhancing patient and physician satisfaction
Improving health outcomes
Promoting collaboration and partnership (relationship-centred care)

The choice of skills has also been influenced by the five principles of effective communication described in Box 1.4. Applicable to any setting, these principles help us to understand what exactly it is that constitutes effective communication (Kurtz 1989).

Box 1.4 Principles that characterise effective communication

Effective communication is characterised by the following principles.

1. **It ensures an interaction rather than a direct transmission process.** If communication is viewed as a direct transmission process, the senders of messages can assume that their responsibilities as communicators are fulfilled once they have formulated and sent a message. However, if communication is viewed as an interactive process, the interaction is complete only if the sender receives feedback about how the message is interpreted, whether it is understood and what impact it has on the receiver.

Just imparting information or just listening is not enough – giving and receiving feedback about the impact of the message becomes crucial. The emphasis moves to the interdependence of sender and receiver, and the contributions and initiatives of each *become more equal in importance* (Dance and Larson 1972). The aim of communication becomes the establishment of mutually understood common ground (Baker 1955). Establishing common ground and confirmation both require interaction.

2. **It reduces unnecessary uncertainty.** Uncertainty distracts attention and interferes with accuracy, efficiency and relationship building. Unresolved uncertainties in any area can lead to lack of concentration or anxiety, which in turn can block effective communication. For example, patients may be uncertain about what to expect during a given interview, about the significance of a line of questioning, about the role of a particular member of the healthcare team, or about the attitudes, intentions or trustworthiness of the other individual. Reducing uncertainty about diagnosis or expected outcomes of care is obviously important although living with some uncertainty is often a necessity in medical situations. However, even then, openly discussing areas where knowledge is lacking or no one is certain what the best choice is can help to reduce uncertainty by establishing mutually understood common ground.

3. **It requires planning and thinking in terms of outcomes.** Effectiveness can only be determined in the context of the outcomes you and or the patient are working toward. If I am angry and the outcome I seek is to vent emotion, I proceed in one direction. However, if the outcome I want is to resolve any problem or misunderstanding that may have caused my anger, I must proceed in a different way to be effective.

4. **It demonstrates dynamism.** What is appropriate for one situation is inappropriate for another – different individuals' needs and contexts change continually. What the patient understood so clearly yesterday seems beyond comprehension today. Dynamism underscores the need not only for flexibility but also for responsiveness and involvement, for engaging with the patient.

5. **It follows the helical model.** The helical model of communication (Dance 1967) has two implications. First, what I say influences what you say in spiral fashion, so that our communication gradually evolves as we interact. Second, reiteration and repetition, coming back around the spiral of communication at a little different level each time, are essential for effective communication.

Skills and individuality

Each process skill listed in the guides is only a clue to learners and facilitators that this is an area where specific behaviours and phrases need to be developed. The list by itself is not enough – each learner has to discover his own way to put each skill into practice. The guides identify the skills that have emerged from research and practice as being of value in doctor–patient communication, but they do not attempt to specify exact or recommended ways of accomplishing these skills. An important task of communication skills teaching is to give participants the opportunity to try out phrases and behaviours that fit their own individual personalities and to extend the repertoire of skills with which each participant is comfortable.

- **Structure**: where am I in the consultation and what do I and the patient want to achieve?
- **Specific skills**: how do I get there with the patient?
- **Phrasing or behaviour**: how can I incorporate these skills into my own style and personality?

A second task of communication teaching is to develop the individual's capacity for *flexibility* such that the individual can apply the skills and relate to the patient in different ways at different times as appropriate. Flexibility requires development not only of communication skills and various ways to apply them but also of the individual's capacity for mindfulness, including their ability to be fully present with each patient, to reflect with accuracy on what is needed at any given moment and to decide on how to apply the needed skills most appropriately. What is called for will vary from patient to patient, across time, and even within a single visit depending on the nature of the problem and the context, the needs and preferences of the patient, and the needs of the clinician (Lussier and Richard 2008).

Going beyond specific skills into individuality is the real challenge of experiential learning (Skelton 2005). Indeed, Salmon and Young (2011) and Skelton (2011) have highlighted the potential conflict between skills teaching and the aim of creativity. We cannot and should not be prescriptive about the best way to proceed in any circumstance. We must recognise that there are enormous variables that influence what is best for you as an individual in a given situation. However, we must also recognise that we can now advocate certain skills that are likely to be more effective than others (Silverman *et al.* 2011).

It is the repeated trying out of alternatives in rehearsal, role-playing with other learners or practising with simulated or real patients that allows us to reconcile the two concepts of skills and individuality. The list of skills is in itself only a start. To learn how to use each skill requires practice and further feedback and through this process of repeated practice, feedback and rehearsal, each learner stamps his own individuality on the communication process.

Relating specific issues to core communication skills

The skills collated in the guides provide the foundations for effective doctor–patient communication in a variety of different medical contexts. There are many highly challenging situations for doctors when they communicate with patients – for example, in breaking bad news, bereavement, revealing hidden depression, gender and cultural issues, communicating with older patients, prevention and motivation. These issues clearly deserve special attention in our teaching and we shall be exploring them further in Chapter 8. However, we stress that the skills delineated in the guides are the *core* communication skills required in all these circumstances, providing a secure platform for tackling these specific communication issues. Although the context of the interaction changes and the content of the communication varies, the process skills themselves remain the same – the challenge is to deepen our understanding of these core skills and the level of mastery with which we apply them.

Summary

In this chapter, we have defined the broad types of skills that constitute medical communication. We have described the individual skills to be included in communication curricula and the theoretical and research bases that validate the choice of these particular skills. We have presented the curriculum of skills in the form of the enhanced Calgary–Cambridge Guides, which not only list the skills but also provide a structure or conceptual framework that enables facilitators and learners to make sense of the individual skills and how they relate to the consultation as a whole.

We shall now explore the individual skills in more detail. What is the rationale for using each skill in the consultation? How is each skill used in practice? And what is the research and theoretical evidence that validates each individual skill? The next six chapters examine these areas in depth. This book is organised to follow the structure of the Calgary–Cambridge Guides, each of the following six chapters describing the process skills that pertain to one task of the basic framework. We start by looking at the skills required for beginning the interview.

Chapter 2

Initiating the session

Introduction

The beginning of the interview is a particularly rich area to explore in communication skills teaching. In these opening minutes, we make our first impressions, begin to establish rapport, attempt to identify the problems that the patient wishes to discuss and start to plan a course for the interview. The scene is set for the rest of the consultation. Yet we know from research that many problems in communication occur in this initial phase of the interview. As we shall see, physicians frequently even fail to discover the most important reason for the patient's attendance!

Doctors tend to underestimate the potential difficulties and opportunities of these brief first minutes. For example, in almost every postgraduate teaching course that we have run, the participants' own agenda at the start of the course emphasises problems in ending the consultation and in keeping to time. Yet so often it becomes apparent as the course proceeds that it is the beginning rather than the end of the interview that is the root cause for many of their perceived difficulties.

Consultations in medicine occur in widely differing contexts – from new to review appointments, from hospital to general practice, from the consulting room to the bedside, from the hospice to the home. Although at first sight there are many differences between the beginnings of interviews in these very diverse settings, the overall objectives and individual skills required are remarkably consistent. The problems that both doctors and patients face in the initial stages of an interview are very similar wherever they meet.

The specific communication skills that doctors choose to demonstrate at the beginning of the consultation are not merely social niceties: they have an important impact on the accuracy and efficiency of the interview and on the nature of the doctor–patient relationship. We therefore set initiation apart as a separate task, devoting a whole chapter to discussing what will take at most only a few minutes to achieve in real time.

Problems in communication

One of the aims at the beginning of the consultation is to identify what the patient wishes to discuss. Here the research evidence extending over more than 30 years reveals some particularly salutary lessons:

- Stewart *et al.* (1979) showed in primary care in Canada that 54% of patients' complaints and 45% of their concerns were not elicited.
- Starfield *et al.* (1981) recorded that in 50% of primary care visits the patient and the doctor did not agree on the nature of the main presenting problem.

- Burack and Carpenter (1983) found that patients and doctors agreed on the chief complaint in only 76% of somatic problems and in only 6% of psychosocial problems in primary care visits in the United States.
- Beckman and Frankel (1984) showed that primary care doctors in the United States frequently interrupted patients so soon after they began their opening statement – after a mean time of only 18 seconds! – that they failed to disclose other equally significant concerns.
- Byrne and Long (1976) identified that interviews in general practice in the UK were particularly likely to become dysfunctional if there were shortcomings in that part of the consultation relating to 'discovering the reason for the patient's attendance'.
- Rhodes *et al.* (2004), in a study in an emergency department in the United States, demonstrated that residents introduced themselves in only two out of three encounters, rarely indicating their training status (8%). Despite a tendency for doctors to start with an open-ended question, (63%), only 20% of patients completed their presenting complaint without interruption. The average time to interruption was 12 seconds.
- Low *et al.* (2011) demonstrated the considerable extent of unvoiced needs and concerns by primary care patients in Malaysia.

Clearly, there is little point in being an excellent diagnostician or possessing great factual knowledge if you are not dealing with the patient's most important problems!

Objectives

We begin our exploration of what to teach and learn in this first section of the interview by looking at our objectives – at what we are hoping to achieve. One of the principles of effective communication that we outlined in Chapter 1 is that *communication requires planning and thinking in terms of outcomes*. It is therefore important in communication to consider our objectives. Objectives make us think about 'Where do we want to get to?', whereas work on individual skills provides strategies for 'How do we get there?'

Objectives include the following:

- establishing a supportive environment and initial rapport
- developing an awareness of the patient's emotional state
- identifying as far as possible *all* of the problems or issues that the patient has come to discuss
- establishing with the patient a mutually agreed agenda or plan for the consultation
- developing a partnership with the patient, enabling the patient to become part of a collaborative process.

These objectives encompass many of the tasks and checkpoints mentioned in other well-known guides to the consultation:

- Pendleton *et al.* (1984, 2003):
  - to understand the reasons for the patient's attendance
  - to establish or maintain a relationship with the patient that helps to achieve the other tasks.
- Neighbour (1987):
  - connecting – establishing rapport with the patient
  - summarising – 'Have I sufficiently understood why the patient has come to see me?'
- AAPP Three-Function Model (Cohen-Cole 1991):
  - gathering data to understand the patient's problems
  - developing rapport and responding to the patient's emotions.
- Bayer Institute for Health Care Communication E4 model (Keller and Carroll 1994):
  - engaging the patient.
- The Four Habits Model (Frankel and Stein 1999; Krupat *et al.* 2006):
  - investing in the beginning.
- The SEGUE Framework for teaching and assessing communication skills (Makoul 2001):
  - setting the stage.
- The Maastricht Maas Global (van Thiel and van Dalen 1995):
  - introduction
  - clarification.
- Essential Elements of Communication in Medical Encounters: Kalamazoo Consensus Statement (Participants in the Bayer-Fetzer Conference on Physician–Patient Communication in Medical Education 2001):
  - open the discussion
  - build a relationship.
- Patient-centred medicine (Stewart *et al.* 2003):
  - exploring both the disease and the illness experience.
- The Model of the Macy Initiative in Health Communication (Kalet *et al.* 2004):
  - prepare
  - open
  - gather.
- The Six Function Model (de Haes and Bensing 2009):
  - fostering the relationship
  - gathering information.

Skills

Having established the objectives of the initiation phase, we can turn our attention to the skills which help us to achieve these goals. The following list of skills is taken from the Calgary–Cambridge Guides (*see* Chapter 1).

Box 2.1   Skills for initiating the session and building the relationship

---

Preparation
- Puts aside last task, attends to self-comfort
- Focuses attention and prepares for this consultation

Establishing initial rapport
- Greets patient and obtains patient's name
- Introduces self, clarifies role and nature of interview, obtains consent if necessary
- Demonstrates interest and respect, attends to patient's physical comfort

Identifying the reason(s) for the consultation
- Identifies the patient's problems or the issues that the patient wishes to address with appropriate opening question (e.g. 'What problems brought you to the hospital?' or 'What would you like to discuss today?' or 'What questions did you hope to get answered today?')
- Listens attentively to the patient's opening statement without interrupting or directing the patient's response
- Confirms list and screens for further problems (e.g. 'So that's headaches and tiredness; anything else …?' or 'Do you have some other concerns you would like to discuss today?')
- Negotiates agenda taking both patient's and physician's needs into account

---

'What' to teach and learn about the initiation: the evidence for the skills

PREPARATION

As we have seen in Chapter 1, *unresolved uncertainties and anxieties can lead to lack of concentration, which in turn can block effective communication*. In clinical practice, it is easy for your mind to still be on the last patient or telephone call, the growing queue of patients still to be seen or your own personal needs. You may find yourself still calling up records on the computer or completing the records as you greet the next patient. These thoughts, feelings and actions can so easily get in the way of providing full concentration at the beginning of the consultation. The alternative is to prepare yourself so that you can give your full attention to the patient and are not distracted by other issues at this critical moment. Although this may be just one of many routine consultations of the day for the doctor, for the patient it may be a far more important and significant occasion. The patient is usually entirely focused on the interview to come – it is clearly helpful if the doctor reciprocates with his full attention.

Suggestions for preparation and achieving full concentration include:

- **putting aside the last task** – making sure that the last consultation will not impinge on the next, making arrangements to return to unresolved issues later

- **attending to our personal needs and comfort** – ensuring that hunger, heat or sleepiness do not disturb your concentration in the next interview
- **shifting focus to the consultation at hand** – preparing as necessary by reading the written or computerised records, searching for results or thinking about the patient's history
- **concluding these activities before greeting the patient** – being free to concentrate in as relaxed and focused a way as possible.

This kind of preparation and focus goes deeper than common courtesy and respect. A study looking at family physicians' perceptions of the causes of their self-admitted clinical errors (Ely *et al.* 1995) showed that hurrying and distraction were among the most common causes to which physicians attributed their mistakes.

ESTABLISHING INITIAL RAPPORT

There has been little research into the value of greetings in the medical setting – presumably because it seems so obvious – but the following elements deserve consideration:

- greeting the patient
- introducing yourself
- clarifying your role
- obtaining the patient's name
- demonstrating interest and respect, attending to the patient's physical comfort.

Introductions are a fascinating insight into doctors' practices, particularly as they so often seem to be completely omitted! Patients frequently complain that the doctor did not introduce himself, that they weren't sure who they were seeing or what the doctor's role was within the team.

Greeting the patient and introducing yourself

If you have not met the patient before, it is relatively easy to welcome and introduce yourself to the patient using a combination of appropriate non-verbal approaches such as handshake, eye contact and a smile plus a suitable verbal greeting:

> *'Hello, I'm Dr Jones, do come and sit down.'*

Experienced doctors often know their patients well and do not need to introduce themselves to every patient. However, they sometimes assume that patients know who they are without any evidence that this is so and inappropriately omit a verbal introduction. They assume that if they have seen a patient before, the patient will remember who they are and therefore there will be no need to introduce themselves again. They may also feel uncomfortable about introducing themselves to patients who they may have met before but cannot now remember. We need to develop ways of overcoming such problems:

> *'Hello, my name is Dr Jones. Am I right in thinking we haven't met before?'*

Clarifying your role and the nature of the interview

For the patient, the uncertainty of not knowing who the doctor is or how she fits into their care can be very unsettling. Yet in a study of 50 medical students, Maguire and Rutter (1976) reported that 80% failed to introduce themselves adequately and to explain their intentions. Would it not be helpful for students to explain their position within the team, the length of time that they have for interviewing the patient, what they will do with the information obtained and how they will relate this information to the doctor in charge of the patient? Would it not be best to state from the outset that the interview is for the prime benefit of the student rather than the patient if that is the case, or, conversely, if this is the only opportunity the patient will have to give their story and ask questions? Similarly, obtaining genuine consent should be seen as an essential part of the introductory process for medical students:

> *'Hello, my name is Catherine Singh, I am a student doctor working with Dr Ko. I am learning how to interview patients. I think Dr Ko suggested to you that I might spend 15 minutes talking to you before he joins us and tries to help you with your problem. Would that still be all right?'*

It might be argued that this is superfluous for experienced doctors, especially in some settings such as family practice, where both patient and doctor understand the nature of the consultation and the cultural rules of the encounter. However, consider the situation in teaching hospitals, health maintenance organisations, interdisciplinary teams and emergency departments. In such settings, where many different clinicians may relate to each individual patient, doctors can prevent confusion by carefully explaining their role and the nature of the interview and obtaining consent rather than letting things go unsaid and be ripe for possible misinterpretation. Yet, as mentioned earlier, Rhodes *et al.* (2004) demonstrated that emergency department residents introduced themselves in only two out of three encounters, rarely indicating their training status (8%). These clarifications are also important when meeting new patients or when circumstances dictate that anyone is changing roles.

> *'Hello, I'm Dr Ko. May I sit here? I'm one of the specialist surgeons attached to the hospital. Your family doctor, Dr Jones, has asked me to see you. May I spend 20 minutes with you now discussing your problems and examining you?'*

Obtaining the patient's name

In circumstances where you know the patient well, this is clearly an unneces-sary step, but whenever there is a possibility of confusion it is always advisable to check that you have the correct name and pronunciation and that the patient's name matches that on the chart. Avoid making assumptions about marital status or preferred form of address.

> 'Hello, I'm Dr Jones, I'm one of the four partners who make up this family practice. Please sit down. Can I just check – is it Mrs Mary French? (pause) I don't think we've met before – what do you prefer that I call you?'

Demonstrating interest and respect, attending to the patient's physical comfort

We cannot emphasise enough the importance of taking steps to build the relation-ship from the very beginning of the interview. Demonstrating interest, concern and respect for the patient and demonstrating appropriate non-verbal behaviour are so important in laying the groundwork for a productive and collaborative relationship.

The doctor's behaviour and demeanour here are vital in enabling the patient to feel welcomed, valued and respected. Taking steps to establish trust and develop the relationship early on will set the scene for efficient and accurate information exchange as the interview unfolds. Eide *et al.* (2003) have demonstrated how very brief informal discussion helps build rapport early on in the consultation and increases patient satisfaction with very little investment of time. Beach *et al.* (2006) showed that when physicians had respect for particular patients, patients were able to perceive this and physicians were more positive in affect and provided more information.

Because this vital area requires attention throughout the whole interview and not just at the beginning, we devote all of Chapter 5 to building the relationship. There we shall explore the research evidence for the importance of rapport-building skills and non-verbal communication in detail.

Virtually everything that we discuss about initiating the interview in this chapter contributes to relationship building by encouraging the patient's contributions and promoting a collaborative approach. However, before leaving our consideration of the skills associated with establishing initial rapport, we would like to comment on one particularly important item: attending to the patient's physical comfort.

Environmental factors affect physical and psychological comfort. They influence position, posture and eye contact, our perception and attitudes and our ability to attend. Are room temperatures set so patients waiting in dressing gowns are com-fortable? Is lighting neither glaring nor too dim? Are the patient and the doctor positioned so that neither must look into the glare of uncurtained windows? In waiting areas, are diversions such as written materials, aquariums or patient edu-cation materials available?

Unless problems such as pain, nausea and injury dictate otherwise, most of us are more comfortable talking while sitting in a chair rather than lying down or dangling our legs over the side of an examining table. All the better if the doctor is also seated, as this puts both participants on a more equal footing, makes unobtrusive note-taking easier, and gives the impression that the doctor is willing to take the time that is needed to give full attention to the patient. In fact, Swayden *et al.* (2012) showed in a randomised controlled study that postoperative surgical patients perceived physicians who sat rather than stood at their bedside as being present longer, even though the actual time the physician spent at the bedside did not change significantly. Patients with whom the physician sat reported a more positive interaction and a better understanding of their condition.

Placing furniture so that doctor and patient can sit at a knee-to-knee angle rather than side by side or directly across from each other is helpful. Positioning communicators on opposite sides of a desk has been found to have an intimidating, competitive or barrier effect (Sommer 1971). People want easy eye contact but not so direct that they cannot readily 'escape'.

As much as possible, talk with patients while they are fully dressed. If sensitive or private matters will be discussed, close doors, draw curtains between beds or, if no privacy is possible, at least reassure the patient and be aware that environment-induced uneasiness may inhibit or distract the patient to the point of giving inaccurate or incomplete information. Finally, keep in mind that all these aspects of environment are as likely to influence the doctor as the patient.

IDENTIFYING THE REASON(S) FOR THE CONSULTATION

Having exchanged introductions and established initial rapport, the next step is to determine what issues the patient wishes to discuss. What is the patient's agenda for the interview? Why has the patient come today? In the context of seeing patients in hospital, clinic or at home, doctors need to clarify the problems that the patient wishes to address, as well as the doctor explaining their own reasons for coming to see the patient.

McKinley and Middleton (1999), for instance, have shown in a study of general practice in the UK that almost all patients had specific preformed requests they wished to make of their doctors. Almost half had specific questions they wished to ask: 55% wanted specific treatment, 60% had their own ideas about why they had developed their problems and 40% had specific concerns about their symptoms. Patients undoubtedly come to the doctor with well thought out agendas that they want to have addressed.

Perhaps this all seems so obvious as to be hardly worth mentioning, but in fact it's more complicated than we might think. Remember the evidence provided at the beginning of this chapter that showed how often doctors fail to detect problems or issues that patients wish to discuss, and how frequently doctors and patients disagree after the interview about the nature of the main presenting problem. In a qualitative study of general practice in the UK, Barry *et al.* (2000) discovered that only four of 35 patients voiced all of their agendas in the consultation. In all of the 14 consultations with problem outcomes, at least one of the problems was related to an unvoiced agenda item. Clearly, there are issues here that need to be addressed. In fact, the doctor's behaviour and approach in the initiation phase can have profound effects on the rest of the consultation, causing differences not only in the structure and timing of what occurs in the consultation but also, indeed, in the very problems that are discussed.

It is interesting to compare the evidence from research with some of the common assumptions that doctors make at the beginning of the interview.

- Several investigators have shown that patients often have more than one concern to discuss. In a variety of settings including primary care, paediatrics and internal medicine, the mean number of concerns ranged from 1.2 to 3.9 in both new and return visits (Starfield *et al.* 1981; Good and Good 1982; Wasserman *et al.* 1984; Greenfield *et al.* 1985). These studies warn of the danger of premature and limited hypothesis testing before identifying a wider spectrum of concerns.
- In a study of internal medicine residents and physicians in primary care, Beckman and Frankel (1984) have shown that:
  - the serial order in which patients present their problems is not related to their clinical importance: the first concern presented is no more likely than the second or third to be the most important as judged by either the patient or the doctor
  - doctors very often assume erroneously that the first complaint mentioned is the only one that the patient has brought
  - in follow-up visits, doctors often assume that the consultation is a direct continuation of the last interview and omit the opening solicitation entirely, proceeding directly to questions about concerns elicited in previous visits.

If the first complaint mentioned is not necessarily the most important, why do we behave as if it is the only one likely to be offered? We all can recall consultations that have suffered from this approach, with the real problem concerning the patient surfacing very late in the interview after our precious allotted time has been used on a less important topic (Robinson 2001). Sometimes it is even worse – we may not discover the main reason for the consultation at all, and the interview may end without the patient plucking up courage to mention their second more important agenda item. Even more fundamentally, why do we often explore the first symptom mentioned by the patient without first discovering all the other symptoms that the patient has noticed even when, as we shall see in Chapter 3, this can lead to significantly less effective clinical reasoning?

How can we overcome these problems? How do we make a route plan of the consultation rather than blindly setting off down the first road that we come across? Here we discuss three related skills that can help the doctor to understand not only why the patient has come but also as many as possible of the patient's reasons for attendance and their relative importance. These skills are as follows:

1. the opening question
2. listening
3. screening and agenda setting.

The opening question

New consultations

Near to the beginning of the interview, it is important to ask the patient an open question such as 'What would you like to discuss today?' We all tend to have a favourite stock question that we use repeatedly. Here are some examples of phrases that participants on our courses say they use time and time again:

> *'How can I help?'*
> *'Tell me what you have come to see me about.'*
> *'What would you like to talk about today?'*
> *'What can I do for you?'*
> *'How are you doing?'*
> *'How are things?'*
> *'What's up?'*
> *'Fine, so, off you go ...'*
> Nothing said (all implied in body language with appropriate pause).

The opening question of an inexperienced medical student on the ward may need to be different from that of the doctor responsible for the patient. The student's task may be to discover, primarily for their own benefit, *'What problems brought you to the hospital?'* from a patient who was admitted some time ago and is therefore already 'in the system'. However, the doctor is more often working in a diagnostic capacity and needs to use phases such as *'Tell me what problems you have been having'*, *'How can I help you?'* or *'I have a helpful letter from your family doctor, Dr Patel, but please start by telling me what the problems are from your perspective'*.

The exact words that we use can become a mantra that we repeat without thought, but in fact the phrasing of this simple task can make a considerable difference to the nature of the rest of the interview. The format of the question we use can subtly change the type of response that the patient provides.

More general enquiries such as *'How are you doing?'* allow the patient to state in broad terms how they are feeling but might not discover the actual problem that the patient has come to see the doctor about (Frankel 1995). For example, *'I'm fine but my arthritis is terrible at the moment'* might be the response, although the patient has actually come to discuss worsening migraines. This ambiguity might be apparent to a specialist neurologist but not to a general internist who does not have such a focused territory. The doctor needs to be aware of the type of question that she has asked and not assume the reason for the visit until she has asked a more specific follow-up: *'Is that why you have come to see me this morning?'*

'How can I help you?' is more explicit, implying that you want to know what the patient wishes to discuss today, although it might limit the patient to medical matters that the doctor can 'help' with.

'Tell me what you have come to see me about' is less medical, more open and might signal your willingness to listen to a wider agenda.

'What's on your agenda today?' certainly implies that you would like to encourage the patient to make a list of all the problems that they would like to discuss, but it might not be understood by all patients unless you explain, at least the first time you ask.

'Fine', *'Yes'* or using body language alone and saying nothing at all are extremely open methods of starting and giving the patient the floor. However, they give little initial direction to the patient whether to tell you about one problem in great detail or list all of their problems.

We are not suggesting that there is one correct opening method to be used on all occasions. However, there is a need for doctors to raise their awareness and think more carefully about the consequences of how they start each consultation (Robinson 2001; Gafaranga and Britten 2003).

Heritage and Robinson (2006) used conversation analysis to explore the effect of various opening questions in primary, acute and outpatient visits. When compared with confirmatory questions in which the physician asks whether the patient has come for a particular reason (e.g. 'I understand you have some sinus problems today'), general open-ended inquiries were associated with significantly longer problem presentations that included more discrete symptoms. In another study, open-ended enquiries were positively associated with patients' evaluation of physicians' listening and relational communication (Robinson and Heritage 2006). Heritage (2011) has also looked at the evidence from conversation analysis in everyday non-medical conversations and explains how normal conversation differs from medical consultations. He explores why doctors have to put aside their normal conversational approach of assuming pre-existing shared understanding with the patient based solely on information from the record or from another health practitioner (such as the triage nurse in primary care) and instead use highly open general enquiries at the beginning of the interview.

White *et al.* (2013) undertook a small study involving conversation analysis to look at the impact of the referral process during the initiation phase of surgeon–patient consultations in New Zealand. In these referred consultations a central task of the opening activities was 'for the participants to establish a shared understanding of the reason for the visit incorporating not only their own understanding but also that of the referring doctor'. Here the authors suggest that overt recognition of the referral process by the surgeon (by for instance explicitly mentioning the referring doctor and/or the referral letter) and the discussion that followed is important for accurately determining the agenda and organising the surgical consultation, providing patients with opportunity to participate in the opening activities of the visit, helping patients to overcome concern about telling the surgeon something they already know, and progressing to appropriate exploration of the problem. In this study, problems arose when there was no recognition of the referral process (although this occurred in only one consultation), when the referral letter was unclear or when the surgeon's understanding of the referral – e.g. regarding the presenting problem or the goal of the consultation – did not align with the patient's and/or the referring doctor's understanding.

We suggest that some of these same issues may arise during the initiation of the visit in primary care, emergency departments, teaching hospitals or other settings where someone other than the doctor handles an intake interview or triage, be it a nurse, nurse practitioner or physician's assistant, medical student or resident. Or in settings like hospitals where patients are moved from one service to another or group practices where, for example, different physicians may see chronic care patients on different occasions. Even though in these contexts the time elapsed may be only minutes or hours, the issues – e.g. inaccuracy or incompleteness in the 'handover', incomplete or unclear records, unchecked assumptions, and patients' uncertainty or reluctance to repeat some important fact or sequence of events that they think their doctor already knows – may be similar. More research is needed on this aspect of initiation.

Follow-up visits

Follow-up visits have much more in common with new consultations than is often believed. The key here is not to make the assumption that you know the reason for the visit until you have actually asked the patient. It is so easy to assume that the patient has come for their routine check and move straight into *'How are you getting along with your new pills?'*, when in fact the patient has a more pressing or at least a second agenda to discuss. Yet it can sound as if you do not remember the patient at all if you start as in a new appointment with *'What would you like to discuss today?'* Perhaps instead, you might start with your understanding of the reason for the visit, as in *'Am I right in thinking that you have come for your routine check'* or *'I've come to see how you're doing and check your incision'*, and then ask the patient to confirm by adding, *'Is there anything else you would like to talk about today?'*

Listening to the patient's opening statement

Learning how to listen at the beginning of the consultation is the first step to an efficient and accurate consultation

It seems at first glance that giving the patient time, space and encouragement to have the floor while the doctor deliberately sits back and listens might not be the most efficient way of beginning an interview. Often, doctors are under so much pressure from time constraints that they feel the need to force the pace by quickly moving into questioning mode and taking the initiative (Levinson and Pizzo 2011). This approach often leads doctors to explore the first item offered by the patient, which, as we have seen, can be counterproductive. So how do we address this problem? How do we establish that listening to the patient early on in the consultation is rewarded by a far more efficient and accurate interview overall?

Listening rather than questioning allows doctors and patients to achieve more of their objectives for this part of the consultation

Reviewing the objectives for this first part of the consultation helps us to find our bearings. Our objectives fall into three broad categories. The first is to understand what the patient wants to discuss today, to add in anything else that you as the doctor wish to discuss, and to plan with the patient how to approach the rest of the consultation. The second is to make the patient feel comfortable, welcomed and an important part of the proceedings – to establish initial rapport. The third is to gauge how the patient is feeling – to be aware of the patient as a person.

How do we achieve all of these simultaneously and with the greatest ease? As we will see in Chapter 3, as soon as the doctor moves into detailed questioning, the patient tends to become a passive contributor. The doctor has to follow each closed question with another, his mind is forced away from the patient's responses into diagnostic reasoning and the interview focuses prematurely on one particular area. In contrast, following an open-ended initial statement or question with attentive listening allows the doctor to discover more of the patient's agenda, to hear the story from the patient's perspective, to appear supportive and interested and, by concentrating on the patient, to pick up cues to the patient's feelings and emotional state that could otherwise be missed.

What is the evidence to support listening?

The importance of doctors' listening skills at the beginning of the consultation has been beautifully demonstrated by two of the most quoted papers in the communication literature, those of Beckman and Frankel (1984) and Beckman *et al.* (1985).

We have known for a long time from Byrne and Long's work in primary care (Byrne and Long 1976) that many dysfunctional consultations arise because of difficulties in discovering why the patient has come to see the doctor. One of the problems here lies with the patient's tendency to withhold psychosocial and other important concerns until later in the visit, when they have tested the water and gained confidence in the doctor. Anxiety or embarrassment about a symptom or a serious worry might make the patient delay mentioning it until late in the day. These late announcements have been termed 'hidden agendas' (Barsky 1981).

This approach to thinking about the interview focuses attention on the patient's apparent decision to withhold, delay or share information. However, another strand of research has concentrated on the role that the doctor plays. It has looked at the influence that doctors' behaviour has on the placement and flow of information provided by the patient and has discovered that doctors' own words and actions have a startling effect on whether (or when) they discover the full reasons for the patient's attendance. The doctor's behaviour may well be more influential here than that of the patient.

Byrne and Long (1976) showed that many doctors are not good listeners and have fixed routines of interviewing patients that demonstrate little capacity for variation to meet an individual's needs. In their key research, Beckman and Frankel (1984) have taken this further, by analysing exactly how doctors' use of words and questions can so easily and inadvertently direct the patient away from disclosing their reasons for wishing to see the doctor. A host of revealing facts have been uncovered by their research.

- Doctors frequently interrupted patients before they had completed their opening statement – after a mean time of only 18 seconds!
- Only 23% of patients completed their opening statement.
- In only one out of 51 interrupted statements was the patient allowed to complete their opening statement later.
- In total, 94% of all interruptions concluded with the doctor obtaining the floor.
- The longer the doctor waited before interruption, the more complaints were elicited.
- Allowing the patient to complete the opening statement led to a significant reduction in late-arising problems.
- Clarifying or closed questions were the most frequent cause of interruption, but any utterance by the doctor that specifically encouraged the patient to give further information about any one problem could also cause disruption: this, perhaps surprisingly, included echoing of the patient's words.
- In 34 out of 51 visits, the doctor interrupted the patient after the initial concern, apparently assuming that the first complaint was the chief one.
- The serial order in which the patients presented their problems was not related to their clinical importance.
- Patients who were allowed to complete their opening statement without interruption mostly took less than 60 seconds and none took longer than 150 seconds, even when encouraged to continue.

Beckman and Frankel have shown us that it is the early pursuit by closed questioning of the first problem mentioned that prevents doctors from discovering all the issues that a patient wishes to discuss. The emphasis quickly shifts from a patient-centred to a physician-centred format. Once this is done, the patient tends to remain in a more passive role, trying to comply by giving short answers, perhaps assuming that if the competent doctor needs to know something he will ask. Inefficient and inaccurate information gathering ensues. Not only does the interview steam ahead before the main concern has necessarily been discovered but hypothesis testing proceeds without patients having a chance to tell their story or to provide information which closed questioning may well never discover.

Beckman and Frankel clearly demonstrate that even minimal interruptions to patients' initial statements can actually prevent other concerns from appearing at all, or can make important complaints arise late in the consultation. By asking patients to start telling you more about any one problem, you restrict their options, preventing them from expanding on other information that they would like to tell you. The patient is in fact faced with a practical problem when the doctor moves in with an interruption. Say the patient has mentioned headaches but is interrupted before they can mention their recent palpitations and marital problems. *'Tell me more about your headaches'* or, worse, *'Where do you get the pain?'* restricts the discussion to the headaches and limits both the patient's options and the efficiency of the interview as a whole.

Marvel *et al.* (1999) repeated and extended Beckman and Frankel's work. In a study of experienced family physicians, they found that, 15 years later, the mean time to interruption was still very short (23.1 seconds) with only 28% of patients completing their opening statement. And although physicians may well intend to return later to let the patient finish, this happened in only 8% of interviews. Gratifyingly, the study found that fellowship-trained physicians who had previous training in communication and counselling skills were more likely to solicit patient concerns and allow patients to complete their initial statements of concerns. Interestingly, they discovered that an alternative approach to encouraging patients to disclose their full agenda was to follow each solicitation with a focused open-ended question such as 'Tell me more about the leg pain' before reverting to another open-ended solicitation such as 'Is there anything else we need to take care of today?' They conclude that models of medical interviewing need to allow for flexibility as long as the desired outcome of a complete agenda and adequate problem definition is achieved.

In a study by Rhoades *et al.* (2001), patients spoke on average for only 12 seconds before being interrupted by family practice or internal medicine residents. In 25% of occasions, residents interrupted patients before they finished speaking.

Ruiz Moral *et al.* (2006), in a study of third-year family physician residents in Spain, showed that patients mentioned new problems at closure ('Oh, by the way …') more frequently when physicians redirected the focus of the interview before patients completed an initial statement of concerns in the early moments of the visit. More than half of the trainees directed the focus of the interview before the patient had completed an initial statement of concerns. Early redirection did not save overall consultation time but, rather, made closures longer and more dysfunctional, as patients raised new problems at the end of the interview.

Langewitz *et al.* (2002) followed up the work of Marvel *et al.*, but conducted their study in the internal medicine outpatient clinic of a Swiss tertiary referral centre, a setting characterised by 'difficult patients with complex histories'. Suggesting that physicians may interrupt so frequently because they assume that patients will interfere with the time schedule if allowed to talk as long as they wish, Langewitz *et al.* wanted to know if this in fact would happen. The sample consisted of 335 patients who were making first contact with this clinic, and 14 experienced internists who were trained to listen actively without interrupting until the patient indicated that his or her list of complaints was complete. Patients did not know they were being timed. Despite the complexities inherent in this tertiary referral setting, patients' mean spontaneous talking time was only 92 seconds and 78% or all patients finished within two minutes. Seven patients talked longer than five minutes, but their doctors felt the information they were giving was important and should not be interrupted.

Rabinovitz *et al.* (2004), in a study in Israeli general practice with consultations about a new clinical problem, demonstrated that the number of completed patient uninterrupted monologues at the beginning of the consultation doubled from 32% when doctors were handed a written note saying, 'when the patient starts speaking, please do not interrupt him or her until you are satisfied that he or she has finished.'

Interestingly, Dyche and Swiderski (2005) showed that it was the initial solicitation of the patient's agenda that was most important in discovering the full range of the patient's concerns as judged by exit interviews. In 37% of interviews in an inner-city health centre in the United States there was no enquiry for the patient's agenda, and under these circumstances there was considerable reduction in identification of concerns. However, if such an initial enquiry did occur, interruption of the patient did not curtail the physician's ability to identify concerns.

Li *et al.* (2004) explored the concept of interruption in more detail. They found that when Canadian primary care physicians attempted to interrupt patients, they were unsuccessful in only 6% of occasions and the interruptions were predominantly intrusive in nature. When patients interrupted physicians, they were unsuccessful in 32% of occasions, and most of their interruptions were cooperative in nature.

Wissow *et al.* (1994) have shown that paediatricians' use of attentive listening is positively associated with parents' disclosure of psychosocial problems; Putnam *et al.* (1988) have shown that it is possible to teach medical residents the skills of attentive listening and that such teaching leads to a significant increase in patient exposition without any associated increase in the length of the interview.

What are the specific skills of attentive listening?

Listening is often equated with 'sitting and doing nothing', a passive rather than active approach. Yet as Egan (1990) says in *The Skilled Helper*:

> *How many times have you heard someone exclaim, 'You're not listening to what I'm saying!'. When the person accused of not listening answers, 'I am too; I can repeat everything you've said', the accuser is not comforted. What people look for in attending and listening is not the other person's ability to repeat their words. A tape recorder would do that perfectly. People want more than physical presence in human communication; they want the other person to be present psychologically, socially and emotionally.*

In fact attentive listening is both active and highly skilled. There are four specific skill areas that can help us to develop our ability to listen attentively:

1. wait time
2. facilitative response
3. non-verbal skills
4. picking up verbal and non-verbal cues.

1. **Wait time.** Making the shift from speaking to listening at appropriate moments in the consultation is not easy. Inadvertently, we often find ourselves preparing our next question rather than focusing attention on what the patient is saying. We may become so involved in formulating our next question that we divert our own attention from hearing the patient's message and, by interrupting, fail to give the patient adequate time to respond. Evidence from the world of education rather than medicine helps to illuminate the value to both doctor and patient of allowing the patient more space to think before answering or to go on after pausing.

   Over 20 years, Rowe (1986) studied non-medical teachers in a wide variety of classroom settings. She found that when teachers asked questions, they waited one second or less for a reply. Similarly, they only waited one second after a student stopped speaking before they responded. However, if the teachers were trained to increase their pauses at each of these key points to three seconds, remarkable changes occurred in the student's behaviour in class. The students contributed more often, spoke for longer, asked more questions, provided more evidence for their thinking and failed to respond less often. Difficult or 'invisible' students started to contribute successfully. In turn, teachers asked their students fewer questions but of a more flexible nature and they increased their expectations of their students.

   In the medical interview, using wait time effectively allows the patient time to think and to contribute more without interruption and the doctor to have time to listen, think and respond more flexibly.
2. **Facilitative response.** Some doctors clearly have a greater ability than others to encourage their patients to say more about a topic, to indicate to patients that they are interested in what they are saying and that they would like them to continue. This is often achieved very efficiently with minimal or no interruption and it is worth considering exactly what these minimal clues are that seem to be such powerful indicators to the patient that we are listening and wish to hear.

   We will look in more detail at facilitation skills in Chapter 3, but at this point we would like to consider which specific facilitative responses are of value in this opening phase of the consultation. Research has clearly shown that the skills employed in attentive listening are different at different stages in the consultation and that facilitation skills known to be helpful later on in the consultation are in fact counterproductive when used early on in the interview.

   Beckman and Frankel's (1984) work has provided clear guidance here. They looked specifically at which facilitative interventions by physicians allowed patients to continue and complete their initial statement of concerns and which interrupted the patient, encouraged early exploration of one specific area and prevented the physician from discovering more of the concerns that the patient wished to discuss. They showed that repetition (echoing), paraphrasing and interpretation, which are all valuable facilitative skills later on in the interview, potentially act as interrupters at the beginning of the interview whereas other more neutral facilitative phrases such as *'uh-huh'*, *'go on'*, *'yes'*, *'um'* or *'I see'* serve to encourage the patient to continue along his or her own path.

3. **Non-verbal skills.** We shall explore non-verbal skills in more detail when we look at 'building the relationship' in Chapter 5. Here, however, we would like to flag some issues about non-verbal communication that are particularly relevant to the beginning of the consultation.

    Much of our willingness to listen is signalled through our non-verbal behaviour, which immediately gives the patient strong clues as to our level of interest in them and in their problems. Many individual components are involved in non-verbal communication, including posture, movement, proximity, direction of gaze, eye contact, gestures, affect, vocal cues (tone, rate, volume of speech), facial expression, touch, physical appearance and environmental cues (placement of furniture, lighting, warmth). All of these skills can assist in demonstrating attentiveness to patients and facilitate the formation of a supportive relationship. Ineffective attending behaviour in contrast both closes off the interaction and prohibits relationship building (Gazda *et al.* 1995).

    Among the most important of all the non-verbal skills is eye contact. We can easily be distracted from providing this by the notes or the computer as we grapple to comprehend our patient's problem, yet poor eye contact can be readily misinterpreted by patients as lack of interest and can inhibit open communication (Goodwin 1981; Ruusuvuori 2001; Nordman *et al.* 2010). First impressions are very important here.

    Communication research has shown that non-verbal messages tend to override verbal messages when the two are inconsistent or contradictory (Koch 1971; McCroskey *et al.* 1971). If you provide the verbal message that you want the patient to tell you all about their problem while at the same time you speak quickly, look harassed and avoid eye contact, your non-verbal message will usually win out. The patient will correctly construe that time is at a premium today and may not tell you about the problem in sufficient detail.

    The importance of both verbal and non-verbal facilitation skills lies in the message that they impart to the patient. Two of the principles of communication that we outlined in Chapter 1 concerned reducing uncertainty and establishing mutually understood common ground. Facilitation skills are effective in encouraging patients to tell us their story because they directly signal to our patients something about our attitude to them, our interest in them and their story, and our helpful intentions. In the absence of these skills, the patient remains uncertain about our interest in what they are saying and our need for the patient to continue with their account. We might be clear in our own minds that we wish the interview to proceed in a certain way but is our verbal and non-verbal behaviour skilful enough for the patient to share that understanding?

4. **Picking up verbal and non-verbal cues.** Another important listening skill is that of picking up patients' verbal and non-verbal cues. This requires both listening and observation. Often patients' ideas, concerns and expectations are provided in non-verbal cues and indirect comments rather than overt statements (Tuckett *et al.* 1985). These cues often feature very early in the patient's exposition of their problems and the doctor needs to look out specifically for

them from the very beginning of the interview. The danger lies in either missing these messages altogether or assuming we know what they mean without checking them out with the patient now or later in the interview. We take up this aspect of attentive listening in greater detail in Chapter 3.

What are the advantages of attentive listening?

Full attention through active listening allows you to:

- signal your interest to the patient
- hear the patient's story
- prevent yourself from making premature hypotheses and chasing down blind alleys
- reduce late-arising complaints
- hear both 'disease' and 'illness', as discussed in Chapter 3
- not have to think of the next question (which blocks your listening and renders the patient passive)
- calibrate the patient's emotional state
- observe more carefully and pick up verbal and non-verbal cues.

Listening attentively without interruption is also extremely helpful to the patient whose ideas and feelings about their health or whose problems are relatively undefined. Giving space to such patients allows them time to clarify what it is that they wish to discuss with the doctor. Not all patients have clear-cut agendas.

With so much to hear and see at the beginning of the interview, why not consciously set aside the first minute or two for the patient and concentrate on listening and facilitating rather than questioning? Listening attentively instead of moving immediately to a series of questions about the history allows us to achieve more of our objectives – although it requires very little time, using these early moments of the consultation wisely pays off handsomely.

Screening

In the discussion here, we have seen how using an appropriate opening question combined with attentive listening and specific facilitation skills allows the physician to discover more of the patient's agenda in the early part of the consultation. Now we would like to explore how making a further deliberate attempt to discover all of the patient's problem *before* actively exploring any one of them can further increase the accuracy and efficiency of consultations.

Screening is the process of deliberately checking with the patient that you have discovered all that they wish to discuss by asking further open-ended enquiries. Rather than assuming that the patient has mentioned all of their difficulties, double-check:

> *'So you've been getting headaches and dizziness lately. Has anything else been bothering you?'*

If the patient continues, resume listening until the patient stops again. Then repeat the screening process until eventually the patient says that they have finished:

> '*So you've also been feeling very tired and irritable and were wondering if you might be anaemic. Anything else at all?*'

At the end of this process when the patient says '*No, that's about it*', you might wish to confirm your understanding and give the patient an opportunity to know what you have heard:

> '*So as I understand it, you've been getting headaches and dizziness but have also been feeling tired, rather irritable and a bit low, and your concern was that you might be anaemic. Did I get that right?*'

Often this method of checking reveals symptoms and concerns relating to the initial complaint but the patient might not yet have revealed a totally separate problem. You might wish to perform one last check here:

> '*I can see these symptoms must have been worrying to you and we'll need to explore them further in a minute; first, let me just check whether there are some other areas that you hope I might be able to help you with today as well.*'

The patient might then produce a second problem area, '*Well, I've also got this terrible cough*' or a social problem, '*Well I'm really terribly worried about my daughter*'. Without this check, you might first discover these issues at the end of the consultation and not have any time or patience left to deal with them.

Interestingly, recent work by Heritage *et al.* (2007) in the United States demonstrated that using the phrase '*Is there something else you want to address in the visit today?*' was more effective in screening than the phrase '*Is there anything else you want to address in the visit today?*' Using 'something' or 'some other concern' strongly reduced the incidence of patients' unmet concerns without significantly increasing visit length. In contrast, using 'anything' or 'any other' was relatively ineffective in eliciting additional concerns and in reducing unmet concerns. This is as predicted by the field of linguistics, which would suggest that the word 'any' is negatively polarised (with a subtle communication of an expectation of a 'no' response) and the word 'some' is positively polarised. It is not clear whether this result is generalisable outside of the United States and how much effect non-verbal communication has in ameliorating the differences between these words.

The four-part approach to identifying the patient's agenda, namely:

1. opening question
2. listening
3. screening
4. confirming

offers many advantages to the doctor and the patient over the more traditional alternative of:

1. asking
2. assuming
3. proceeding.

For the doctor, there is a better chance of discovering the patient's full agenda, negotiating how best to use the time available and pacing the interview appropriately. Screening also provides a way for doctors to check out their expectations and assumptions about why the patient may have come or what the patient wants to talk about, helping the doctor to keep an open mind.

For the patient, screening establishes mutually understood common ground and provides the reassurance that you are really interested in their problems and thoughts – both in turn enhance trust and disclosure. Helping the patient reveal their most important problems early on prevents the patient's attention from remaining focused on how and when to introduce their unstated concern rather than on the agenda in progress (Korsch *et al.* 1968; Mehrabian and Ksionsky 1974). Screening helps prevent uncertainty in the patient's mind leading to distraction and blocking effective communication.

Patients may of course still reveal their underlying problem, their 'hidden agenda', later in the interview when they have tested the water and gained confidence in the relationship. Screening encourages but does not guarantee early problem identification and we must still remain open to late-arising complaints and be sensitive to the reasons that the patient might have in delaying their introduction. Indeed, Peltenburg *et al.* (2004) has demonstrated that some agenda items that emerge as the consultation proceeds were not anticipated by either patient or doctor prior to the interview – this emerging agenda appears to relate to the ability of the doctor to pick up affective cues.

Several North American texts now propose the following sequence for the early part of the consultation (Riccardi and Kurtz 1983; Lipkin 1987; Cohen-Cole 1991; Baker *et al.* 2005):

- encouraging the patient to discuss their main concerns by attentive listening without interruption or premature closure
- confirming the list identified so far by summarising
- checking repeatedly for additional concerns (*'Is there something else you wish to discuss today?'*) until the patient indicates that there are none
- negotiating an agenda for the consultation.

We shall look more closely at the skills of checking and summarising in Chapter 3.

The balance between listening and screening

Having discovered the importance of screening for the full range of problems, learners often identify a dilemma about when exactly to screen and when to listen. A balance has to be achieved in the use of these two complementary skills that will be determined in part by the context of each interview.

In certain interviews, it is possible and beneficial to be quite up front about screening and to explain your plan to the patient straightaway. So, as an example, the patient referred to a specialist might receive the following introduction:

'Hello, I'm Dr Smith. I've got a letter from your GP so I've got some idea of why you've come today, but I'd like to hear the story from you first hand and then try to help as best I can. I'd like to start, if you agree, with us making a list of all the problems you've been having or things you'd like help with and then we can explore them together in more detail.'

This approach makes the structure very clear to the patient. It makes it apparent that the doctor wants to understand the whole of the patient's agenda from the start and will then attend to all of their concerns. Otherwise, the patient may not know if they are expected to steam ahead with one problem or to mention them all briefly.

At the other extreme, a patient who enters the room and immediately breaks into a story that they clearly need to tell, or a patient who on sitting down dissolves into tears because her father has just died, deserves our full attention now. Here listening takes priority over screening. It would be inappropriate to interrupt and say, *'We'll come back to that – is there anything else that you would like to discuss today?'*!

Some patients come with their pre-written list giving the doctor a perfect opportunity to screen the agenda and negotiate what is possible in the time today. Other patients come with a well-rehearsed speech that they have nervously prepared – the telling of it is essential for the patient's peace of mind before the doctor and patient can settle down to work together. Often this opening statement can be so rich in feelings, thoughts, ideas, concerns and expectations and give such clues to the patient's life-world that it would be a mistake not to give the patient the floor to express their story. If you do not listen first, you might well miss clues that could be important in helping the patient with their problem.

This dilemma can be resolved by another of the principles of communication that we have already discussed: *dynamism*. What is appropriate for one situation is inappropriate for another and we have to continually monitor how best to approach the consultation as we proceed. Knowing that it is helpful to both listen and screen and being flexible enough to use both appropriately in differing situations is the key.

Agenda setting

Screening naturally leads on to negotiating and setting an agenda, taking both the patient's and the doctor's needs into account (Kaplan *et al.* 1997; Manning and Ray 2002; Robins *et al.* 2011). In keeping with our emphasis on developing a partnership between patient and physician – a collaborative relationship – this is an overt and involving approach to clarifying how the interview should proceed.

We look in more detail at how to structure an interview in Chapter 3 when we consider summary and signposting. We will describe how these methods encourage the doctor to consider where he or she has got to so far in the interview, what exactly he or she is trying to achieve next and how to verbalise these thoughts to the patient. There are many advantages to this over simply moving forward without explaining the process to the patient. For the doctor, organisation of thought prevents aimless or unnecessary questioning and incomplete data gathering. For the patient, the structure of the interview is made overt and an opportunity is provided for more involvement and more responsibility in what is taking place.

Agenda setting is another example of structuring the consultation. Priorities can be established and negotiated:

> *'Shall we start with the new problems, the diarrhoea and the fever, and then move on to the problems you have been having with your medication?'*

The doctor's agenda can also be added:

> *'OK, let's think about your headaches and then look at the rash. I wouldn't mind checking on your blood pressure and your thyroid tablets too, later on, if that's all right'*

Problems with time can be acknowledged and negotiated:

> *'That's quite a list for us to get through and I'm not sure that we are going to have enough time to do it all justice. How about ...?'*

In negotiating priorities, a balance may need to be struck between the patient's personal hierarchy of concerns and the doctor's medical understanding of which problems might be more immediately important:

> *'I can see that the arthritis is the thing that's really bothering you most today but if you don't mind, I'd rather we started by checking out those chest pains you had last week.'*

Interestingly, Levinson *et al.* (1997) showed that primary care physicians who educated the patient about what to expect and the flow of the visit were less likely to have suffered malpractice claims.

Notice that in agenda setting and negotiating, you are not just telling the patient what to do but are inviting the patient to participate in making an agreed plan. One of the principles of communication that we discussed in Chapter 1 was that *effective communication promotes an interaction rather than a process of direct transmission*. Cassata (1978) explained how crystallising agendas at the beginning of the consultation promotes just such an interaction, a two-way communication that encourages the patient to be a more active, responsible and autonomous participant throughout the consultation. Another of our five principles concerned *reducing uncertainty* – here, overt agenda setting does just that by establishing mutually understood common ground. Joos *et al.* (1996) provide research validation of this approach. They taught internal medicine residents and physicians the skills of eliciting the patient's full concerns and negotiating an agreed agenda, and they demonstrated that doctors who received this training not only subsequently discovered more of their patients' concerns but also, and equally as important, achieved this without any increase in the length of the visit.

Haas *et al.* (2006) similarly taught primary care physicians the skills of agenda eliciting and negotiation in a brief workshop. Patients' post-workshop ratings of medical visits demonstrated an increase in whether all problems were addressed in the visit. Rodriguez *et al.* (2008) taught practising physicians the skill of 'agenda-setting', eliciting the full set of concerns from the patient's perspective and using that information to prioritise and negotiate which clinical issues should most appropriately be dealt with and which should be deferred to a subsequent visit. The intervention resulted in statistically significant improvement in physicians' ability to explain things in a way that was easy to understand and marginal but significant improvement in the overall quality of physician–patient interactions compared with control group physicians. Brock *et al.* (2011) found that patients of physicians trained in agenda setting were more likely to indicate agenda completion and raised fewer concerns later in the encounter with no increase in visit length. Mauksch *et al.* (2008) undertook a literature review to explore the determinants of efficiency in the medical interview. Three domains emerged from their review that can enhance communication efficiency: (1) rapport building, (2) upfront agenda setting and (3) picking up emotional cues.

Summary

In this chapter, we have examined the skills of initiating the consultation, one of the most important parts of any interview. The skills involved in establishing initial rapport, identifying the reasons for the patient's attendance and agreeing an agenda set the scene for the rest of the interview. These skills directly influence whether three important goals of medical communication – *accuracy, efficiency and supportiveness* – are achieved throughout the interview as a whole.

The skills of initiation are very different from the skills of gathering information, as we have shown in the Calgary–Cambridge Guides. Yet so often we do not separate out these tasks in our minds and they merge together with deleterious results. Clearly, having in mind a structure for the consultation as we progress through the interview is of vital importance. Before going on to explore the patient's problems in detail, it is helpful to ask, 'Have I achieved my objectives for this first part of the interview? Have I established a supportive environment and initial rapport? Have I discovered all the problems that the patient has come to discuss. Have I established mutually understood common ground regarding the problem list and developed a mutually agreed plan for the consultation? Have I enabled the patient to become part of a collaborative process?' Once these tasks have been completed, the doctor can then move on to gathering information about each problem.

Chapter 3

Gathering information

Introduction

Having seen how vital the beginning of the interview is to successful doctor–patient communication, we now turn our attention to the next section of the interview – gathering information.

For many years, we have known of the overriding importance of history taking to diagnosis. Clinical studies have shown repeatedly that the history contributes 60%–80% of the data for diagnosis. In Hampton's study in medical outpatients, the history alone was sufficient to make the diagnosis in 66 out of 80 patients (Hampton *et al.* 1975; Sandler 1980; Kassirer 1983, Peterson *et al.* 1992).

Yet the way that many doctors have been taught to take a history in medical school can lead to inaccuracy and inefficiency. Traditional questioning methods do not encourage comprehensive history taking or effective hypothesis generation. Fortunately, developments in communication theory and research have greatly improved our understanding of the *process* of gathering information.

They have also opened up a whole new *content* area of history taking – namely, the patient's perspective of their illness (McWhinney 1989). Traditional medical interviewing has concentrated on pathological disease at the expense of understanding the highly individual needs of each patient. As a consequence, much of the information required to understand our patients' problems remains hidden. Studies of patient satisfaction, adherence, recall and physiological outcome all validate the need for a broader view of history taking that encompasses the patient's life-world as well as the doctor's more focused biological perspective.

Both the content and process skills of gathering information are central to effective medical interviewing and in this chapter we shall explore each of these areas in turn.

Problems in communication

There is considerable evidence of communication problems in the gathering information phase of the consultation.

- Byrne and Long's (1976) classic work studying 2000 consultations in British primary care showed that doctors used a remarkably uniform style despite differences in the problems presented to them or in their patients' behaviour. They often pursued a 'doctor-centred' closed approach to information gathering that discouraged patients from telling their story or voicing their concerns.
- Platt and McMath (1979) observed 300 encounters in hospital internal medicine in the United States and showed that both a 'high control style' [process]

and premature focus on medical problems [content] lead to an over-narrow approach to hypothesis generation [perceptual] and to limitation of the patients' ability to communicate their concerns [content]. These in turn lead to inaccurate consultations.

- Research by Tuckett *et al.* (1985) on information giving in general practice in the UK, which we shall explore more fully in Chapter 6, demonstrated the central importance of eliciting patients' beliefs about their illness in enabling patients to understand and recall information. Yet these researchers' efforts were hampered by the very few examples that they were able to find of doctors asking patients to volunteer their ideas, or even of doctors asking the patient to elaborate on their ideas if they did spontaneously bring them up.
- Kleinman *et al.* (1978) used cross-cultural work to show how undiscovered discordance between the health beliefs of patient and physician can lead to problems in patient satisfaction, adherence, management and outcome.
- Maguire *et al.* (1996) showed that less than half of health professionals before a communication workshop were able to identify a minimum of 60% of their patients' main concerns.
- Levinson *et al.* (2000) found that patients gave verbal and non-verbal cues throughout the interview but that physicians only responded positively to patient cues in 38% of cases in surgery and 21% in primary care.
- Rogers and Todd (2000) discovered that oncologists preferentially listened for and responded to certain disease cues over others – they ignored patients' cues about pain unless it was pain that was amenable to specialist cancer treatment. Other pains were not acknowledged or were dismissed.
- Kuhl (2002) demonstrated that doctors who trivialise or disregard patients' views or fail to take into account patients' concerns may inadvertently cause what he terms 'iatrogenic suffering' – that is, pain and suffering inflicted by another unintentionally. Citing a number of compelling examples based on cancer patients' stories of their experiences, Kuhl suggests that iatrogenic suffering 'occurs when patients bear the burden of a doctor's own unresolved psychological and emotional issues about death, suffering, pain, and relationship.'
- Agledahl *et al.* (2011) in a qualitative study observed a consistent pattern in the consultations of hospital clinicians in Norway. The doctors were primarily concerned with their patients' biomedical health. This medical focus often overrode other important aspects of the consultations, and doctors actively directed the focus away from their patients' concerns, rarely addressing the personal aspects of a patient's condition. Although doctors incorporated a polite and friendly approach, they did not pick up and explore the patient's cues to their underlying concerns and feelings.
- Mjaaland *et al.* (2011) demonstrated quantitatively the lack of exploration by hospital physicians in Norway of negative emotions expressed as cues and concerns.
- Ruiz-Moral *et al.* (2006) demonstrated how most Spanish specialty physicians showed a limited range of communication skills, adopting a doctor-centred style with no exploration of patients emotions, expectations or psychosocial aspects.
- Maguire and Rutter (1976), more than 30 years ago, showed serious deficiencies in senior medical students' information-gathering skills. Few students managed to discover the patient's main problem, to clarify the exact nature of the problem and explore ambiguous statements, to clarify with precision, to elicit the impact of the problem on daily life, to respond to verbal cues, to cover

more personal topics or to use facilitation. Most used closed, lengthy, multiple and repetitive questions.

Objectives

When gathering information in medical interviews, the physician's objectives go beyond just extracting information from a passive patient. We also need to make our patients feel listened to and valued, ensure mutual understanding and sustain an ongoing collaborative relationship. Our objectives for this part of the interview therefore include:

- exploring the patient's problems to discover the biomedical perspective, the patient's perspective and the background information
- ensuring that information gathered is accurate, complete and mutually understood (establishing common ground)
- ensuring that patients feel listened to, that their information and views are welcomed and valued (confirmation)
- continuing to develop a supportive environment and a collaborative relationship
- structuring the consultation to ensure efficient information gathering and to enable the patient to understand and be overtly involved in where the interview is going and why.

Again these objectives encompass many of the tasks and checkpoints mentioned in other well-known guides to the consultation:

- Pendleton *et al.* (1984, 2003):
  - to understand the reasons for the patient's attendance
    (1) the nature and history of the problems
    (2) their aetiology
    (3) the effects of the problems
    (4) the patient's ideas, concerns and expectations
  - to establish or maintain a relationship with the patient that helps to achieve the other tasks.
- Neighbour (1987):
  - connecting – establishing rapport with the patient
  - summarising – 'Have I sufficiently understood why the patient has come to see me?'
- AAPP Three-Function Model (Cohen-Cole 1991):
  - gathering data to understand the patient's problems
  - developing rapport and responding to the patient's emotions.
- Bayer Institute for Health Care Communication E4 model (Keller and Carroll 1994):
  - engaging the patient
  - empathising with the patient.
- The Four Habits Model (Frankel and Stein 1999; Krupat *et al.* 2006):
  - eliciting the patient's perspective.
- The SEGUE Framework for teaching and assessing communication skills (Makoul 2001):
  - eliciting information.

- The Maastricht Maas Global (van Thiel and van Dalen 1995):
  - exploration
  - clarification
  - summarisations
  - emotions.
- Essential Elements of Communication in Medical Encounters: Kalamazoo Consensus Statement (Participants in the Bayer-Fetzer Conference on Physician–Patient Communication in Medical Education 2001):
  - gather information
  - understand the patient's perspective.
- Patient-centred medicine (Stewart *et al.* 2003)
  - exploring both the disease and the illness experience.
- The Model of the Macy Initiative in Health Communication (Kalet *et al.* 2004)
  - gather
  - elicit and understand the patient's perspective.
- The Six Function Model (de Haes and Bensing 2009):
  - gathering information.

Our objectives, along with those of several other models, make it clear that both content and process skills are significant elements of information gathering. We would like first to explore the content related to this part of the medical interview and next to look closely at the process skills for gathering information. Towards the end of this chapter, we shall discuss the influence of clinical reasoning and the focused history on both the process and content of medical interviewing.

The content of information gathering in medical interviews

So what information is it that doctors need to discover by the end of the interview? What information should they present on ward rounds and write in patients' records? Once this is defined, we can turn our attention to how best to approach this section of the interview and consider what process skills enable accurate, efficient and supportive information gathering.

We start by exploring two contrasting approaches to information gathering, the traditional medical history and the disease–illness model.

The traditional medical history

The traditional method of history taking is so firmly established in medical practice that it is easy to assume that it is the correct approach. Yet often in medicine we make such assumptions without considering the origins of what we do and their relevance to modern-day practice. McWhinney (1989) has eloquently traced the origins, strengths and weaknesses of the traditional clinical method which we briefly précis here.

Origins of the traditional method

At the beginning of the nineteenth century, a new method of clinical medicine began to emerge, pioneered in post-revolutionary France. Prior to this, medicine had lacked any scientific basis – patients' symptoms had been the focus of doctors' attention and there had been little understanding of underlying disease processes.

Innovations such as the stethoscope now revealed a whole new range of clinical information. At the same time, physicians began to examine the internal organs after death and tried to correlate physical signs in life to post-mortem findings in death. From here on, the physical expression of the patient's illness became central to the profession's approach – it became the aim of the diagnostician to interpret the patient's symptoms in terms of specific diseases and to provide a scientific explanation. This change was to herald the incredible advances in diagnosis and treatment of the twentieth century.

By 1880, a fully defined clinical method had become established. This is apparent from hospital clinical records where the structured method of recording the history and examination that we are all so familiar with today had already taken root (Tait 1979; Roter 2000). The history of present complaint, history of past illness, medication and allergy history, family history, personal and social history and systems review provided a standard method of recording clinical enquiries and forged an ordered approach to history taking (*see* Chapter 1, Box 1.2).

This method still dominates medicine today and has been consolidated by the incorporation of powerful new methods of investigation that have further enhanced our ability to interpret the patient's problems in terms of underlying physical pathology. Imaging, microbiology, biochemistry and haematology are the essentials of our trade – they have taken our understanding of the disease process to the cellular level and beyond.

Strengths

It is the scientific approach to the patient that is the traditional clinical method's greatest strength. There is no doubt that the development of a method of classification of the underlying cause of disease paved the way for the advances in medical science that have followed. It provided the first real possibility of precise clinical audit with the pathologist giving clinicians feedback on their diagnostic skills. It gave a common language to unify the 'medical approach'.

It also provided physicians with a clear method of taking and recording the clinical history, supplying a carefully structured template with which to arrive at a diagnosis or to exclude physical disease. It simplified and unified a very complex process, prevented the omission of key points and enabled the data extracted from the patient to appear in a standard assimilable form.

Weaknesses

The strength of the traditional clinical method is also its weakness. As the profession has embraced the objectivity required to diagnose disease in terms of underlying pathology, it has increasingly concentrated on the individual parts of the body that are malfunctioning and has honed this process down to a cellular and now molecular level. Yet this very detached objectivity so easily misses the patient as a whole. As Cassell (1985) has put it, 'the patient's individual concerns are brushed aside to support the function of their organs'.

The scientific method does not aim to understand the meaning of the illness for the patient or place it in the context of his life and family. Subjective matters such as beliefs, anxieties and concerns are not the remit of the traditional approach. Science deals with the objective, that which can be measured, whereas the patient's feelings, thoughts and concerns are unquantifiable and subjective, and are therefore deemed less worthy of consideration.

Medical students have been traditionally brought up in this world of the objective and the technological – at the expense of understanding the sick person, they have been taught to concentrate on the underlying disease mechanism and thereby to avoid the patient's perceptions and feelings. Unsupervised and undervalued forays into the uncharted territory of the patient's ideas and emotions only serve to reinforce the need for objectivity.

There is a further problem with the classical method of history taking. As we have seen in Chapter 1, students often erroneously perceive that the format in which they present their findings or document information in the case records is that in which they should obtain the information. They mistake the content of the traditional medical history for the process of medical interviewing. The way that doctors have been taught about the symptoms that we need to explore in order to make a diagnosis suggests that if we ask the 15 questions we have learned about the functioning of a particular organ system, we will gather all the information that we need. However, as we shall see later, this closed approach to questioning actually encourages an inefficient and inaccurate method of history taking (Evans *et al.* 1991). In fact, it is the premature search for scientific facts that stops us from listening, that prevents us from both taking an accurate history and picking up the cues to our patient's problems and concerns. Disease-centred medicine so quickly turns into doctor-centred medicine to the detriment of us all.

The disease–illness model

McWhinney (1989) and his colleagues at the University of Western Ontario proposed a 'transformed clinical method' to replace the traditional content of medical history taking. This approach, which requires doctors to understand their patients as well as their patients' diseases, has also been called 'patient-centred clinical interviewing' to differentiate it from the 'doctor-centred' approach that attempts to interpret the patient's illness only from the traditional perspective of disease and pathology (Stewart *et al.* 1995, 2003; Stewart 2001). The term 'patient centred' can be misinterpreted to mean consumerism, but this is clearly not what the authors intended.

More recently, Tresolini *et al.* (1994) suggested a somewhat different conceptualisation of the healthcare process, 'relationship-centred care', in an attempt to recognise that the nature and the quality of relationships are central to healthcare and the broader healthcare delivery system and to the well-being of both patient and physician. Taking this paradigm further, Beach *et al.* (2006) identified four principles of relationship-centred care: (1) relationships in healthcare ought to include the personhood of the participants, (2) affect and emotion are important components of these relationships, (3) all healthcare relationships occur in the context of reciprocal influence and (4) the formation and maintenance of genuine relationships in healthcare is morally valuable. In relationship-centred care, relationships between patients and clinicians remain central, although the relationships of clinicians with themselves, with each other and with the community are also emphasised. Relationship-centred care and patient-centred care are complementary paradigms.

Returning to our explication of McWhinney's clinical method, patient-centred medicine encourages doctors to consider *both* the doctor's agenda and the patient's agenda in each interview (Mischler 1984; Campion *et al.* 1992; Epstein 2000; Barry *et al.* 2001). The disease–illness model (*see* Figure 3.1) attempts to provide a practical way of using these ideas in everyday clinical practice:

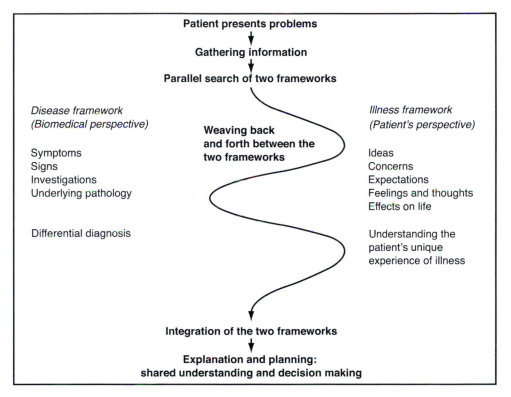

Figure 3.1 The disease–illness model. After Levenstein *et al.* (1989) and Stewart *et al.* (2003).

Definition of disease and illness

The beauty of this analysis of gathering information is the clarity with which it demonstrates how we need to explore both 'disease' and 'illness' to fulfil our unique role as medical practitioners. *Disease* is the biomedical cause of sickness in terms of pathophysiology. Clearly it is the doctor's role to search for symptoms and signs of underlying disease. Discovering a diagnosis for the patient's 'disease' is the doctor's traditional and central agenda. *Illness* in contrast is the individual patient's unique experience of sickness – how each patient perceives, experiences and copes with their illness. The patient's perspective is not as narrow as the doctor's and it includes the feelings, thoughts, concerns and effect on life that any episode of sickness induces. It represents the patient's response to events around them, the patient's understanding of what is happening to them, and the patient's expectations of help.

Patients can be ill but have no disease. Often we cannot find a root cause for symptoms in any underlying pathological disease. For instance, consider the patient with a bereavement reaction and the symptoms that grief can produce, or the businessman with tension headaches, or the young child with problems at school leading to abdominal pain. On the other hand, patients can have a disease but not be knowingly ill – for example, those with asymptomatic disease such as ovarian cancer or hypertension.

Disease and illness normally coexist but one of the great fascinations of medicine is how the same disease can cause remarkably different illness experiences in every individual. Imagine for a moment all the patients you have seen with any one condition. The variation between patients' reactions to their similar symptoms or to their common diagnosis is enormous. Their thoughts, feelings, ideas, concerns, expectations, support systems and previous life experiences influence not only their ability to cope but also the physical effect of the disease itself. One person with a sore throat is happy to wait for nature to provide a cure and does not go to the doctor at all, while another wants antibiotics because he remembers how awful it was when he had a peritonsillar abscess. One woman with breast cancer presents with a tiny lump, while another is discovered by chance to have a hidden fungating mass.

Why doctors need to explore both perspectives

Doctors have always attempted to separate out these two contrasting perspectives of sickness but in the past have tended to discard the patient's illness framework as simply a collection of confounding variables that get in the way of discovering the underlying diagnosis. A patient's fear, anxiety and pain threshold can all encroach on our ability to find out, say, if this abdominal pain is appendicitis or not. We only consider the patient's unique response so as to prevent it from clouding our technological judgement. All too often, the result is that we then focus only on the body, discard the understanding that we have obtained about our patient, and thereby fail to consider the patient as a person (Cassell 1985).

Mischler (1984) has explained how the doctor, in her desperation to make a diagnosis, selectively listens to patients' comments that help her interpret their problems from the technological perspective. The doctor does not hear or pursue comments that give her insight into their world. Mischler describes this as 'two parallel monologues' in which patient and doctor talk at cross purposes in different languages.

Whereas doctors have discarded the information that they have obtained from the illness framework, healers, practitioners of alternative medicine and counsellors who have not been brought up in the tradition of Western disease-centred medicine have tended to place less emphasis on information from the disease framework and have concentrated instead on 'illness' (Kleinman *et al.* 1978).

Doctors in fact have a *unique responsibility* to do both – to listen to the disease and illness frameworks and not discard either (Smith and Hoppe 1991). The disease–illness model does not in any way negate our scientific disease approach but adds a patient-centred arm as well. We are not counsellors whose sole aim is to help patients to become aware of how their thoughts and feelings are influencing their lives and their illness – we have the extra responsibility and burden of diagnosing and treating disease. However, if we consider our role as purely that of discovering disease, we will not fully help our patients with their very individual needs.

We need to take into account both our own traditional disease agenda and our patient's very personal illness agenda. When a patient presents with joint pains, the doctor may see his role in terms of diagnosis and treatment of any underlying disease. However, the patient's main concern may be the possibility of loss of future independence – the patient's agenda may concern discussing prognosis more than diagnosis. These two agendas overlap but without addressing the patient's beliefs and concerns as well as diagnosing the disease process, the doctor will not have fully served the patient as an individual. The patient-centred approach enlarges the doctor's agenda to take account of both disease and illness. Interestingly, in the study by O'Keefe *et al.* (2003) of medical student interviews in paediatrics, clinical competence was a more significant determinant of maternal evaluations of medical student interviews than was patient-centredness. However, high levels of both patient-centredness and clinical competence were associated with the highest maternal satisfaction.

The advantages of taking a history that includes both arms of the disease–illness model are numerous.

1. **Supporting, understanding and building a relationship.** Taking only a traditional disease-centred history of chest pain in a 55-year-old man may well allow you to diagnose angina and plan investigation and treatment. Although this is an absolutely necessary task, failing also to understand the meaning of the chest pain to the patient and the implications that your diagnosis might have to that individual may well limit your effectiveness as a doctor. The patient may become agitated at the mention of angina because his father died suddenly from a heart attack at the same age. Or the patient may have been very fit and active up until now and may be devastated that heart disease might prevent the active future that he had planned. He may be a commercial traveller whose livelihood depends on his ability to drive. His wife may be ill and he might not want to burden her with his problems. Your ability to help him depends on your ability not only to diagnose effectively but also to understand your patient's perspective and support him through adversity.

2. **The traditional disease model does not explain everything about a patient's problems.** There may not be a 'disease' in terms of the traditional medical model to explain our 55-year-old man's chest pain and his feelings of illness. It may have roots in personal unhappiness, in stress at home or at work, or in anxiety about health. Although it is clearly our responsibility to exclude physical disease, however hard we try we will not find a disease in all our patients. Even if we do, it may not explain why the patient has come to see the doctor on this occasion – a muscular pain may well be tolerated when the patient is comfortable with his life but be cause for concern when he is under stress.

   We need to extend our interviewing to include not only the disease but also the illness framework. Using just the disease approach, our man's chest pain may not sound ischaemic and his ECG may be normal. However, if he keeps returning with unexplained pain, we may feel forced to investigate further. Exploring the illness perspective as well may allow him to talk about his marital difficulties or his unresolved grief which in itself may well lead to resolution of his symptoms (Epstein *et al.* 1999). Searching both frameworks can make the consultation more accurate and efficient as well as supportive. In a study by Stewart *et al.* (1997) in family practice, patient-centredness and the patient's perception of finding common ground regarding both frameworks resulted in fewer follow-up appointments, investigations and referrals.

   There is considerable research evidence to support the lack of organic disease to explain much about our patients' problems. In 50% of patients presenting to general practitioners with chest pain, the cause was unproven after six months of follow-up (Blacklock 1977). Similar statistics are available for tiredness, abdominal pain and headache. But it would be a mistake to think that this is a problem that is restricted to family medicine – what about the globus of ENT or the irritable bowel syndrome of gastroenterology or the non-organic chest pain of cardiology? All specialists see patients whose symptoms are not necessarily caused by disease.

3. **Discovering the patient's perspective can aid diagnosis and make for more effective and efficient interviews.** Asking for the patient's ideas can aid diagnosis. Discovering that the pain started after a fall may be an important clue to the cause of the problem, which might otherwise never have been discovered. Discovering that the patient's agenda is simply to obtain a sickness certificate, as their back pain is resolving, may save time and money by preventing unnecessary disease-centred questioning or uncalled-for prescribing. As in the earlier Stewart *et al.* (1997) study, Epstein *et al.* (2005) have demonstrated that patient-centred communication is associated with fewer diagnostic testing costs.

4. **Groundwork for explanation and planning.** When we explore explanation and planning in Chapter 6, we shall look at the research that demonstrates the central importance of eliciting and understanding the patient's unique perspective of their illness in this later stage of the consultation. We shall see that without an explanation that addresses our patients' individual ideas, expectations and concerns, our patient's recall, understanding, satisfaction and compliance are all likely to suffer.

Tuckett *et al.* (1985) have shown that consultations go wrong where there is an incongruity between the patient's and the doctor's explanatory frameworks. Our 55-year-old man with chest pain might well think that he has lung cancer, as his friend has recently died from the disease. You might be perfectly happy that it is musculoskeletal and of no consequence. Unless you have discovered your patient's ideas and explained why you think that it is not due to cancer, he may leave the consulting room with the nagging doubt that you may not have considered the possibility. This doubt may block the patient's understanding and commitment to your explanations and undermine his acceptance of your diagnosis or treatment plan. Similarly, an elderly woman with arthritis of the knee may not wish any active treatment for a pain that she can easily tolerate. Her concern may be that she is developing rheumatoid arthritis like her mother, and she might just want reassurance that she is not. Without understanding her expectations, the doctor might use the word 'arthritis' and not explain the difference between osteo- and rheumatoid arthritis. The doctor might prescribe an anti-inflammatory drug that the patient might not wish to take. It is surprisingly easy to treat the disease rather than the patient.

So, as well as splitting the two arms of disease and illness apart, the physician has to put the two back together again. This is the stage labelled *integration* in the disease–illness model. Without this step it is impossible to achieve a shared understanding with the patient about the nature of the problem and its management and it is difficult to enable the patient to participate in shared decision making.

Basing our negotiation on an open understanding of our respective positions and reaching mutually understood common ground is the final aim. However, as we shall see later in this chapter and in Chapter 6, understanding the patient's perspective does not mean abrogating our responsibility as doctors and promoting an entirely consumerist approach. Consider the person who attends with a viral sore throat that the doctor thinks does not require antibiotics. Discovering the patient's expectations first, rather than assuming that all patients wish to be prescribed antibiotics, is helpful in itself. A treatment plan can then be negotiated that is based on a true understanding of the patient's position. If, as is so often the case, the patient would prefer not to have antibiotics if at all possible, a comfortable negotiation is assured from the outset. If the patient would prefer antibiotics, eliciting and addressing that expectation and explaining your position in relation to their views is vital. Only then can the patient understand your rationale and feel that their position has at least been taken into consideration. As a study by Steihaug *et al.* (2012) demonstrates, overtly recognising the patient's perspectives makes it easier to tolerate disagreement, and conflict and dissatisfaction can be anticipated and defused.

An alternative template for the content of the information-gathering section of the interview

The disease–illness model provides the foundation upon which we have developed an alternative template for the content of information gathering. This template retains all the elements of the traditional medical history but in addition includes the 'new' content of the patient's perspective (Kurtz *et al.* 2003).

This template explicitly demonstrates how the discrete elements of the traditional medical history and the components of the disease–illness model can seamlessly work together in clinical practice.

Content to be discovered

Biomedical perspective - disease
  Sequence of events
  Symptom analysis
  Relevant systems review

Patient's perspective - illness
  Ideas and beliefs
  Concerns
  Expectations
  Effects on life
  Feelings

Background information - context
  Past medical history
  Drug and allergy history
  Family history
  Personal and social history
  Review of systems

Figure 3.2   An alternative template for the content of information gathering.

It is important that this template makes intuitive sense to practising physicians, clinical faculty who teach on the wards or in history-taking courses, and those who teach in communication courses. All of these groups need to be able to embrace the same template with enthusiasm so that students, whether in the formal communication course or on the wards or clinics, can receive a consistent message about the content of the medical interview. The template we provide here fits beautifully with what happens in real-life clinical practice. Clinicians readily see how the new and traditional content fit together and also how this content model relates to the process skills of information gathering that we shall discuss shortly.

This template forms the backbone of how physicians can record information in the medical records and present their findings to others, as we have described in Chapter 1 (*see* Figure 1.4). This provides a more appropriate approach to record-keeping in the modern era. Interestingly, the Health Informatics Unit, Royal College of Physicians (2008) in the UK has produced documentation on standards for the structure and content of medical records for patients admitted to hospital. Their standards for medical records specifically include all of the elements mentioned here, including the patient's concerns, expectations and wishes.

The biomedical perspective

The information that the physician needs to discover about the 'disease' aspect is identical to that of the traditional medical history. We have divided this into three equally important parts.

1. **Sequence of events.** Before analysing the symptoms in depth, it is useful for the doctor to discover the exact sequence of events over time in relation to the problem areas that the patient has identified. We shall discuss the process skills that enable this to be achieved in the most effective fashion in the next section of this chapter.
2. **Symptom analysis.** The doctor also needs to analyse each symptom in depth. We would like to emphasise at this point the importance of a thorough analysis of each symptom, an approach that the traditional methodology of history taking has always stressed. The following are two examples of aide-memoirs that list the content required to investigate a symptom and thereby help us to be systematic in our approach.

WWQQAA plus B

1. **Where** – the location and radiation of a symptom
2. **When** – when it began, fluctuation over time, duration
3. **Quality** – what it feels like
4. **Quantity** – intensity, extent, degree of disability
5. **Aggravating and alleviating factors**
6. **Associated manifestations** – other symptoms
7. **Beliefs** – the patient's beliefs about the symptoms

Macleod's Clinical Examination (Munro and Campbell 2000)

1. Site
2. Radiation
3. Character
4. Severity
5. Duration
6. Frequency and periodicity
7. Special times of occurrence
8. Aggravating factors
9. Relieving factors
10. Associated phenomena

---

3. **Relevant systems review.** A further essential element consists of the components of the systems review that are relevant to the particular part of the medical history that is being discussed. If a patient has explained that the problem that they have come to the doctor with is abdominal pain, then after determining the sequence of events and the analysis of this symptom, the most appropriate next step in exploring the biomedical perspective is to work through the gastrointestinal system review, even if this only reveals important 'relevant negatives'.

It is important to bring this part of the systems review forward rather than leave it to near the end of the interview as part of the full systems review. Doing so fits better with the clinical reasoning process – in real life, clinicians start to problem solve early on in the interview and therefore require information about relevant systems to be juxtaposed as closely as possible.

The patient's perspective

The doctor also needs to gain information and understanding about the patient's illness perspective, the 'new' content of the medical history:

- **ideas and beliefs** – beliefs or thoughts about the causation or effect of the illness, and about health and what influences or contributes to it
- **concerns** – worries about what the symptoms might mean
- **expectations** – hopes of how the doctor might help, and outcomes that the patient wants from the visit
- **effects on life** – the effect the illness has on day-to-day living
- **feelings** – emotions that the problems induce.

Background information: context

Of course, the doctor also needs to discover the background information that has always been carefully delineated in the traditional medical history. This information provides important insights into the context within which current problems or symptoms are occurring. Such information is necessary to make a fully informed interpretation of current events. The level of detail required here will depend on whether a complete or focused history is being taken. Background information includes:

- past medical history
- family history
- personal and social history
- medications and allergies
- systems review.

Further information concerning the exact questions that constitute the individual elements of this background information is well described in many medical textbooks (Seymour and Siklos 1994; Munro and Campbell 2000; Seidel 2003).

The process skills of information gathering

We now turn our attention to the communication process skills of gathering information. How do we go about gathering all the information from the patient we have discussed earlier? What impact do communication process skills have on the content that is gathered? What communication skills can we employ to be most effective in this phase of the medical interview?

Box 3.1 delineates the communication process skills needed for gathering information effectively. We would like to stress that, used appropriately, these process skills apply equally to taking a complete or focused history and in all settings, whether in hospital, in the clinic or on the wards, or in family practice.

Box 3.1   Gathering information

Exploration of the patient's problems
- **Patient's narrative**: encourages patient to tell the story of the problem(s) from when first started to the present in own words (clarifying reason for presenting now)
- **Questioning techniques**: uses *open and closed questioning techniques*, appropriately moving from open to closed
- **Listening**: listens attentively, allowing the patient to complete statements without interruption; leaves space for the patient to think before answering or go on after pausing
- **Facilitative response**: facilitates the patient's responses verbally and non-verbally, e.g. use of encouragement, silence, repetition, paraphrasing, interpretation
- **Cues**: picks up the patient's verbal and non-verbal cues (body language, vocal cues, facial expression, affect); checks them out and acknowledges as appropriate
- **Clarification**: checks out statements that are vague or need amplification (e.g. *'Could you explain what you mean by light-headed?'*)
- **Time-framing**: establishes *dates and sequence* of events
- **Internal summary**: periodically summarises to verify own understanding of what the patient has said; invites the patient to correct interpretation and provide further information.

- **Language**: uses concise, easily understood questions and comments; avoids or adequately explains jargon

Additional skills for understanding the patient's perspective
- Actively determines and appropriately explores:
  - patient's ideas (i.e. beliefs regarding cause)
  - patient's concerns (i.e. worries) regarding each problem
  - patient's expectations (i.e. goals, what help the patient expects for each problem)
  - effects of each problem on the patient's life
- Encourages expression of feelings

Next we examine in detail each of the process skills for gathering information listed in Box 3.1, and we explore the evidence from theory and research that validates their use in the consultation. We shall look at each skill separately and then put them together into a practical approach that physicians can use in everyday practice.

EXPLORATION OF THE PATIENT'S PROBLEMS

In Chapter 2 we examined the beginning of the interview and saw the advantages of initiating the consultation carefully and making a route plan of the consultation rather than blindly setting off down the first road that appears. We now turn to the skills associated with in-depth exploration of the patient's problems.

We start by exploring the central importance of questioning techniques to information gathering. Readers will note that we recommend in Box 3.1 that eliciting the patient's narrative in chronological sequence is the first approach to consider after initiation. However, the skill of discovering the patient's narrative is a specific application of the use of open questioning techniques and is easiest to consider after we have discussed questioning in more depth.

Questioning techniques

It is easy to assume at this point in the consultation that the doctor's influence on events is limited, that the patient will tell their prepared story whatever the doctor does or says. However, our own actions and utterances profoundly influence our patients' replies and the type of responses that they provide. How we ask questions plays a central role in the quality and quantity of information that we obtain.

We should remember that doctors exert considerable control over the interview. We direct the patient to an area for further exploration and by the nature of our questions and responses impose certain limits to the patient's freedom to elaborate. Yet very often we are not consciously aware of the effect that we are having. How can we make this process more intentional so that we can more adeptly choose to use different questioning approaches as and when required? Let's start with some definitions.

What are open and closed questions?

Closed (convergent) questions are questions for which a specific and often one-word answer, such as yes or no, is expected. They limit the response to a narrow field set by the questioner. The patient usually provides a response of one or two words without elaboration.

Open (divergent) questioning techniques in contrast are designed to introduce an area of enquiry without unduly shaping or focusing the content of the response. They still direct the patient to a specific area but allow the patient more discretion in their answer, suggesting to the patient that elaboration is both appropriate and welcome.

Here are some simple examples of these questioning styles:

- **open** – *'Tell me about your headaches'*
- **more directive but still open** – *'What makes your headaches better or worse?'*
- **closed** – *'Do you ever wake up with the headache in the morning?'*

We would like to emphasise that both open and closed questions are valuable. In our efforts to demonstrate that doctors tend to use closed questions too often, at the wrong time and at the expense of open questions, we do not mean to imply that doctors should not use closed questions at all. Both are essential but achieve very different ends. Their use at different times in the interview needs to be chosen with care.

Because asking questions is not the only way to gather information, the term 'question' is something of a misnomer here. More accurate would be the broader open and closed 'questioning techniques'. Many open techniques are in fact not questions at all but, rather, directive statements:

'Start at the beginning and take me through what has been happening ...'
'Tell me more about that ...'
'Tell me how you have been doing since your operation yesterday ...'

as opposed to questions:

'What has been going on from when you first noticed the pain up until now?
'Why did your doctor admit you to the hospital today?'
'How have you been feeling since your operation ...?'
'What were your thoughts ...?'

When should we use open and closed methods: the open-to-closed cone

Understanding how to intentionally choose between open and closed questioning styles at different points in the interview is of key importance. Starting with open questions and later moving to closed questions is called the *open-to-closed cone* (Goldberg *et al.* 1983). The doctor uses open questioning techniques first to obtain a picture of the problem from the patient's perspective. Later, the approach becomes more focused with increasingly specific although still open questions and eventually closed questions to elicit additional details that the patient may have omitted. The use of open questioning techniques is critical at the beginning of the exploration of any problem – their power as an information-gathering tool here cannot be overemphasised. The most common mistake is to move to closed questioning too quickly. A second mistake is to use open techniques only at the beginning of the consultation. Using multiple open-to-closed cones throughout the interview – for example, whenever you begin exploration of a new issue or topic – is more appropriate.

What are the advantages of open questioning techniques?

Why does staying open before moving to closed questions provide maximum efficiency in information gathering? Look at what might happen if we were to use two very different approaches to the same scenario.

A consultation relying on closed methods might go like this:

Doctor:	*'Now about this chest pain – where is the pain?'*
Patient:	*'Well, over the front here.'* (Pointing to the sternum)
Doctor:	*'What are the pains like – are they a dull ache or a sharp pain?'*
Patient:	*'Quite sharp, really.'*
Doctor:	*'Have you taken anything for it?'*
Patient:	*'Just some antacids, but they don't seem to help much.'*
Doctor:	*'Do the pains go anywhere else?'*
Patient:	*'No, just there.'*

An initially more open-ended questioning style might reveal very different information:

Doctor:	*'Tell me about the chest pain that you have been having.'*
Patient:	*'Well, it's been building up over the last few weeks. I've always had a little indigestion, but not as bad as this. I get this sharp pain right here* (pointing to sternum) *and then I belch a lot and get a really horrible acid taste in my mouth. It's much worse if I've had a drink or two and I'm not getting much sleep.'*
Doctor:	*'I see. Can you tell me more about it?'*
Patient:	*'Well, I was wondering if it was brought on by the tablets I've been taking for my joints – they've been much worse and I took some ibuprofen. I need to keep going at the moment, what with John and all.'*

Why is there such a difference in the information obtained with open questioning? The advantages of open questioning methods are that they:

- encourage the patient to tell their story in a more complete fashion
- prevent the stab-in-the-dark approach of closed questioning
- allow the doctor time and space to listen and think and not just ask the next question

- contribute to more effective diagnostic reasoning
- help in the exploration of both the disease and the illness frameworks
- set a pattern of patient participation rather than physician domination.

1. **Encouraging the patient to tell their story in a more complete fashion.** Closed questions give the doctor more control over the patient's responses but limit the possible information that can be obtained. Open questions, in contrast, encourage the patient to answer in an inclusive way and may well provide much of the information that is being sought. By asking an open question, information about a problem can be obtained quickly and efficiently. In the previous examples, more useful information about the chest pains was discovered with two open questions than with four closed questions.

2. **Preventing the stab-in-the-dark approach of closed questioning.** In the closed approach, all the responsibility rests with the interviewer. He has to consider which areas might be worth enquiring about and then frame appropriate questions to ask. Clearly, the information obtained will only relate to those very areas that the doctor thinks are likely to be relevant, and the doctor may well forget to ask about key areas of importance. Each question is like a stab in the dark, potentially a very inefficient process. In the open method, the patient can mention areas that the interviewer might not have considered – in the earlier example of closed questioning, the doctor may not have thought to ask about alcohol and would have missed an important clue. This does not decry the value of closed questioning later on in the interview process. Closed questions are essential to clarify points or screen for areas not yet mentioned, but this is more efficiently achieved after first eliciting a wider view of the problem and hearing more of the patient's narrative.

3. **Allowing the doctor time and space to listen and think and not just ask the next question.** In the closed method, the doctor has to follow each closed question with another. Instead of listening and thinking about the patient's replies, the doctor is formulating the next question to keep the flow of the interview going which in turn stops him from hearing important information. The open method allows the doctor time to more carefully consider replies and pick up cues as they emerge.

4. **Contributing to more effective diagnostic reasoning.** Unless doctors use open questioning techniques at the beginning of their information gathering, it is all too easy to restrict diagnostic reasoning to an over-narrow field of enquiry. We know that doctors start the process of problem solving very early on in the consultation. They quickly attempt to match the initial information presented by the patient to their underlying knowledge of individual diseases and to organisational frameworks that they have previously developed to aid problem solving. They then direct their further questioning to prove or disprove their initial thoughts (Kassirer and Gorry 1978; Barrows and Tamblyn 1980; Gick 1986; Mandin *et al.* 1997; Groopman 2007). Open methods allow doctors more time to generate their problem-solving approach and provide them with more information on which to base their theories and hypotheses. Closed questioning, in contrast, quickly leads to the exploration of one particular avenue that may well prove inappropriate and lead inexorably to a dead-end. The doctor may have to start again and generate a different problem-solving strategy – inefficient and inaccurate information gathering ensues. In our examples

given earlier, listening to the patient's story with the use of open questions has allowed the doctor to avoid the trap of early questioning about the possibility of ischaemic heart disease and has enabled the expression of further symptoms and concerns that will help to form a more accurate working hypothesis.

5. **Helping in the exploration of both the disease and the illness frameworks.** Closed questions as explained earlier are not an efficient initial method of exploring the disease aspects of a problem. They are even less helpful in discovering the illness framework. Because closed questions by their nature follow the doctor's agenda, they will tend to concentrate on the clinical aspects of the problem and omit the patient's perspective. Open questions, in contrast, encourage patients to talk about their illness from their unique point of view, to tell their story in their own way using their own vocabulary. Patients can choose what is important from their own perspective and the doctor can better understand the patient's personal experience of illness. Most important, open questions allow the patient time to order their stories into a more logical framework and to make them more understandable, not only to the doctor but also to the patient. There are several advantages to this method, in that patients who can make sense of their stories with the help of their doctors often 'feel' better too; this contributes to the doctor's therapeutic effect and also helps to build the relationship between doctor and patient (Launer 2002).

6. **Setting a pattern of patient participation rather than physician domination.** As we discussed in Chapter 2, 94% of all interruptions conclude with the doctor obtaining the floor (Beckman and Frankel 1984). The early pursuit of one problem by closed questioning shifts the whole emphasis from a patient-centred to a physician-centred format and once this is done, the patient tends to remain in a more passive role. Once you begin closed questioning, patients will often not volunteer anything that is not explicitly asked – most patients defer to your lead. Open questions allow the patient to participate more actively, signal that is it appropriate to elaborate, and make the doctor's willingness to listen apparent.

Why is it important to move from open to closed questioning techniques?

As the interview proceeds it is important for the doctor to become gradually more focused. He needs to use increasingly specific open questions and eventually move to closed questions to elicit fine details. He needs to use closed questions to investigate specific areas if they do not emerge from the patient's account, to analyse a symptom in detail and to take a functional enquiry (though even this can begin openly, e.g. *'Tell me about any problems with your skin …'*).

In Chapter 4 we explore how to move from open to closed questioning with the use of clear and explanatory transitional statements and shall see how summary and signposting can help overcome the perceived loss of control and potentially more disordered information gathering inherent in the use of open questioning. In Chapter 5, we will also look at the importance of non-verbal communication to the success of question asking and see how even closed questions asked in a facilitating manner can encourage the patient to tell more of their story – good non-verbal communication can turn closed questions into open ones.

What is the evidence for the value of open and closed questioning techniques?

Roter and Hall (1987) investigated the association between primary care physicians' interviewing styles and the medical information that they obtained during consultations with simulated patients. They found that physicians on average elicited only 50% of the medical information considered important by expert consensus, with a worrying range of 9%–85%! They found that the amount of information elicited was related to the use of both appropriate open and closed questions. However, open questions prompted the revelation of substantially more relevant information than closed questions.

Stiles *et al.* (1979) have shown that patients at a hospital-based medical walk-in clinic were more satisfied with the information gathering phase of the interview if they were allowed to express themselves in their own words rather than provide yes/no or one-word answers to closed questions.

Goldberg *et al.* (1983) investigated the ability of family practice residents in the United States to detect emotional and psychiatric problems in their patients. They looked at which aspects of residents' interview styles determined their ability to detect psychiatric disorders. Two of the skills that they found to be related to the accuracy of the residents' assessments were the open-to-closed cone and open directive rather than closed questions.

Maguire *et al.* (1996b) have shown that cancer patients disclose more of their significant concerns if their doctors use open rather than leading questions.

Further evidence of the relative value of open and closed questioning comes from the detailed studies of Cox *et al.* (Cox *et al.* 1981a, 1981b; Rutter and Cox 1981; Cox 1989). They studied interviews with parents of children referred to a child psychiatric clinic. In the first phase of their study, they observed the interviews of trainee psychiatrists in order to determine the effect that certain interview behaviours had both on the gathering of factual information and on the expression of emotions and feelings. Their research showed that:

- the ratio of open to closed questions was significantly correlated with parents' talkativeness and contributions, and the more talkative the parents, the more likely they were to bring up problems spontaneously
- the amount of talk by the interviewer, the number of topics raised by the interviewer and the number of floor-holdings were negatively correlated with parents' amount of talk and duration of utterances
- open questioning and longer utterances, encouraged by the interviewer talking less, facilitated both the expression of emotions and the gathering of sensitive data.

In the second phase of their study, experienced psychiatrists were trained to use different styles of interviewing to demonstrate that the findings from the first arm of the study could be reproduced experimentally. They were able to reproduce the earlier findings and also showed that:

- if mothers were encouraged to express their concerns freely, they mentioned most but not quite all of the key issues without the need for closed questioning; many of the items not raised turned out to be normal or unremarkable

- in less probing styles, patients mentioned more symptoms or problems that had not been previously raised or considered by the interviewer, while in more probing styles, symptoms thought to be relevant by the interviewer were slightly less likely to be missed.

Their conclusion was 'that it is desirable to begin clinical diagnostic interviews with a lengthy period with little in the way of detailed probing and in which informants are allowed to express their concerns in their own way'.

The research of Cox and colleagues has also shown the value of closed questioning:

- the number of topics raised by the interviewer directly was significantly associated with a larger number of symptoms being discovered to be definitely absent, which can be very important information
- more information was obtained when interviewers used more specific requests for detailed information and more specific detailed probes per topic.

Their conclusion here was that 'if psychiatrists are to obtain sufficient detail about family problems and child symptoms for them to make an adequate formulation on which to base treatment plans there must be some systematic and detailed probing and questioning.'

Takemura *et al.* (2007) found significant positive relationships between three particular interview behaviours and the amount of information obtained in real family medicine interviews: (1) the open-to-closed cone, (2) facilitation and (3) summarisation.

Eliciting the patient's narrative

Listening is just as important in information gathering as it is at the beginning of the consultation. But before you can start to listen, how do you set the patient off in the right direction? How do you ask the patient to give you further information about each problem?

From the discussion here, it is clear that open rather than closed questioning techniques at the beginning of problem exploration will pay dividends.

> *'Tell me about your headaches'*

will be far more advantageous than

> *'You mentioned headaches. Where exactly are they?'*

One particularly useful method of gathering information in an initially open way is the 'patient's narrative', encouraging the patient to tell the story of their problem from when it first started up to the present in their own words.

> *'Tell me all about it from the beginning.'*

This is a natural way to find out about the patient's experience and to gather all the information that you need in an orderly fashion. It allows the patient to tell their story to you chronologically in much the same way as they would tell it to a friend – people will usually have discussed their problem with several people before they come to see the doctor (Stimson and Webb 1975). From a medical standpoint, it provides the doctor early in the interview with a clear picture of the sequence of events. This important component of the biomedical perspective (disease history) enhances accuracy. Asking the patient to tell their story chronologically provides you with an organisational framework that contributes to clinical reasoning and helps you as well as the patient keep details of the history in mind more easily. In contrast, consider how difficult it is to elicit the sequence of events using closed questioning, which may explain why this valuable component of the history is sometimes overlooked.

This method offers all the advantages of open questioning while providing the patient with a simple method of telling their story chronologically. It is an excellent way to understand the patient's perspective and it helps prevent Mischler's 'two parallel monologues', in which patient and doctor talk at cross purposes in different languages (Mischler 1984). The role of the doctor is to listen carefully and, if necessary, guide the patient through their storytelling, possibly seeking brief clarification but quickly returning to *'Then what happened?'* The device of the patient's narrative allows the doctor to make some interruptions without necessarily taking the floor from the patient – he can return control to the patient by asking the patient to continue their story. However, this should be done sparingly, because once the doctor has interrupted it is all too easy for him to continue in control with closed questions and forget to re-establish the patient's narrative.

Open questioning and the patient's narrative are ideal ways to enter the arenas of the biomedical and the patient's perspectives simultaneously. High-quality information can be obtained about both.

Attentive listening

As the patient tells their story, the doctor needs to listen attentively without interrupting. We have already covered the importance of attentive listening in depth in Chapter 2 when we looked at the beginning of the interview. As we have seen, attentive listening is a highly skilled process, requiring a combination of focus, facilitation skills, wait time and picking up cues. More recently this skill has been referred to as 'mindful listening' or 'deep listening'.

If we look again at the advantages of attentive listening listed in Chapter 2, we can see how many features are shared with the advantages of open questions mentioned earlier in this chapter. This similarity is because attentive listening is a direct consequence of the use of open questions – it is almost impossible to employ active listening and closed questioning together.

Facilitative response

As well as listening, it is important to actively encourage patients to continue their storytelling. Closed questioning is so predominant that patients may well initially respond even to excellent open questions with only a word or two unless they are encouraged to continue. Any behaviour that has the effect of inviting patients to say more about the area that they are already discussing is a facilitative response. When we began our discussion of facilitative responses in Chapter 2, we looked at the research evidence showing that certain skills, such as echoing or repetition, could be counterproductive when used too early in the interview. At the beginning of the interview, our objective is to obtain as wide as possible a view of the patient's whole agenda before exploring any one problem in detail. Now let's turn our attention to the use of facilitative responses in the information gathering phase. What are the skills that are useful here when we are trying to encourage patients to talk about each of their problems in greater depth?

The facilitative response involves both verbal and non-verbal communication skills. In this chapter we focus primarily on verbal communication and we also discuss selected non-verbal skills. We explore non-verbal communication in greater depth in Chapter 5.

The following skills can be used to facilitate the patient to say more about a topic, indicating simultaneously that you are interested in what they are saying and that you are keen for them to continue:

- encouragement
- silence
- repetition (echoing)
- paraphrasing
- sharing your thoughts.

Encouragement

Along with non-verbal head nods and the use of facial expression, doctors practising attentive listening use innumerable verbal encouragers, which signal the patient to continue their story. This is often achieved very efficiently with minimal or no interruption and yet it provides the patient with the necessary confidence to keep going. Such neutral facilitative comments include *'uh-huh'*, *'go on'*, *'yes'*, *'um'*, *'I see'* – we all have our own particular favourites.

Use of silence

Most verbal facilitation is ineffective unless immediately followed by non-verbal attentive silence. In Chapter 2, we discussed the work of Rowe (1986) on wait time and how the use of brief silence or pause can very easily and naturally facilitate the patient to contribute more. Longer periods of silence are also appropriate if patients are having difficulty expressing themselves or if it seems that they are about to be overwhelmed by emotion. The aim of providing a longer pause is to encourage patients to express out loud the thoughts or feelings that are occurring inside their head. There is a delicate balance here between comfortable and uncomfortable silence, between encouraging communication and interfering with it by creating uncertainty and anxiety – the doctor must attend carefully to accompanying non-verbal behaviour. However, remember that the clinician feels anxiety more often than the patient does – patients usually tolerate silence better than doctors!

If the clinician does feel that a silence is producing anxiety or the patient eventually needs further encouragement to speak, particular attention must be given to how the silence is broken. For instance:

> *'Can you bear to tell me what you are thinking?'*

acts to allow the patient to stay with his or her thoughts and further facilitates the process – as does repetition of the patient's last words, as we shall see shortly.

Repetition or echoing

Repeating the last few words that the patient has said encourages the patient to keep talking. Doctors often worry that this 'echoing' will sound unnatural, but again it is remarkably well accepted by patients. Note how repetition encourages the patient to continue with their last phrase and is therefore slightly more directive than encouragement or silence. This explains Beckman and Frankel's (1984) findings, as discussed in Chapter 2, which showed that echoing could act as a possible interrupter at the beginning of the interview by forcing the patient down a specific path before the doctor had discovered the full spectrum of concerns.

Following through the example used earlier, we can see the skills mentioned here in action to explore the biomedical and patient's perspectives of a problem:

Doctor: *'Tell me about the chest pain that you have been having.'* (open question)
Patient: *'Well, it's been building up over the last few weeks. I've always had a little indigestion, but not as bad as this. I get this sharp pain right here* (pointing to sternum) *and then I belch a lot and get a really horrible acid taste in my mouth. It's much worse if I've had a drink or two, and I'm not getting much sleep.'*
Doctor: *'Yes, go on'* (encouragement)
Patient: *'Well, I was wondering if it was brought on by the tablets I've been taking for my joints – they've been much worse and I got some ibuprofen from the chemist. I need to keep going at the moment, what with John and all.'*
Doctor: (silence – accompanied by eye contact, slight head nod)
Patient: *'He's really going downhill, doctor, and I don't know how I'm going to cope at home if he gets any worse.'*
Doctor: *'How you're going to cope?'* (repetition)
Patient: *'I promised him I wouldn't let him go into hospital again, and now I'm not sure if I can do it.'*

Paraphrasing

Paraphrasing is restating in your own words the content or feelings behind the patient's message. It is not quite the same as checking or summarising – it is intended to sharpen rather than just confirm understanding, and therefore it tends to be more specific than the original message. Paraphrasing checks if your own *interpretation* of what the patient actually means is correct. Continuing our example:

> Doctor: *'Are you thinking that when John gets even more ill, you won't be strong enough to nurse him at home by yourself?'* (paraphrase of content)
>
> Patient: *'I think I'll be OK physically, but what happens if he needs me day and night? There's only me, and I can't call on Mary, since she has a job'*
>
> Doctor: *'It sounds as if you're worried that you might be letting John down.'* (paraphrase of feeling)

Paraphrasing combines elements of facilitation, summarising and clarification. It is particularly helpful if you think that you understand but are not quite certain, or you think that there might be hidden feelings behind a seemingly simple message. Paraphrasing is a very good facilitative entry point into the patient's perspective.

Sharing your thoughts

Sharing why you are asking questions is another excellent way to encourage the patient to be more inclusive in their answer and it acts as a very effective facilitative tool:

> *'Sometimes, chest pains can be brought on by stress – I was wondering if you felt that might be true for you?'*

This is ostensibly a closed question, but the fact that the patient can understand the reasoning behind your request allows her to answer and then elaborate. The more direct *'Are you under a lot of stress at present?'* is far more likely to produce a one-word response containing little information. We shall discuss the issue of sharing your thoughts with the patient further in Chapter 5.

What is the theoretical evidence for facilitation?

The facilitative skills enumerated earlier are the key skills of non-directive counselling. They have been extensively discussed by Rogers (1980), Egan (1990) and others and are widely accepted as crucial elements of any communication in which the aim is to encourage the client to talk more about their problem without undue professional direction.

Levinson *et al.* (1997) showed that primary care physicians who used more facilitation statements (soliciting patients' opinions, checking understanding, encouraging patients to talk, paraphrasing and interpretation) were less likely to have suffered malpractice claims. This association was not found for surgeons in the same study. Takemura *et al.* (2007) found facilitation to be positively related to the amount of information obtained in family medicine interviews. In a further study in 2008, they reported a significant positive association between reflection or legitimisation and patient satisfaction in hospital outpatients.

Collectively facilitation skills form a major part of the patient-centred interviewing style of Henbest and Stewart (1990a, 1990b), which, as we discuss in the next section, has been demonstrated to favourably affect many measurable parameters of communication. Patient-centredness in these studies was scored by a combination of open-ended questions, facilitative expressions and specific requests for patients' expectations, thoughts and feelings in response to patients' comments.

Picking up verbal and non-verbal cues

Through attentive listening and verbal and non-verbal facilitation, we make patients feel comfortable and welcomed, indicate that we are interested in what they are saying and encourage them to continue and elaborate even further. Surprisingly, however, although we may be listening and give the impression that we are taking in everything that the patients are telling us, we may not have actually heard what our patients are saying! We may be eliciting the information beautifully but failing to register it. This is akin to measuring a patient's blood pressure but instantly realising after removing the cuff that you did not register the reading mentally, something that all physicians have experienced.

Hearing what the patient is saying is a vital ingredient in information gathering. This relates not only to what the patient is telling us overtly but also to what they are telling us indirectly or perhaps even unintentionally through verbal and non-verbal cues. Patients are generally eager to tell us about their own thoughts and feelings but often do so indirectly through verbal hints or changes in non-verbal behaviour (body language, vocal cues such as hesitation or a change in volume, facial expression, affect). Picking up these cues is an essential skill for exploring both the biomedical (*'and I've had this ... sort of ... it's not really a pain ...'*) and patient's perspectives (*'things haven't been easy ...'* or *'I'm alone ...'*) (Tuckett *et al.* 1985; Branch and Malik 1993; Cegala 1997; Suchman *et al.* 1997; Lang *et al.* 2000). Levinson *et al.* (2000) found in both primary care and surgical office settings that over 50% of interviews included one or more clues, with mean numbers of 2.6 in primary care and 1.9 in surgery. Salmon *et al.* (2004) explored psychosocial cues expressed by patients with unexplained symptoms. Contrary to common belief, almost all patients expressed opportunities for doctors to address psychological needs through explicit questions and cues. Mjaaland *et al.* (2011a) demonstrated similar findings when they looked at videotaped physician–patient encounters across the specialties in a Norwegian general hospital. In their study patients expressed negative emotional cues and concerns in more than half of the consultations, with a mean of 1.69 per consultation.

And hearing the cue in itself is still not enough. We need to respond, to check out each cue with the patient and acknowledge it as appropriate (Suchman *et al.* 1997). Levinson *et al.* (2000) found that patients gave cues throughout the interview from the opening to the closing minute, but that physicians only responded positively to patient cues in 38% of cases in surgery and 21% in primary care, and in the remainder entirely missed the opportunity to respond to the patients' cues. Where the cue was missed, half of the patients brought up the same issue a second or third time and in all of these cases, the physician again missed these further opportunities to respond. In a follow-up to the earlier study by Mjaaland *et al.* (2011a), the authors demonstrated that when patients expressed negative emotions or cues, physicians tended to move away from emotional communication without follow up or exploration, particularly if the emotion was expressed as an explicit concern (Mjaaland *et al.* 2011b).

The danger is therefore twofold – either missing the message altogether or having heard it, assuming we know what it means without checking it out with the patient. Patients' cues and the assumptions we make about them need to be explored and acknowledged either now or later in the interview. Although it can be appropriate to hear a cue and decide to leave your response to later, there is a danger to this course of action. First, there is a considerable chance that you will forget your mental note. Second, an immediate response and acknowledgement of the patient's cue acts as confirmation to the patient that you are interested and helps to ensure an atmosphere conducive to even more disclosure.

The study by Levinson *et al.* (2000) also showed that picking up and responding to cues *shortens* visits. Primary care visits that included at least one cue were longer when the physician missed the opportunity to respond than when physicians demonstrated a positive response (mean time, 20.1 minutes vs. 17.6 minutes). Findings were similar in surgery (14.0 minutes vs. 12.5 minutes). Visits in which patients repeatedly brought up emotional issues after the physician missed an opportunity to respond were longer than visits where physicians made at least one positive response (18.4 vs. 17.6 minutes in primary care and 15.5 vs. 12.5 minutes in surgery visits). Levinson *et al.* concluded that these two aspects of the medical encounter – patient cues and physician response – were 'a key to building a trusting patient-physician relationship, thus ultimately improving outcomes of care'.

Later in this chapter, when we investigate techniques for exploring the patient's perspective, we shall look at some of the ways in which patients' cues can be picked up and responded to.

Clarification of the patient's story

Clarifying statements that are vague or need further amplification is a vital information-gathering skill. After an initial response to an open-ended question, doctors may need to prompt patients for more precision, clarity or completeness. Often patients' statements can have two possible meanings – it is important to ascertain which one is intended.

Clarifying is often open in nature:

> 'Could you explain what you mean by light-headed?'

but may also be closed:

> 'When you say dizzy, do you mean that the room seems to actually spin round?'

If the patient does not provide dates for important events in their history, ask for them. Check that you understand the sequence of events correctly if you are uncertain. And to improve accuracy, learn to time-frame your own questions. Compare:

> *'Have you experienced depression?'* (undated)
> *'Have you ever experienced depression?'*
> *'Have you experienced depression in the last two weeks since you hit your head?'*

Too often we ask the first when we mean the third. When patients answer 'occasionally', which question are they answering?

Internal summary

Summarising is the deliberate step of making an explicit verbal summary to the patient of the information gathered so far and is one of the most important of all information-gathering skills. Used periodically throughout the interview, it helps the doctor with two significant tasks – namely, ensuring accuracy in the consultation and facilitating the patient's further responses.

Accuracy

With respect to accuracy, summarising is a highly effective practical test of whether you have understood the patient correctly, enabling the patient to confirm that you have understood what they have said or to correct your misinterpretation. It is a means of ensuring that you and the patient have attained *mutually understood common ground*. Platt and Platt (2003) liken the process to two authors passing drafts of a work back and forth until both are satisfied. Takemura *et al.* (2007) found a significant positive relationship between summarisation and the amount of information obtained in real family medicine interviews.

Remember to summarise both the disease and illness aspects of the patient's story. Summarising both helps to fulfil two of our previously stated objectives for this phase of the interview, namely:

- exploring and understanding the patient's perspective so as to understand the meaning of the illness for the patient
- exploring the biomedical perspective or disease framework so as to obtain an adequate 'medical' history.

Summarising tells you whether you have 'got it right'. If you have, the patient will confirm your picture with both verbal and non-verbal signs of agreement. However, if your understanding is inaccurate or incomplete, the patient will tell you or provide non-verbal signals of being unhappy (Neighbour 1987). Without overt verbal summary, we rely on conjecture and assumption that we have understood our patients correctly.

Quilligan and Silverman (2012) urged a slight note of caution here, finding that use and effect of summary was more complex than might be thought. In a study of medical students working with simulated patients, summary did appear to aid accuracy. However, the patient's perspective was summarised less frequently than the biomedical perspective. Also, when summaries were repeatedly incorrect, the simulated patients felt they were not being listened to, particularly if the purpose of summary was not carefully introduced.

Facilitation

Summarising not only makes for greater accuracy, it also expands your understanding of the patient's problems. Summary acts as an excellent facilitative opening. Followed by a pause and attentive listening, it is an important method of enabling the patient to continue their story without explicit direction from the doctor. It acts as a facilitative tool by inviting and making space for the patient to go further in explaining their problems and thoughts.

Doctor: *'Can I just see if I've got this right? – You've had indigestion before, but for the last few weeks you've had increasing problems with a sharp pain at the front of your chest, accompanied by wind and acid. It's stopping you from sleeping, it's made worse by drink and you were wondering if the painkillers were to blame. Is that right?* (Pause ...)

Patient: *'Yes, and I can't afford to be ill now with John being so ill. I don't know how I'm going to cope.'*

The advantages for patients are numerous – internal summary:

- clearly demonstrates that you have been listening
- demonstrates that you are interested and care about getting things right – it confirms the patient
- offers a collaborative approach to problem solving
- allows the patient to check your understanding and thoughts
- gives the patient an opportunity to either confirm or correct your interpretation and add in missing areas
- invites and allows the patient to go further in explaining their problems and thoughts by acting as a facilitative opening
- demonstrates the doctor's interest in the illness as well as the disease aspects of the patient's story.

The advantages for the doctor are also significant – internal summary:

- maximises accurate information gathering by allowing you to check the accuracy of what you think the patient has said and rectify any misconceptions; it promotes mutually understood common ground
- provides a space for you to review what you have already covered
- allows you to order your thoughts and clarify in your mind what you are not sure about and what aspect of the story you need to explore next
- helps you to recall information later
- allows you to distinguish between and consider both disease and illness.

We shall explore summarising in more depth and discuss the evidence for its use in Chapter 4.

Language

The use of concise, easily understood questions and comments, without jargon, is important throughout the interview. We shall be concentrating on this aspect of communication when we explore explanation and planning in Chapter 6.

ADDITIONAL SKILLS FOR UNDERSTANDING THE PATIENT'S PERSPECTIVE

The skills of problem exploration outlined here will enable the doctor to discover information about all three elements of the medical history – the biomedical perspective, the patient's perspective and background information.

As the story unfolds, information about both disease and illness will flow from the patient, and the skilled interviewer will be able to weave between these two vital aspects of the patient's problems. However, the skills of understanding the patient's perspective – namely, determining and acknowledging the patient's ideas, concerns and expectations and encouraging the expression of feelings and thoughts – have a different intrinsic quality, which requires additional expertise from the doctor. Here we shall explore the particular skills necessary to complete this aspect of information gathering.

What is the evidence to support exploring the patient's perspective of their illness?

Earlier in this chapter, we looked in detail at the disease–illness model and the importance of exploring both the doctor's and the patient's frameworks in the consultation. We would now like to examine the research evidence that validates the importance of understanding the patient's perspective of their illness.

As noted earlier in this chapter, the patient's perspective or illness framework includes:

- ideas or beliefs (about the causation or effect of the illness, about health and what influences or contributes to it)
- concerns (worries about what symptoms might mean)
- expectations (hopes of how the doctor might help)
- thoughts and feelings (emotions and thoughts that the illness induces)
- effects on life (the effect the illness has on day-to-day living).

Anthropological and cross-cultural studies

Many of the concepts that helped to formulate the disease–illness model came originally from anthropological and cross-cultural studies. The seminal review paper by Kleinman *et al.* (1978) brought together the lessons from qualitative anthropological research and explained how the results of this work can be applied to everyday medical interviews. The authors explore how patients' explanatory frameworks of their illness are culturally shaped. Our social, cultural and spiritual beliefs about health and illness influence our perception of our symptoms, our expectations about our illness and our help-seeking behaviour (from families, friends and professionals). Illness behaviour is governed by cultural rules with marked cross-cultural variations in how disorders are both defined by society and dealt with by the individual. These differences also exist within a culture across class and family boundaries. Sultan (2007) explores these issues in the context of a rural Iraqi community.

It is not only patients' beliefs that are culturally determined but also doctors' beliefs! Even within modern Western medical practice itself, there are large cultural differences that determine what is perceived as 'clinical reality'. We have all noticed marked differences in explanations and treatment that physicians from other parts of the world have given our patients during holidays abroad. The biomedical viewpoint is also 'culture specific and value laden' rather than as we so often think 'objective'.

Kleinman *et al.* (1978) quotes examples of the wide range of explanatory frameworks of illness in ethnic minorities living in the United States. For instance, Chinese and Guatemalan patients' understanding of illness differs markedly from the biomedical perspective of their US-trained doctors. Often cultural minorities will not respond to illness in the way expected by their professional advisors. In Chinese cultural settings, for example, mental illness is highly stigmatised and minor psychiatric disorders are commonly manifested by somatisation. The authors then proceed to explore the relevance of differences between the explanatory models of doctor and patient within a single culture. In their model, multicultural interviews simply represent an extreme example of all medical encounters. In all patient–doctor interactions, there is potential for differences in explanatory models which can inhibit effective communication.

In a study of health beliefs related to culture in a multicultural urban setting, Chugh *et al.* (1994) showed clearly that beliefs *within* a cultural group are often as diverse as beliefs *between* cultural groups. Understanding the diversity of health beliefs related to culture is important, but it is still essential to discover the health beliefs of each individual patient.

Claramita *et al.* (2011) explored the perceived ideal communication style for doctor–patient consultations and the reality of actual practice in a Southeast Asian context in Indonesia. Patients, doctors and medical students appear to be in favour of a partnership style of communication that was in sharp contrast to observed communication styles where a paternalistic style prevailed, irrespective of patients' educational background. Patients were unprepared and hesitant to participate in consultations despite their preference to do so and doctors concluded therefore that this style was not required. Doctors also were not equipped to use a partnership style. Moore (2009) reported similar findings in Nepal.

Kleinman *et al.* (1978) recommend that doctors should not only elicit their patients' explanatory model but also openly compare and discuss the patient's and doctor's conflicting ideas. This they see as an essential step to improving compliance with medical advice, which is likely to be poor if the doctor has not explained his recommendations in relation to his patient's beliefs and if the doctors' advice does not seem to help with the problem as the patient sees it.

This is the stage labelled 'integration' in the disease–illness model (*see* Figure 3.1). Only by discovering the patient's illness framework can we explain and plan in terms the patient can understand and accept. The patient's ideas and beliefs, concerns and expectations need to be built into our explanation of the disease process so that we cover the questions that are most important from the patient's perspective and together reach some degree of common ground. It is important to get to a position where our explanations and recommendations make sense in the patient's world.

Therefore, exploring the patient's beliefs involves a three-stage process:

- **identification** – discover and listen to the patient's ideas, concerns and expectations
- **acceptance** – acknowledge the patient's views and their right to hold them, without necessarily agreeing with them; then pause so as to make space for the patient to say more if they wish
- **explanation** – explain your understanding of the problem in relation to the patient's understanding and reach mutually understood common ground.

We discuss acceptance in greater depth in Chapter 5 and explore this three-stage model further in Chapter 6 when we look at the work of Tuckett *et al.* (1985) on the influence that eliciting the patient's explanatory framework has on our patients' recall and understanding of our explanations.

Wright *et al.* (1996) add further depth to our understanding of the patient's perspective. In their book on beliefs in healthcare, they substantiate the point that what patients believe about their illness – treatment, aetiology, prognosis, the role of health in their lives, relationships between spirituality and health – has more influence on how they cope with illness than any other factor. The authors also explore the positive role clinicians can play in understanding, building on and influencing those beliefs. These objectives are central to narrative-based medicine (Launer 2002; Haidet and Paterniti 2003). In this model, the clinician encourages the patient to tell his or her story using questioning techniques commonly used by family therapists. The language used by the patient and physician in the consultation is the basis for helping the patient 'change their story' and for healing to occur.

To gain additional insight into the nature and value of carefully eliciting the patient's perspective, we encourage you to look at some of the narratives that patients have published about their own experiences in healthcare, as well as some of the studies in which researchers have collected and analysed the narratives of others. Both kinds of literature are worth exploring – looking at patients' stories written from their own point of view deepens our understanding of the patient's perspective and the significant role it plays in healthcare and healing. The text by Geist-Martin *et al.* (2003) provides compelling and useful examples of both kinds of work.

Outcome studies

What evidence do we have that eliciting patients' own perspectives about their illness actually effects disease outcome?

The Headache Study Group of the University of Western Ontario (1986) performed a one-year prospective study of 272 patients presenting to family physicians with a new complaint of headache. The purpose of the study was to describe the natural history of headache in primary care and to assess the importance of possible variables to the successful resolution of the headaches after one year. The group looked at many different variables, including physician diagnosis, organic or non-organic diagnosis, the presence of certain symptoms, treatment, investigation, referral, age, sex and the presence of psychosocial problems. While treatment, investigation and referral made no impact on symptom resolution at a year, the most important of all the possible variables was the patient's perception that they had been able to discuss their headaches and the problems surrounding them fully at the first visit (3.4 times more likely to have full resolution). An organic diagnosis (3.2) and lack of visual symptoms (2.2) were the other two most important factors. This paper clearly demonstrates the importance of doctor–patient communication to the outcome of chronic headache. Indeed, it raises communication to a procedural level where we can begin to talk about communication as a treatment option that anyone can use.

Orth *et al.* (1987) showed that reduction of blood pressure was significantly greater in hypertensive patients who, during visits to the doctor, were allowed to express their health concerns in their own words without interruption, as opposed to answering yes/no questions.

Brody and Miller (1986) looked at recovery from upper respiratory infections in patients attending a hospital walk-in clinic. Whereas symptom type and severity, initial level of health concern, findings on examination, culture result and therapy appeared to be unrelated to speed of recovery, recovery was related to reduction in concerns after the visit (particularly about the seriousness of the problem and its consequences for the future) and to satisfaction of the patient with the helpfulness of time spent discussing concerns.

Roter *et al.* (1995) showed in a randomised controlled trial that training physicians in primary care in 'problem-defining and emotion-handling skills' (which included many of the skills of exploring the illness framework) not only improved the detection and management of psychosocial problems but also led to a reduction in patients' emotional distress for as long as six months.

Kinmonth *et al.* (1998) employed a randomised controlled trial to assess the effect of additional training of UK practice nurses and general practitioners in patient-centred care on the lifestyle and psychological and physiological status of patients with newly diagnosed type 2 diabetes. They discovered that patients reported better communication with the doctors and greater treatment satisfaction and well-being. Differences in lifestyle and glycaemic control were not significant. However, patients' body mass index was significantly higher, as were triglyceride concentrations, whereas knowledge scores were lower. The authors suggest that trained practitioners showed greater attention to the consultation process than to preventive care and that those committed to achieving the benefits of patient-centred consulting should not lose the focus on disease management. It may well be that the training intervention in this trial was insufficient to enable learners to consider *both* the doctor's and the patient's perspectives in each interview – as we have said before, the patient-centred approach enlarges rather than replaces the doctor's agenda to take into account both disease and illness. The ability to attend to both simultaneously is one of the key skills that need to be adopted as practitioners change their approach to a more patient-centred style of medical interviewing (Roter 2000).

Stewart *et al.* (2000a) showed that patient-centred communication in primary care visits as judged by patients' perceptions of patient-centredness was associated with better recovery from discomfort and concern, better emotional health two months later and fewer diagnostic tests and referrals.

Alamo *et al.* (2002) compared usual practice vs. a patient-centred approach in a small, randomised controlled trial with patients with chronic pain and fibromyalgia in Spanish general practice. They demonstrated that patient-centredness led to greater improvement in psychological distress and number of tender points.

Croom *et al.* (2011) explored adolescents' and parents' perceptions of patient-centred communication in managing type 1 diabetes. Higher levels of patient-centred communication were associated with greater perceptions of control and competence for both adolescents and parents, and mediation analyses indicated that patient-centred communication was indirectly related to subsequent adherence and metabolic control.

Satisfaction and compliance studies

Many studies document the relationship between a patient-centred approach and patient satisfaction and compliance. Korsch *et al.* (1968) and Francis *et al.* (1969), in their seminal study of 800 visits to a paediatric walk-in outpatients in Los Angeles (Korsch *et al.* 1968; Francis *et al.* 1969), were the first research to tackle the doctor–patient interaction using rigorous methods. Satisfaction and compliance with the consultation was shown to be reduced if doctors demonstrated:

- lack of warmth and friendliness
- failure to take concerns and expectations into account
- use of jargon
- lack of clear explanations of diagnosis and causation.

Korsch *et al.* showed that mothers' expectations were often not elicited by the paediatrician and that only 24% of mothers' main worries were mentioned. Lack of heed of mothers' expressed worry or expectation led them to 'click off' from the interview and give little further information. On the other hand when the needs that mothers perceived to be urgent were met, mothers appeared attentive and amenable to the doctors' ideas and plans. The highest incidence of dissatisfaction on follow-up occurred in those visits where neither expectations nor main concern received attention. No further time was taken when expectations were discovered.

Joos *et al.* (1993) and Kravitz *et al.* (1994) have also shown, both in patients with chronic medical conditions and in those attending internal medicine outpatients, that patients were significantly more satisfied if their prior expectations of help were fulfilled in the interview. However, many patients' desires for further information about their disease or medication or for help with emotional and family problems remained unmet. Bell *et al.* (2002) showed that, in office visits in family practice, internal medicine and cardiology, patients with unexpressed desires were less satisfied by the visit and achieved less symptom improvement.

Eisenthal and Lazare in a series of classic studies on the 'customer approach' to patients in a psychiatric walk-in clinic (Eisenthal and Lazare 1976; Eisenthal *et al.* 1979, 1990; Lazare *et al.* 1975) studied patients' expectations extensively by looking specifically at 'how the patient hoped the doctor might help them', as well as at their presenting symptoms. They clearly demonstrated that patients' expectations are often not obvious from the chief complaint, that clinicians need to make a specific enquiry to discover their patients' expectations and that doctors do not routinely ask for patient's expectations. Their research showed that if physicians did ask for patient's expectations, patients were more likely to feel satisfied and helped and also to adhere to a negotiated plan. Most important, their research clearly demonstrated that this increased satisfaction was apparent regardless of whether or not the request was granted. This is a very significant finding: in Korsch's and Joos' work, the positive relationship between expectations and satisfaction related to patient's expectations being fulfilled rather than just elicited. This is perhaps not surprising – if patients get what they wanted, they feel happier. But the real question left begging by Korsch is this: if expectations are elicited and discussed but not eventually granted, is the fact that the expectation is still unmet still a cause for dissatisfaction or is the process of discovery and negotiation helpful in itself?

Eisenthal and Lazare have shown that eliciting and addressing the expectation is, indeed, of value in itself, that a negotiated treatment plan based on an understanding of the patient's expectations is helpful. In other words, it is not finding out whether the patient wants antibiotics for their cough and going along with their wishes that is important but finding out their expectations and explaining your position in relation to their views. This fits in with the three-stage plan of exploring beliefs outlined earlier. Basing our negotiation on an open understanding of our respective positions and reaching mutually understood common ground is the final aim.

Interestingly, Mangione-Smith *et al.* (1999, 2006) showed that paediatricians' perceptions of parental expectations for antimicrobials was the only significant predictor of inappropriate prescribing of antimicrobials for conditions of presumed viral aetiology; in contrast, paediatricians' antimicrobial prescribing behaviour was not associated with actual parental expectations for receiving antimicrobials. In other words, doctors made assumptions about parental expectations and prescribed accordingly, without discovering or negotiating around their true expectations. Again, it is not that physicians have to fulfil the patient's expectations. In these studies, meeting parental expectations *regarding communication* during the visit was the only significant predictor of parental satisfaction. Failure to provide expected antimicrobials did not affect satisfaction.

Britten *et al.* (2000) identified 14 categories of misunderstanding relating to patient information unknown to the doctor, doctor information unknown to the patient, conflicting information, disagreement about attribution of side effects, failure of communication about the doctor's decision, and relationship factors. All the misunderstandings were associated with lack of patients' participation in the consultation in terms of the voicing of expectations and preferences or the voicing of responses to doctors' decisions and actions. They were all associated with potential or actual adverse outcomes such as non-adherence to treatment. Doctors seemed unaware of the relevance of patients' ideas about medicines for successful prescribing. On the other hand, in a study of patients using treatment suboptimally and having poor clinical control, Dowell *et al.* (2002) showed that extended consultations using a structured exploration of patients' beliefs about their illness and medication and specifically addressing understanding, acceptance, level of personal control, and motivation led to 14 out of 24 patients having improved clinical control or medication use three months after intervention ceased.

Little *et al.* (1997), in an open randomised trial of the management of sore throat in primary care, showed that satisfaction with the consultation predicted the duration of illness and was strongly related to how well the doctor dealt with patient concerns.

Stewart (1984) audiotaped 140 consultations in primary care and analysed the physician behaviour to determine how 'patient-centred' they were in terms of seeking the patients' views and facilitating the patient's self-expression and asking of questions. Patients were then interviewed in their homes ten days later. Stewart demonstrated that a high frequency of patient-centred behaviour was related to higher compliance and satisfaction.

Henbest and Stewart (1990a, 1990b) took this work further by developing a specific tool for measuring the degree to which physicians allowed the patient to express their feelings, thoughts and expectations. Patient-centredness in these studies was scored by a combination of open-ended questions, facilitative expressions and specific requests for patients' expectations, thoughts and feelings. Patient-centredness was found to be significantly related to the doctor ascertaining the patient's reason for coming to see them and to resolution of the patient's concerns.

Arborelius and Bremberg (1992) showed in a study in general practice that successful consultations where both doctor and patient rated the interview positively were characterised by increased efforts being made to establish the patient's ideas and concerns, with more time being spent on the tasks of shared understanding and involving the patient in their own management.

Kinnersley *et al.* (1999) showed that for patients presenting for new episodes of care in general practice, the general practitioner's consulting style, specifically the patient-centredness of the consultation, was positively and statistically significantly associated with patient satisfaction.

Little *et al.* (2001b) showed that patients in general practice expressed a strong preference for a patient-centred approach and if they did not receive it they were less satisfied and less enabled.

Abdel-Tawab and Roter (2002) studied the feasibility, acceptability and effectiveness of patient-centred models of communication in 31 family planning clinics in Egypt. Consultations between 34 physicians and 112 clients requesting family planning methods were audiotaped and analysed for physician communication style. Two-thirds of physician consultations were characterised as physician-centred and one-third as client-centred. A client-centred consultation was associated with a threefold increase in the likelihood of client satisfaction and continuation of contraception method at seven months. The study findings suggest that in Egypt, as in more developed countries, patient-centred models of communication are likely to produce better client outcomes than provider-centred models.

Margalit *et al.* (2004) demonstrated that a teaching intervention in general practice to promote a biopsychosocial approach led to a reduction in medications prescribed, fewer investigations ordered and improved patient satisfaction, without changing markedly the duration of the encounter.

Matthys *et al.* (2009) also found an association between the expression of patients' concerns and expectations and less medication prescribing.

Understanding and recall studies

The research of Tuckett *et al.* (1985) on information giving, which we shall explore more fully in Chapter 6, demonstrates the great importance of eliciting patients' beliefs and views of their illness in enabling them to understand and recall information provided by the doctor. Their research efforts were hampered by the very few examples that they were able to find at all of doctors asking for patients to volunteer their ideas, or even of doctors asking the patient to elaborate on their ideas if they were spontaneously brought up. Doctors often evaded their patients' ideas and positively inhibited their expression. This behaviour led to a considerably increased likelihood of failure of understanding and recall.

Doctors' understanding is also enhanced by patient-centred interviewing. Peppiatt (1992) showed in a study of 1000 interviews undertaken by one family physician that 77% of patients either spontaneously offered or responded to requests to express a cause for their condition and that 20% of patients' ideas of causation helped the doctor decide on a cause with 9% enabling the doctor to actually make a diagnosis.

Are patient-centred interviews longer?

Stewart (1985) looked at 133 interviews in primary care and compared their 'patient-centredness' score with the length of the consultation. Low scores for patient-centredness produced interviews of (on average) 7.8 minutes, intermediate scores produced interviews of 10.9 minutes and high scores produced interviews of 8.5 minutes. Stewart concluded that doctors can expect to take longer while they learn the skills. However, doctors who have *mastered* the patient-centred approach took little extra time compared with doctors who did not employ these techniques.

Roter *et al.* (1995) also found no increase in the length of interviews in primary care following training in the skills of 'problem-defining and emotion-handling'.

Levinson and Roter (1995) showed that primary care physicians with more positive attitudes to psychosocial aspects of patient care used more appropriate communication skills and as a consequence their patients had more psychosocial discussions and were more involved as partners in their own care. Yet these same physicians did not have longer interviews than colleagues with less positive attitudes.

Roter *et al.* (1997) found five distinct communication patterns in primary care visits in the United States:

1. 'narrowly biomedical', characterised by closed-ended medical questions and biomedical talk
2. 'expanded biomedical', like the restricted pattern but with moderate levels of psychosocial discussion
3. 'biopsychosocial', reflecting a balance of psychosocial and biomedical topics
4. 'psychosocial', characterised by psychosocial exchange
5. 'consumerist', characterised primarily by patient questions and physician information giving.

They found no evidence that patient-centred consultations took any longer then strictly biomedical interviews.

Levinson *et al.* (2000) showed that primary care and surgical office visits where physicians missed opportunities to pick up patients' emotional cues tended to be longer than visits with a positive response.

In the aforementioned study by Abdel-Tawab and Roter (2002), patient-centred consultations were only one minute longer than physician-centred consultations, despite markedly improved patient satisfaction and adherence.

Epstein *et al.* (2005) found somewhat different results. They found that patient-centred communication was associated with increased visit length but it was associated with fewer diagnostic testing costs.

Mauksch *et al.* (2008) undertook a literature review to explore the determinants of efficiency in the medical interview. Three domains emerged from their study that can enhance communication efficiency: (1) rapport building, (2) upfront agenda setting and (3) picking up emotional cues.

A recent review by the Cochrane collaboration (Lewin *et al.* 2012) summarised the effect of interventions for providers to promote a patient-centred approach in clinical consultations. They conclude that there is fairly strong evidence to suggest that some interventions to promote patient-centred care in clinical consultations may lead to significant increases in the patient-centredness of consultation processes, and that there is also some evidence that training healthcare providers in patient-centred approaches may have a positive impact on patients' satisfaction with care. However, not many studies were found that examined an impact on healthcare behaviour or health status outcomes.

How to discover the patient's perspective

There are two alternative ways of exploring the patient's illness framework as the interview proceeds. The first is by directly asking for the patient's ideas, concerns, expectations and feelings. The second is by picking up cues (i.e. verbal and non-verbal hints) provided by the patient during the course of the consultation.

Maguire *et al.* (1996b) have demonstrated the value of both directly asking and picking up cues. Cancer patients disclosed more of their significant concerns and feelings if doctors asked them questions about psychological aspects of their care (*'How has that made you feel?'*) rather than concentrating solely on physical aspects of their disease. They also disclosed more concerns if doctors specifically clarified psychological cues that arose (*'You say that you have been worrying ...'*). As predicted, the use of open questions, summarising and empathic statements also promoted disclosure of concerns.

One recent high-quality stream of research is based on the Verona Coding Definitions of Emotional Sequences, a consensus-based system for coding patient expressions of emotional distress in medical consultations (Zimmermann *et al.* 2011). Here a cue is defined as a verbal or non-verbal hint that suggests an underlying unpleasant emotion that lacks clarity, whereas a concern is defined as a clear and unambiguous expression of an unpleasant current or recent emotion that is explicitly verbalised. Please note that the term 'concern' has a slightly different meaning in this research context than we have used earlier. Del Piccolo *et al.* (2007) concluded that listening, together with supporting and emotion-centred expressions, activates cue emission by encouraging the patient to add new information or to direct the physician's attention to issues of importance, whereas physicians' closed questions tend to suppress cue expressions. On the other hand, soliciting a patient's expression of personal needs by open enquiry and active listening, acknowledging and sensitively handling their expressions will satisfy these very needs and lower cue offers. Bensing *et al.* (2010) demonstrated that physicians' facilitative communication, eye contact and psychosocial questions are related to more disclosure of both cues and concerns. Interestingly Eide *et al.* (2011) noted a difference in the relationship between clinician empathy and the expression of cues or concerns. Looking at nurse specialists working with fibromyalgia patients, they discovered that lack of empathic responding led to increased numbers of expression of cues, whereas high levels of empathic responding led to increased expressions of concerns. This fits with the hypothesis that cues escalate if not acknowledged by the clinician.

Cegala and Post (2009) demonstrated that physicians engage in significantly more exploration of patients' disease and illness when interacting with high-participation patients than when interacting with low-participation patients. Active participation in medical interviews by patients influenced physicians to adopt a more patient-centred style.

Floyd *et al.* (2005) explored the flexibility that might be required from physicians in either asking directly for the patient's perspective or picking up cues, depending on the language used by the patient in their opening statement.

Picking up and checking out cues

Patients are keen to tell us about their own thoughts and feelings. In Tuckett *et al.*'s (1985) research, 26% of patients spontaneously offered an explanation of their symptoms to the doctor. However, when patients did express their views, only 7% of doctors actively encouraged their patients to elaborate, 13% listened passively and 81% made no effort to listen or deliberately interrupted. Half of patients' views were expressed covertly rather than overtly, with overt cues being picked up far more readily than covert cues. The conclusion here is that many patients provide cues that we unfortunately ignore! Butow *et al.* (2002) have demonstrated that doctors effectively identify and respond to the majority of informational cues. However, they are less observant of and less able to address cues for emotional support. This study also showed that cues can be addressed without lengthening the consultation or increasing patient anxiety. Zimmermann *et al.* (2007) undertook a systematic review, documenting 58 original quantitative and qualitative research articles demonstrating patient expressions of cues and/or concerns, all based on the analysis of audio- or videotaped medical consultations. Yet again, their overall conclusion was that physicians missed most cues and concerns and adopted behaviours that discouraged disclosure. Communication training improved the detection of cues and concerns. Kale *et al.* (2011) discovered that expression of cues and concerns in immigrant patients in Norway is dependent on the patient's language proficiency.

Gill *et al.* (2010) used conversation analysis to explore how patients explain ideas about causation in a subtle way, by raising the potential for relatively benign interpretations of their symptoms followed by enumerating circumstances that undermine these simple explanations. In this way, patients hint at more serious hypotheses without pressing for them outright.

We have already described the work of Cox *et al.* (Cox *et al.* 1981a, 1981b; Rutter and Cox 1981; Cox 1989), who showed that open questioning and attentive listening facilitated both the expression of emotions and the gathering of sensitive data with a high emotional significance. If the doctor establishes an atmosphere of interest and openness, many of the patient's feelings and thoughts will appear as cues in the attentive listening stage. It can then be a relatively easy and natural process to pick up and explore these cues further. This often feels more comfortable for both patient and doctor than the asking of direct unprompted questions. Interestingly, Del Piccolo *et al.* (2000) found that in primary care consultations, the proportion of cues given by patients with emotional distress was related to the general practitioner's verbal behaviour, increasing with closed psychosocial questions and decreasing with the use of active interview techniques such as the use of open questions and emotional responses. The authors postulate that patient-centred techniques enable the patient to directly tell their story without the need to make covert signals to the physician.

It should be emphasised that cues do not only appear as verbal comments. Non-verbal cues in body language, speech, facial expression and affect are also highly significant. To ensure accurate interpretation of such non-verbal behaviour, it is important to observe the patient carefully and then sensitively verify your perceptions with the patient.

But why do doctors repeatedly fail to respond to patients' cues? Perhaps it is in part due to issues of control. Doctors have traditionally controlled the interview via closed questions that limit patients' contributions and render them more passive. When we pick up patient cues, perhaps we feel that we are being taken off our pre-planned flight path and are uncertain of where we might be lead – we start to feel out of control. An awkward moment ensues that is all too easy for the physician to sidestep by returning to safer ground (Epstein *et al.* 1998). Paradoxically, cues are usually a shortcut to important areas requiring our attention.

Cocksedge and May (2005) introduced the concept of the 'listening loop', which clinicians can actively choose to employ if they wish to pick up cues. The listening loop offers a simple model of listening that emphasises choice and judgement in response to patients' cues within interactions. Emphasising this choice highlights both picking up cues and pragmatic limits and resistance to attending to them.

We may also fail to pick up cues to the illness framework because we are preferentially listening for cues about disease. If the patient says, *'It's been difficult at home and I've been getting a lot more pains lately'*, it is so easy to preferentially pick up the disease rather than the illness cue and say, *'Tell me about the pains'* without returning to *'You mentioned things have been difficult at home ...'*. Fascinatingly, Rogers and Todd (2000) discovered that oncologists even preferentially listened for and responded to certain disease cues over others – they ignored patients' cues about pain unless it was the 'right kind' of pain, pain that was amenable to specialist cancer treatment. Other pains were not acknowledged or were dismissed.

Box 3.2   Examples of ways to pick up verbal and non-verbal cues

---

Repetition of cues
- *'upset ...?'*
- *'something could be done ...?'*

Picking up and checking out verbal cues
- *'You said that you were worried that the pain might be something serious. What theories did you have yourself about what it might be?'*
- *'You mentioned that your mother had rheumatoid arthritis. Did you think that's what might be happening to you?'*

Picking up and checking out non-verbal cues
- *'I sense that you're not quite happy with the explanations you've been given in the past. Is that right?'*
- *'Am I right in thinking you're quite upset about your daughter's illness?'*

Asking specifically about the patient's illness perspective

Although picking up patient cues might be easier, asking specifically about the illness perspective is still a very necessary task (Platt *et al.* 2001). In a family practice clinic setting, Lang *et al.* (2002) showed that in response to sequenced questioning about the patient's perspective, 44% of patients revealed specific, significant concerns that had not been otherwise disclosed. Among patients without prior contact with their provider, satisfaction with the encounter was significantly higher when such sequenced questions were used than when they were not. Yet in Tuckett's work, only 6% of doctors asked patients directly for their own thoughts about their illness. Direct questions need careful timing, with good signposting of intent and attention to detail in wording. Bass and Cohen (1982) showed that when parents in a paediatric practice were asked, *'What worries you about this problem?'* the majority of patients responded with *'I'm not worried'*, whereas the phrase *'What concerns you about the problem?'* produced previously unrecognised concerns in more than a third of patients.

Box 3.3   Examples of different phrasing required when asking questions about patients' ideas, concerns or expectations

---

Ideas (beliefs)
- *'Tell me about what you think is causing it.'*
- *'What do you think might be happening?'*
- *'Have you any ideas about it yourself?'*
- *'Do you have any clues? Have you any theories?'*
- *'You've obviously given this some thought. It would help me to know what you were thinking it might be.'*

Concerns
- *'What are you concerned that it might be?'*
- *'Is there anything particular or specific that you were concerned about …?'*
- *'What was the worst thing you were thinking it might be?'*
- *'In your darkest moments …'*

Expectations
- *'What were you hoping we might be able to do for this?'*
- *'What do you think might be the best plan of action?'*
- *'How best might I help you with this?'*
- *'You've obviously given this some thought. What were you thinking would be the best way of tackling this?'*

Feelings

Many doctors find entering the realm of patients' feelings particularly difficult. It doesn't fit naturally with the objective approach of the traditional clinical method and it is something that at medical school we were often taught to avoid. Impassive objectivity can be appealing – feelings are often difficult to handle and may be painful to the doctor as well as the patient. Doctors are frightened of 'opening a Pandora's box' of their patients' emotions and feelings. In comparison, it is the area that other professionals such as counsellors and therapists are most encouraged to explore! Maguire *et al.* (1996b) reported doctors using a ratio of three inhibitory behaviours for every one facilitative one. It is therefore particularly important to become aware of and practise the skills involved in discovering and responding to patients' feelings (*see* Box 3.4).

Box 3.4   Skills involved in discovering and responding to patients' feelings

---

Picking up and checking out verbal cues
- *'You said you felt miserable. Could you tell me more about how you've been feeling.'*

Repetition of verbal cues
- *'angry ...?'*

Picking up and reflecting non-verbal cues
- *'I sense that you're very tense – would it help to talk about it?'* or *'You sound sad when you talk about John.'*

Direct questions
- *'How did that leave you feeling?'*

Using acceptance, empathy, concern, understanding to allow the patient to feel that you are interested in their feelings (*see* Chapter 5)
- *'I can see that must have been hard for you.'*

Early use of feelings questions to establish your interest in the subject

Asking for particular examples
- *'Can you remember a time when you felt like that? What actually happened?'*

Asking permission to enter the feelings realm
- *'Could you bear to tell me just how you have been feeling?'*

How to end the discussion of feelings and not sink into a downward spiral with the patient
- *'Thank you for telling me how you have been feeling. It helps me to understand the situation much better. Do you think you've told me enough about how you are feeling to help me understand things?'* or *'I think I understand now a little of what you have been feeling. Let's look at the practical things that we can do together to help.'*

Effect on life

An open question about how the symptoms or illness are affecting the patient's life is an excellent entry into the patient's perspective of the problem and in particular often leads the patient to talk openly about their thoughts and feelings.

PUTTING THE PROCESS SKILLS OF INFORMATION GATHERING TOGETHER

We have now explored each individual process skill of information gathering. But how in practice can we best combine these process skills to negotiate a path through this section of the interview? How can they be used most effectively to discover the content of:

- the biomedical perspective
- the patient's perspective
- background information?

Exploration of both the biomedical perspective and the patient's perspective

Sequence of events
Encourage the patient to tell the narrative, use open questioning methods
Listen attentively
Facilitate
Use more directed open questions
Clarify and time-frame
Pick up and respond to verbal and non-verbal cues, regarding both disease and illness
Summarise the biomedical perspective and the patient's perspective
Signpost to:

Further analysis of each symptom and the relevant systems review
Start with open questions and gradually move to closed ones
Signpost to:

Further exploration of the patient's perspective
Use predominately open questions
Acknowledge patient's views and feelings
Signpost to:

Discovering the background information

Use increasingly directed questions, and eventually closed ones

---

Here we present one practical approach to combining the process skills that physicians can use in everyday practice once they have completed the initiation phase of the interview and identified the list of the patient's problems. Please note that this is only one of many ways to combine these skills. The key is to be flexible and dynamic, responding to the patient's cues and responses as you go.

The continuum of open to closed questioning techniques

In the approach suggested here, there is a continuum of open to closed questioning techniques. The interview gradually moves from open to closed questions as each specific component of the content of the history is explored.

Initially, open questioning techniques are used at the start of the exploration:

> *'Tell me what has been going on from when you first began to feel ill right up until now.'*

As the interview proceeds, you may need to become more directive, guiding the patient to elaborate further on specific areas of both the biomedical and the patient's perspective that have surfaced as they tell their narrative. You can do this by employing more focused verbal encouragement in the form of more directed open statements and questions:

> *'Tell me more about the pain.'*
> *'You mentioned breathlessness. Tell me about that.'*
> *'You said that the pain was frightening. Can you tell me more about how you felt?'*
> *'Did you notice anything else while all this was going on?'*
> *'And what did you do then?'*

As the exploration of the problem progresses, important facets of the biomedical perspective may well not emerge from the patient's account and the gradual movement from open to closed questioning ensures that these areas are explored. Each symptom needs to be explored thoroughly as we have described earlier in this chapter, and more focused questions are essential here. Again these more directive questions can be open at first and then increasingly closed if necessary:

> *'Can you describe what the pain felt like?'*
> *'Was it a sharp pain?'*

You will also want to explore the patient's perspective. As described earlier, open questions are most profitable here, although sometimes more closed questions can be useful:

> *'What are you concerned that it might be?'*
> *'Were you worried about cancer?'*

As the interview proceeds, you will have started the process of clinical reasoning. Your perceptual skills will drive further focused questioning. For example, a patient with non-organic sounding chest pain might not overtly mention stress as possibly contributing to her symptoms. After careful listening and the judicial use of open questions, you might ask the specific closed question:

> Doctor: *'Are you under a lot of stress at the moment?'*
> Patient: *'Well, my daughter's marriage has been breaking up recently.'*

Be careful that your closed questioning is not too focused. It is easy to ask the patient an inappropriate closed question – we think ahead too quickly, think of a possible answer to a question we have posed to ourselves and then test our own premature hypotheses. Instead, ask the question that was in your mind right from the start! A good example of this would be:

> The doctor here wonders if his patient is under any stresses at the moment. Instead of asking a general question such as *'Are there any stresses in your life at the moment?'*, he thinks ahead, wonders if she is having problems at home and asks, *'Are things OK with your husband at present?'* The patient says fine and the doctor moves on without an answer to his original question.

Next you require detailed information about the background information of the patient's past medical history, family history, personal and social history, medication and allergy and full systems review. At this point, increasingly directed questions are used until you arrive at the review of systems, which becomes almost a checklist of closed questions. As we have seen from the work of Cox and colleagues earlier in this chapter, important information is lost if a systematic approach to the exclusion of associated symptoms is not employed. Although this may only discover which symptoms are definitely absent, this is still highly useful diagnostic information that cannot otherwise be assumed. Negative findings can be as important as positive ones.

The complete versus the focused history in information gathering

We would like to emphasise that both the process and the content frameworks outlined here are equally applicable to the complete and the focused medical history.

When medical students are learning how to interview patients, they are initially taught to take a complete medical history that covers all aspects of the content of the medical interview as described here.

The content of the complete medical interview

Patient's problem list
1.
2.
3.
4.

Exploration of patient's problems
Biomedical perspective
Sequence of events, symptom analysis, relevant systems review

Patient's perspective
Ideas, concerns, expectations, effects on life, feelings

Background information – context
Past medical history
Family history
Personal and social history
Drug and allergy history
Systems review

However, in practice they rarely observe doctors interviewing patients in this way. Most doctors, whether in hospital outpatient clinics, in the emergency room or in general practice, take focused histories that are substantially shorter in duration than complete histories. Students in their early clinical years, when asked what the difference is between these approaches, commonly state that in focused histories the doctor simply abandons the initial listening phase and moves quickly into closed questions. They assume that the process skills that we have advocated so far in this book, such as listening, screening, agenda setting, facilitation, using the open-to-closed cone, the narrative thread and summarising, do not apply to the focused history.

Nothing could in fact be further from the truth. It is in reality the content that changes here, not the process. In the focused history, the information obtained is not the same as in the complete history. While the problem list, biomedical history of the patient's problems and patient's perspective are still vital and cannot be truncated, only certain relevant and actively selected parts of the background information are sought. For instance, the full systems review is almost never completed. There is therefore a more selective and judicial approach to the background information.

The contents of the focused medical interview

Patient's problem list
1.
2.
3.
4.

Exploration of patient's problems
Biomedical perspective
Sequence of events, symptom analysis, relevant systems review

Patient's perspective
Ideas, concerns, expectations, effects on life, feelings

Background information – context
  Past medical history
  Family history
  Personal and social history   } Selective application only
  Drug and allergy history
  Systems review

So in both the complete and the focused history, the process skills – including attentive listening and the open-to-closed cone – remain constant. All parts of the history of the patient's problems, including the patient's perspective, continue to be important. It is simply the extent of the closed questioning phase that changes as less background detail is sought.

Why do communication process skills so frequently seem to be a casualty of the transition from complete to focused history taking? Part of the explanation may be that there is a mismatch between what we teach about focused and complete history taking and how we expect students and residents to perform during examinations. This became clear yet again during a discussion we had with a recently graduated resident who at first insisted that the focused history had to be mostly directed towards biomedical information obtained through closed questions. As he talked, the following insight was reconfirmed. All too often when students and residents are asked to perform a focused history in evaluations (or on the ward), what they are really expected to demonstrate is their knowledge of content by saying it out loud in the form of the questions they ask. Almost inevitably that means using closed questions focused on the biomedical history throughout, especially if the exam is a time-truncated OSCE station (such as the stations that frequently appear in local clerkship and residency OSCEs and in high stakes exams such as the LMCC in Canada or medical finals in the UK).

We concluded once again from this discussion that there are really three approaches to interviewing in the 'real world' of students and residents: (1) the complete history, (2) the focused history and (3) the exams-manship history. Unfortunately, learners (and probably some faculty) tend to think of the focused history and the exams-manship history as one and the same thing – a misapprehension that they may hold onto for several years, until the habit of associating focused histories with closed questioning and a too-narrow emphasis on the biomedical history is locked in place. Is it any wonder then that learners tend to lose track of process skills, open questioning techniques, the patient's narrative, relationship and so on as they make the transition from the complete and inclusive medical history of their early training in communication to the focused history that they think is essentially the same thing as the exams-manship history?

This exams-manship history is decidedly different from the focused history that we are talking about in this chapter, where we are trying to help learners and practitioners alike make the transition from complete to focused histories without losing relationship- or patient-centred content and without losing or diminishing the quality of their process skills. In other words, the exams-manship history is a sort of faux focused history that is very different from the real thing, in which physicians elicit information about both biomedical and patient perspectives efficiently, go after relevant background information in a highly selective way, and at the same time continue to develop relationship and use the rest of the process skills effectively. This, of course, is a very strong argument for changing many of the high-stakes and other OSCEs that are currently in place as they inadvertently have a very strong negative educational impact.

The effect of clinical reasoning on the process of information gathering

Just as with the type of history, the effect of different approaches to clinical reasoning should not in any way influence the process skills required for information gathering.

When clinical students start to see patients, they initially use a variation of hypothetico-deductive reasoning to attempt to solve clinical problems. In this approach, all of the information is obtained from the patient first. Then the student

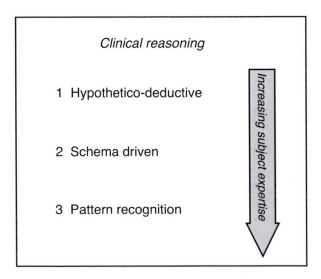

Figure 3.3   Approaches to clinical reasoning.

stands back to consider what the differential diagnosis might be. Students next 'guess' at potential diagnoses and then consider how to rule them in and out. This is a very early approach to clinical reasoning that is generally not used by clinicians in real life unless they are well away from their area of subject expertise. As clinical reasoning is an after-event, it does not interfere with the interviewing process and fits easily with the interviewing framework described here.

As clinicians develop subject expertise, they adopt increasingly more sophisticated approaches to clinical reasoning (*see* Figure 3.3) (Elstein and Schwarz 2002; Dornan and Carroll 2003).

More advanced hypothetico-deductive reasoning

The first approach is a variation on hypothetico-deductive reasoning in which, after the presenting problems are elicited, a number of diagnostic hypotheses (no more than five or six) are formed in the early minutes of the interview and then these hypotheses are validated or rejected by selective questioning ('rule in/rule out'), selective physical examination and selective investigations. Hypothesis generation occurs early and drives the questions that the doctor asks as the interview proceeds.

Schema-driven approach

In the next variation, physicians use preformed schema or mental flow diagrams to help solve the problem (Mandin *et al.* 1997). This approach is only possible with increased subject expertise and knowledge. Schema enable inductive reasoning to occur – highly selective and discriminating questioning can enable large diagnostic areas to be ruled in or out at a time and can allow fast navigation through a well-defined problem area.

Pattern recognition

Highly experienced physicians use a method of clinical reasoning that is not available to medical students. As their career progresses, clinicians continually accumulate details and key features about specific conditions as templates or memory structures known as 'illness scripts' (Schmidt *et al.* 1990). These are often 'pegged' to particular patients. When confronted with a specific problem, the clinician searches her 'bank' of illness scripts to see if a pattern can be recognised. Initial impressions will then be tested for 'goodness of fit' by further inquiry. Such pattern recognition is not a shortcut but, rather, an essential skill that all clinicians use – it is predicated on having seen a large number of patients over many years.

How do these different clinical reasoning approaches influence the process of information gathering?

All three of the different approaches to clinical reasoning described here necessitate doctors starting the process of problem solving early on as the interview proceeds. At first sight, this might suggest that clinicians employing such techniques should move more quickly to closed questioning as they test out hypotheses, schema and recognised patterns, thereby narrowing the field of potential diagnoses.

In fact, the opposite is true. All of these approaches are critically dependent on adopting the same approach to the process of information gathering that we have described earlier in this chapter. The potential danger of all three approaches is starting down a path of clinical reasoning prematurely. Early closed questioning can quickly lead to the exploration of one particular avenue that may well prove inappropriate and lead inexorably to a dead-end. The doctor may have to start again and generate a different problem-solving strategy. Inefficient and inaccurate information gathering ensues.

All three approaches to clinical reasoning in fact depend on a clear and careful listening phase through which the doctor can obtain enough of the picture first so that eventually she can apply the right schema or increase the chance of the right pattern being recognised. Wise use of the process skills of screening, open questioning, attentive listening and discovering the patient's narrative in the opening minutes of the interview allows doctors more time to generate their problem-solving strategies and provides them with more information on which to base their theories and hypotheses. Here we see how perceptual, content and process skills in communication are inextricably linked and cannot be considered in isolation.

Summary

In this chapter, we have looked at both the theory and the practice of gathering information. We have explored the content of information gathering and discussed the strengths and limitations of the traditional method of history taking. We have examined the need for a transformed clinical method that takes into account both the doctor's and the patient's perspectives of the problem being discussed. We have also examined the process of information gathering and demonstrated that accurate and efficient information gathering is not achieved simply by interrogating the patient for symptoms but, rather, that it requires the more effective initial techniques of open questions and listening. And we have looked at the additional skills needed to explore the patient's perspective of their illness.

Before moving on to the physical examination or to the explanation and planning phase of the interview, the doctor needs to think through the skills outlined in the gathering information section of the Calgary–Cambridge Observation Guide and to consider: 'Have I explored the disease aspect of the patient's problems effectively? Have I explored the patient's perspective of their problems and understood the meaning of the illness to the patient? Have I discovered the background information? Have I ensured that the information gathered is accurate and complete? Have I confirmed that I have understood the story correctly? Have I continued to develop a supportive and collaborative environment?'

Chapter 4

Providing structure to the interview

Introduction

In this chapter we explore the communication skills that doctors can employ to structure the interview to the benefit of both doctor and patient. Providing structure is one of two tasks of the interview that we intentionally show in the Calgary–Cambridge Guides as continuous threads throughout the interview, rather than as part of a sequential pattern. Providing structure, like relationship building, is a task that occurs throughout the interview rather than sequentially. It is essential for the five sequential tasks to be achieved effectively.

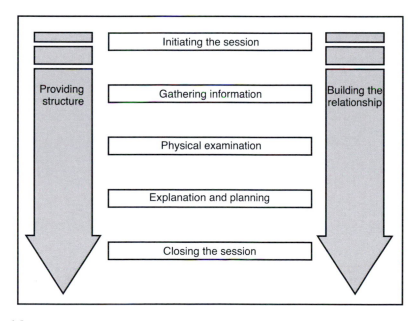

Figure 4.1

The medical consultation is not an aimless or chance meeting, a social chat between two equal friends. It is a highly choreographed discussion between a professional and a client in which both parties often behave in certain stereotypical patterns according to tacit traditions, rules and customs. The interview proceeds along set pathways that both parties may be subliminally aware of but rarely openly discuss.

How is the structure of the meeting determined? Although doctors can all recall interviews with patients in which they have felt completely out of control, the almost invariable pattern is that it is the professional who sets the parameters of the consultation and determines the structure of the interaction. The greater degree of power implicitly rests with the doctor – we can determine the time available for discussion, move the interview to new areas at whim, decide how many topics can be discussed today and terminate the interview when we wish. We exert considerable control over the interview. Our behaviour imposes limits on our patients' freedom whether we like it or not (Pilnick and Dingwall 2011).

Power of course leads to responsibilities. What are our responsibilities in directing the medical interview? What do we want to achieve in structuring the interview? The traditional approach to structure is via a series of closed questions in which the patient is a mainly passive contributor to the consultation. In this book, we have taken a patient- or relationship-centred approach to the medical interview and the skills that we have identified promote a more collaborative partnership between patient and doctor. This is not because of our own subjective opinion but because, in most circumstances, the skills that enable this approach have been shown in both practice and research to produce better outcomes for patients *and* doctors.

The concept of a collaborative partnership implies a more equal relationship between patient and doctor. However, as doctors control the shape of the interview, this shift in power will only occur if doctors structure the interview appropriately – it will not happen on its own simply because we want it to. Physicians in effect determine the level of contribution of the patient, the patient's degree of involvement in the direction that the interview takes and the balance between doctor- and patient-centredness (Robins *et al.* 2011).

An awareness of structure at all times throughout the interview helps the doctor to feel that she has appropriate influence on the overall parameters of the encounter and of her working day. Used appropriately it also enables the patient to become more involved in the consultation and to take part in a more balanced relationship.

Objectives

The task of providing structure involves the following objectives:

- enabling a flexible but ordered interview
- helping the patient to understand and be overtly involved in where the interview is going and why
- encouraging the patient to be part of the structuring process
- encouraging patient participation and collaboration
- enabling accurate information gathering and giving
- using time efficiently.

These objectives encompass some of the tasks and checkpoints mentioned in other well known guides to the consultation:

- Pendleton *et al.* (1984, 2003):
  - to use time and resources appropriately.
- Neighbour (1987):
  - summarising – 'Have I sufficiently understood why this patient has come to see me?'

- AAPP Three-Function Model (Cohen-Cole 1991):
  - gathering data:
    - 〉 survey of problems
    - 〉 negotiate priorities
    - 〉 summarising.
- The Four Habits Model (Frankel and Stein 1999; Krupat *et al.* 2006):
  - investing in the beginning
    - 〉 plan the visit with the patient.
- The Maastricht Maas Global (van Thiel and van Dalen 1995):
  - summarisations
  - ordering.
- Essential Elements of Communication in Medical Encounters: Kalamazoo Consensus Statement (Participants in the Bayer-Fetzer Conference on Physician–Patient Communication in Medical Education 2001):
  - structure, clarify and summarise information.
- Patient-centred medicine (Stewart *et al.* 2003):
  - enhancing the doctor–patient relationship – sharing power
  - being realistic – time.
- The Model of the Macy Initiative in Health Communication (Kalet *et al.* 2004):
  - managing flow.

Skills

In his comments on structuring the interview, Cassata (1978) emphasises the importance of two-way communication in every part of the consultation and in particular stresses the importance of making expectations and agendas overt at the very beginning of the interview. This encourages patient participation, ownership and collaboration. In Chapter 2 we explored how the following three skills can facilitate this collaborative approach and at the same time lead to more efficient consultations:

1. problem identification
2. screening
3. agenda setting.

Here we concentrate on four additional skills that are relevant throughout the interview and enable us to work with the patient to orchestrate an overtly structured interview.

Box 4.1   Additional skills that are relevant throughout the interview

---

Making organisation overt
- **Internal summarising**: summarises at the end of a specific line of inquiry to confirm understanding before moving on to the next section
- **Signposting**: progresses from one section to another using transitional statements; includes rationale for next section

> Attending to flow
> - **Sequencing**: structures interview in logical sequence
> - **Timing**: attends to timing and keeping interview on task

'What' to teach and learn about providing structure: the evidence for the skills

MAKING ORGANISATION OVERT

How can we help patients understand the structure of the interview and become more involved in the consultation? The key here is to make the organisation overt. Robins *et al.* (2011) explore the concept of transparency, of clear signalling to the patient about the process as well as the content of the interview, so that not only the physician but also the patient understands where the interview is going and why. They clarify how this promotes relationship building, reduces uncertainty for the patient and enables a more collaborative consultation. Transparency involves making the organisation of the interview overt to the patient throughout the interview. Robins *et al.* (2011) demonstrate in their study how physicians spent little time using such process-related transparency and in particular did not orient the patient to the progress of their interviews.

Summarising

What is summarising?

Summarising is the deliberate step of providing an explicit verbal summary to the patient. There are two kinds of summary:

1. *internal summary*, which focuses on a specific part of the interview
2. *end summary*, which concisely pulls together the entire interview.

We explore end summary in more detail in Chapter 7.

Why is internal summary a key skill in structuring the consultation?

In Chapter 3, we explored the role of internal summary as one of the most important of the information gathering skills. Here we discuss its equally vital role in structuring the interview. Understanding how to structure a consultation via *agenda setting*, *summarising* and *signposting* is a key area in communication skills teaching.

Traditionally doctors have imposed structure on the consultation via closed questions, which, as we have explained earlier, keep doctors 'in control' at the expense of rendering the patient passive. However, as we have seen, this approach can be highly inefficient, can lead to inaccuracy in obtaining quality information and can feel unsupportive to the patient. But if staying open and using attentive listening is so effective, why do we shy away from it? Perhaps it is because:

- it can feel like we have lost control of the consultation
- we worry we will not need or be able to remember all that we are being told

- information flows out in a less ordered form – we seem to be receiving a cloud of unprocessed information that is not in an order that we can easily assimilate.

These are very genuine concerns – there is no doubt that open methods do seem to produce a less ordered consultation. However, there is a way out of this difficulty. *Structuring the consultation via summary and signposting* provides an alternative method for the doctor to obtain order and appropriate control without sacrificing the benefits of openness.

Summarising as a structuring tool allows you to:

- pull together and review what you have heard so far
- order the information into a coherent pattern
- realise what information you still need to obtain or clarify
- gain space to consider where the consultation should go next
- separate and consider both disease and illness.

Learners grappling with the techniques of open questions and attentive listening find summarising especially useful – when unsure of what to ask next or what the patient has already said, summarise and play for time! The very act of summarising and the patient's response will normally establish the most appropriate path forward without embarrassment or apparent loss of momentum.

Doctor:	*'Can I check that I understood what you said correctly – you've had pain in both feet for several months, especially on walking, and you have also noticed that you have been stiff in all your joints in the mornings and you have been generally tired?'*
Patient:	*'Yes, that's it – and I'm finding it increasingly difficult to cope with my children now.'*

What is the evidence for the value of summarising in the medical interview?

Here we present the evidence for the value of summarising to both 'gathering information' and 'providing structure to the interview'. We have only identified four research papers that validate the importance of summarising.

1. Cox *et al.* (1981a) demonstrated that checking by repetition led parents of children referred to a child psychiatric clinic to be more voluble.
2. Maguire *et al.* (1996b) showed that summarising is one of several skills (along with the use of open questions, focusing on and clarifying psychological aspects, empathic statements and making educated guesses) that facilitate cancer patients to disclose more of their significant concerns.
3. Takemura *et al.* (2007) found significant positive relationships between three particular interview behaviours and the amount of information obtained in real family medicine interviews: the open-to-closed cone, facilitation and summarisation.
4. Quilligan and Silverman (2012) sounded a cautionary note that summary may not always be beneficial and is perhaps more complex than previously described.

In a qualitative study of medical students with simulated patients, the use of summary did appear to improve accuracy; however, if summary was not carefully introduced, inaccurate summaries could make the patient question whether or not they had been heard. Also, the overuse of summary, particularly when paraphrasing very small interactions, could lead the patient to question whether they had been clear and could potentially damage the rapport between patient and doctor. Therefore, summary needs to be used flexibly to suit the patient.

Despite limited direct research on summary in clinical settings, there is impressive theoretical evidence from the discipline of communication to underpin the value of summarising. In Chapter 1 we describe five principles that characterise effective communication. One of these principles is that *effective communication is a helical rather than a linear process – reiteration and repetition are essential.* Summary is an efficient way to build this principle into information gathering.

A second and related principle is that *effective communication ensures an interaction rather than a direct transmission process.* If communication is viewed as direct transmission, the senders of messages assume that their responsibilities as communicators are fulfilled once they have formulated and sent a message. However, if communication is viewed as an interactive process, the interaction is complete only if the sender receives feedback about how the message is interpreted, whether it is understood and what impact it has on the receiver. Just imparting information or just listening is not enough – giving and receiving feedback about the impact of the message becomes crucial and the emphasis moves to the interdependence of sender and receiver in establishing mutually understood common ground (Dance and Larson 1972).

Summarising is the key skill in the information-gathering and structuring phases of the interview that enables this principle to be put into practice. It provides intentional feedback to the patient about what you think you have heard when listening to their story. As we shall see later, additional skills are required in the explanation and planning phase to ensure a similar degree of interaction.

Let us look further at these critical pieces of theory in the context of history taking. Without feedback from the doctor, how do patients know whether they have made themselves understood? You might say that non-verbal cues are being transmitted by the doctor in attentive listening that allow patients to know that the doctor is concentrating on and interested in their story and has understood their message. However, this is an assumption. We cannot assume that exemplary listening by itself leads to correct understanding – communication is complicated and many misinterpretations are possible. The key question to ask yourself as a doctor is: 'How do I know that what I have understood from the patient is an accurate representation of what they wanted to tell me?' From the patient's perspective, the question becomes 'I know that the doctor seems to be listening but how do I know that he has understood me?' How do both patient and doctor know that they have established mutually understood common ground?

There are many possible sources of distortion in communication as any message is sent between two parties. Consider a patient giving their story to a doctor. Possible distortion can occur at the following points:

- what the patient says might be ambiguous
- the patient may have simply forgotten to say something

- the patient may have misunderstood the doctor's question
- having already told their story to one member of the healthcare team, the patient may assume this new individual already knows it
- the patient may have been led off topic and never returned to complete the unfinished comment
- the patient may have inadvertently made a verbal mistake that distorts his meaning
- the patient may give a nonverbal cue such as a laugh that suggests something unintended to the doctor
- the patient may have said exactly what he meant but distortion occurred in the circumstances of transmission of the message (e.g. a noisy printer prevents the doctor hearing fully what was said)
- the doctor hears the correct message but misinterprets what was meant
- the doctor understands what was meant but makes an incorrect assumption about what lay behind the message
- the doctor may have personal biases and prejudices that affect accuracy (e.g. based on gender, race or age of the patient, the doctor's medical training, the location of the interview, or previous experience with the patient).

All of these distortions can lead to inaccurate history taking. The only way to be sure that the message has been formulated properly, received correctly and interpreted and understood is through feedback. In the doctor–patient interview it is unlikely that the patient will feel confident enough to ask the doctor to demonstrate their understanding of the patient's story! Unless we as doctors take responsibility by giving feedback via summary as the interview proceeds, we will leave the patient uncertain as to whether they have been understood and we ourselves will be unsure that we have obtained an accurate account. Importantly, all of these distortions can also lead to inaccuracy and misunderstanding during the explanation and planning phase, especially if you switch the placement of 'doctor' and 'patient' in each point of possible distortion listed above.

Signposting

What is signposting?

Signposting is the twin skill of summarising. A signposting statement introduces and draws attention to what we are about to say. For example, it is helpful to use a signposting statement to introduce our first summary. This announces what we are going to do and invites the patient to think with us, to add in forgotten areas or to correct our interpretation if we got something wrong. For example:

> 'Can I just check if I have understood you – let me know if I've missed something …'

Then the interactive process can continue, as the patient says:

> 'No, that's not quite right …'

After summarising produces a 'yes' response from the patient, use signposting again to:

- make the progression from one section to another
- explain the rationale for the next section.

> *'You mentioned two areas there that are obviously important – first, the joint problems and the tiredness, and second, how you are going to cope with your kids. Could I start by just asking a few more questions about the joint pains that would help me understand what might be causing them, and then we can come back to your difficulties with the children?'*

or

> *'Since we haven't met before, it will help me to learn something about your past medical history. Can we do that now?'*

or

> *'I can see that you are in some discomfort, but I need to ask a few questions about the drugs that your doctor has prescribed and then make a brief examination to be able to help sort out what exactly is going on.'*

Use signposting to move from one section to the next so that:

- the patient understands where the interview is going and why
- you can share your thoughts and needs with the patient
- you can ask permission
- the consultation is structured overtly for you both.

Examples of when to signpost during history taking include when moving:

- from the introduction into the information-gathering stage
- from open to closed questions
- into specific questions about the patient's ideas, concerns or expectations
- into different parts of the history
- into the physical examination
- into explanation and planning
- into closing.

Summarising and signposting together provide an overt structure apparent to the patient – the patient understands and becomes part of the structuring process. This is so much better than structuring via the use of closed questions, where the patient is left in the dark about the process of the interview.

Another of the five principles of effective communication we discussed in Chapter 1 is *reducing unnecessary uncertainty*. Unresolved uncertainties can lead to lack of concentration or anxiety, which in turn can block effective communication. By knowing where the interview is going and why, much possible uncertainty and anxiety is reduced. In the previous case, the patient knows that you have picked up her cue about her children and that there will be an opportunity to explore this in a little while. This will let her concentrate on the next part of the interview without worrying that one of her main concerns might not be addressed. Levinson *et al.* (1997) showed that primary care physicians who used more signposting, which was described in this study as orienting statements, were less likely to have suffered malpractice claims.

Floyd *et al.* (1999), in a study from the United States on assessing HIV risk, have shown that patients are more comfortable answering questions about sensitive issues if signposting (or, as the authors label this skill, a lifestyle bridge question) is used prior to asking direct questions about sexual health.

Summarising and signposting together therefore:

- are key skills promoting a collaborative and interactive interview
- make the structure overt and understood to the patient
- allow you and the patient to know where you are going and why
- allow you to signal a change in direction
- establish mutually understood common ground and reduce uncertainty for the patient.

Signposting and summarising are equally important during the explanation and planning and closing phases of the interview. In Chapters 6 and 7 we shall discuss how to use these two skills in this context, and we offer additional relevant evidence.

ATTENDING TO FLOW

Sequencing

After agenda setting and negotiation have established an overt and agreed plan for the interview, it is clearly the responsibility of the clinician to help to carry out the agreement and maintain a logical *sequence* that is apparent to the patient as the interview unfolds. A flexible but ordered approach to the organisation, with clear transitions via signposting from one section of the interview to the next, helps both the physician and the patient in efficient and accurate data gathering.

One of the key ways in which this can be achieved is for the doctor to have in their head at all times a clear structure to the medical interview, such as the Calgary–Cambridge content and process guides. The ability to take stock at points throughout the consultation and to consider what has and what has not been achieved so far allows the practitioner to regain control over what might otherwise become a meandering interview, confusing to doctor and patient alike. In fact, a clear structure paradoxically enables flexibility. Knowing the steps and how to return to them provides you with the confidence to allow the interview free flow: 'structure sets you free'.

Timing

Another important skill for the doctor to utilise is timing. There is no doubt that time issues are a constant concern in modern medicine and that all physicians feel under pressure of time to complete interviews as efficiently as possible. Achieving all of the different needs of the doctor and the patient is not easy in the time available, although, as we have shown in Chapter 3, patient-centred interviews take little extra time compared with more traditional approaches. Mauksch *et al.* (2008) undertook a literature review to explore the determinants of efficiency in the medical interview. Three domains emerged from their study that can enhance communication efficiency: rapport building, upfront agenda setting and picking up emotional cues. A key skill is being able to manage time effectively in the interview, to pace the session so that balanced amounts of time are taken over each section of the meeting. This is not just about pacing but also about the perception of time.

Thorne *et al.* (2009) in Canada have explored the issue of time on the patient's perspective in the cancer care context. They have elegantly shown that despite the omnipresence of time pressure, some clinicians pay considerable attention to the quality of the patient experience and find communication approaches that manipulate and manufacture time to optimal advantage. Patients reported how some physicians were able to utilise the small amount of time available more effectively by being 'present' for the patient both verbally and non-verbally, negotiating time by offering future appointments or contact, and manufacturing a sense of time even when time was limited by encouraging questions or creating an impression that they were not rushed.

Summary

In this chapter we have looked at the skills involved in providing structure to the interview and how they need to be utilised throughout the medical encounter. We have looked at issues of power, control and ordering within the medical interview, and we have seen how the physician needs to explicitly consider the structure of the interaction that will take place and make this apparent to the patient. We have explored the advantages of developing an overt structure that is clearly signposted and apparent to and agreed with the patient, enabling the doctor to plan a path through a complex situation and the patient to understand and if necessary influence the proposed course of action. The skills of structuring allow doctors to order their interviews, patients to feel more comfortable and clear about what will happen next and both parties to move through the interview with confidence.

Chapter 5

Building the relationship

Introduction

An unmistakeable theme runs throughout this book and our companion volume: relationship matters. It makes a difference to communication in healthcare, to the people who are involved, to healthcare and its outcomes.

As shown in Figure 5.1, five tasks of the interview follow a natural sequence as the consultation evolves. In contrast, both building the relationship and providing structure are continuous threads that occur throughout the interview. Building the relationship runs in parallel to the five sequential tasks. It is the cement that binds the consultation together.

Nearly all of the communication skills we advocate in this book with respect to the sequential tasks also contribute to building a solid relationship with the patient. However, we deliberately include this all-pervasive task as a separate category and devote a chapter to it here to emphasise its significance and to highlight important relationship-building skills that apply throughout the consultation rather than fitting under just one task heading.

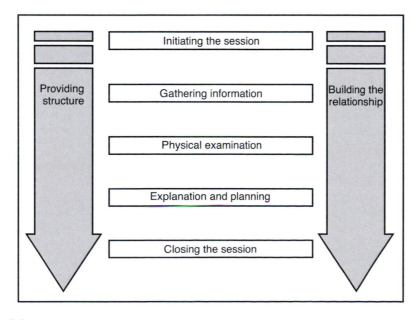

Figure 5.1

Building the relationship is a task that is easily taken for granted or forgotten. The sequential components of the interview often dominate as the doctor moves through the consultation trying to make sense of the patient's illness and disease. Yet without paying specific attention to the skills of relationship building, these more 'concrete' tasks become much more difficult to achieve. Relationship building in the consultation can be an end in itself – the doctor's role is sometimes that of supportive counselling alone. But in the majority of consultations, relationship building contributes substantively to achieving all the goals of medical communication that we have outlined in Chapter 1 – namely, accuracy, efficiency and supportiveness, increased satisfaction for both patient and doctor, and promotion of partnership and collaboration. Relationship building enables the patient to tell their story and explain their own concerns, it promotes adherence and prevents misunderstanding and conflict.

Forging a relationship with the patient is central to the success of every consultation whatever the context. Often, especially in specialist medicine, the relationship between doctor and patient is short term in nature. Here developing rapport is of vital importance – it enables the patient to feel comfortable in discussing problems with an unfamiliar person and to benefit fully from the consultation. Yet the doctor faces the added difficulty of having to accomplish the task of relationship building in a short period of time and often in the face of considerable patient anxiety (Barnett 2001).

Building the relationship is also the entry point to a longer-term view of medical practice than we have considered so far. In many circumstances, the relationship between doctor and patient extends beyond a single interview into a continuing association over many meetings (Leopold et al. 1996). There is a need to maintain a reliable, trusting relationship over time, often without expectation of cure (Cocksedge et al. 2011). Many doctors see the development of relationships over several years as the most rewarding aspect of their work.

Patients wish their doctors to be competent and knowledgeable but they also need to be able to relate to their doctor, to feel understood and to be supported through adversity. Attention to relationship building offers the potential prize of patients who are more satisfied with their doctors and doctors who feel less frustrated and more satisfied in their work (Levinson et al. 1993). Bensing et al. (2011) confirmed the views of patients – laypeople in 32 focus groups throughout Europe were invited to formulate 'tips' for doctors after rating the quality of communication from videotaped consultations. Top tips included the importance of non-verbal communication, personal attention, listening and empathy.

Relationship-building skills are increasingly important not only in the context of physician–patient consultations but also between healthcare providers. In her book reporting on a series of studies that show the power of relationships to achieve high performance in the airline industry, Hoffer Gittel (2003) includes a chapter that discusses a large study (Hoffer Gittel et al. 2000) she and her colleagues conducted comparing the efficiency and outcomes of nine hospitals (located in Boston, New York and Dallas) with respect to joint replacement surgery. Some of these hospitals invested heavily in hiring and subsequent training for 'relational competence' – that is, the ability to interact with others to accomplish common goals. Others looked instead for the most highly qualified individuals – the tendency in this group of hospitals to neglect relational competence was most pronounced in physician hiring. This study found significant differences between hospitals in the strength of relational coordination among their care providers that significantly improved the patient care process. To illustrate, Hoffer Gittel (2003) reported that a 100% increase in relational coordination enabled a 31% reduction in the length of hospital stay, a 22% increase in the quality of service patients perceived, a 7% increase in postoperative freedom from pain and a 5% increase in postoperative mobility. As Hoffer Gittel *et al.* (2000) concluded, those in positions that require high levels of functional expertise also tend to need high levels of relational competence to integrate their work with others. A participant in their study put it this way: 'We've moved from patients experiencing individuals as caregivers to patients experiencing systems as caregivers … It's not just individual brilliance that matters anymore. It's a coordinated effort.'

So in healthcare, relationship-building skills and relational competence are important to the patient–doctor consultation *per se* and also to relationships between healthcare providers. Whether it be with patients or co-workers, we agree with Hoffer Gittel that relational competence is necessary to realise the potential contributions of individual experts. This chapter focuses on building the relationship between physician and patient in the medical consultation, but the skills we present here are also relevant to building relationships throughout the broader contexts of healthcare, for example with co-workers or the patient's significant others.

The paragraphs above give support to relationship-centred care. Drawn from the biopsychosocial paradigm and akin to patient-centred medicine, relationship-centred care has been concerned with bringing a personalised, partnership-oriented approach to medical care (Suchman *et al.* 2002). It is an approach to healthcare and healing that places relationship at the core of the therapeutic process. This way of conceptualising the consultation and the broader context of healthcare helps focus attention on the very basic need for relationships between patients, doctors, family members, other caregivers, their healthcare organisations and their communities (Tresollini and the Pew-Fetzer Task Force 1994; Beach and Inui 2006). It recognises that clinician–patient communication and relationship take place within organisational contexts and are therefore influenced not only by the needs and skills of the individuals but also by the values expressed in the organisation's policies and processes and by the way people within the organisation treat each other and are treated (Suchman 2001). This resonates with the work of Aita *et al.* (2005), which explored primary care settings in the United States. They showed that individual physicians function within personal and professional value systems as well as within practice systems. In their sample of physicians' practices, a key determinant of patient-centred care was physicians' ability to create an environment that emphasised patient-centred values within their practice and surrounding administrative structures. Suchman and his colleagues' recent book on leading change in healthcare offers excellent, in-depth explanations of relationship-centred care and relationship-centred administration along with several detailed case studies demonstrating how to apply these paradigms to promote change and enhance healthcare in a variety of settings (Suchman *et al.* 2011).

The skills and concepts we discuss throughout this chapter, along with those related to relationship building that are specific to the sequential tasks of the consultation, offer the means for physicians to enhance their relational competence and their ability to engage in relationship-centred care. As Hoffer Gittel says, 'The first step is to become a caring person – the second step is to find ways to communicate this caring on an everyday basis as well as in times of extreme crisis.'

David Sluyter, a past officer of the Fetzer Institute and editor of a book on emotional intelligence, adds further insight to this discussion by adding the notion of personal capacity, which may be innate but can be developed. Sluyter suggests that 'it is really necessary to have both the capacity, which can perhaps be developed through personal development and personal growth processes, and the skills to communicate that capacity to others, which is more of a skills training issue and which would probably be taught differently'. He offers the following example: 'a person could be very loving and forgiving (capacities) but not very good at loving and forgiving. That is, they may lack the skills to put [the capacity] into practice.' We find it appealing to think of compassion or caring as capacities rather than as attributes or qualities – somehow capacity suggests more room for growth and development.*

Problems in communication

There are considerable reports in the media of patient dissatisfaction with the doctor–patient relationship. Many articles comment on doctors' lack of understanding of the patient as a person with individual concerns and wishes. Perhaps most striking are those articles written by physicians themselves who have found themselves in the unexpected role of patient. Many such articles are now published in series such as 'Personal View' in the *British Medical Journal*. So often they focus on the sudden revelation of the inhumanity of medicine and with the lack of caring and support offered by their physicians. What a shame that it takes our personal experience of illness to draw this to our attention.

From the very earliest research into medical communication, relationship problems have featured highly as predictors of poor outcome. In the seminal study by Korsch *et al.* (1968) of 800 visits to a paediatric walk-in outpatient clinic in Los Angeles, physician lack of warmth and friendliness was one of the most important variables related to poor levels of patient satisfaction and compliance.

Poole and Sanson-Fisher (1979) have shown that there are significant problems in medical education in the development of relationship-building skills. They demonstrated that we cannot assume that doctors have the ability to communicate empathically with patients or that they will acquire this ability during their medical training. They demonstrated poor skills in empathy in both first- and final-year medical students. They also showed that psychiatric residents who might be thought to develop these skills in their training also demonstrated low empathy skills. More recently, Morse *et al.* (2008) found that doctors missed 90% of the opportunities to express empathy in a study in cancer care, and Hsu *et al.* (2012) found that providers missed most of the opportunities to respond empathically to their HIV patients' emotions.

Many commentators link the poor development of doctor's relationship building skills with the way that students and residents are taught to remain 'uninvolved' during their medical training. As we have seen in Chapter 3, the traditional clinical method is based on scientific reasoning and values clinical detachment. Medical students are brought up in the world of the objective and the technological. At the expense of understanding the sick person, they are taught to concentrate on

---

* Personal communication. David Sluyter, email correspondence with Suzanne Kurtz, 2004.

underlying disease mechanisms. Much is made in traditional medical education of the need to protect ourselves from the powerful emotions of medical practice where feelings are painful for both patient and doctor. Impassive objectivity is recommended as a coping mechanism. In this milieu, relationship-building skills clearly will not flourish.

Suchman and Williamson (2003)[*] offer further insights about how medical schools impact the development of students' relationship skills:

> *Students of medicine learn first and foremost from what they see and experience, rather than from what's written in the syllabus. If they witness respectful and collaborative interactions; if they experience listening, empathy, and support; and if they see difference approached with curious inquiry and dialogue rather than conflict and domination, then these interactions will frame their expectations for the nature of relationships in medicine. But if instead they see powerful figures in medicine routinely entering into non-healing or even negative relationships with one another and their patients; if they see their mentors emphasising the importance of expert technical knowledge above all else, especially above knowledge of self and other; and if they experience hazing or humiliation as standard techniques of medical pedagogy, then they will develop a very different template for their lifelong practice.*

Objectives

The objectives that we seek to accomplish in building the relationship with the patient can be summarised as:

- developing rapport to enable the patient to feel understood, valued and supported
- establishing trust between doctor and patient, laying down the foundation for a therapeutic relationship
- encouraging an environment that maximises accurate and efficient initiation, information gathering and explanation and planning
- enabling supportive counselling as an end in itself
- developing and maintaining a continuing relationship over time
- involving the patient so that he understands and is comfortable with participating fully in the process of the consultation
- reducing potential conflict between doctor and patient
- increasing both the physician's and the patient's satisfaction with the consultation.

These objectives encompass many of the tasks and checkpoints mentioned in other well-known guides to the consultation:

- Pendleton *et al.* (1984, 2003):
  - to establish or maintain a relationship with the patient that helps to achieve the other tasks.

---

[*] Personal communication. Anthony Suchman and Penelope Williamson, email correspondence with Suzanne Kurtz, 2003.

- Neighbour (1987):
  - connecting – establishing rapport with the patient.
- AAPP Three-Function Model (Cohen-Cole 1991):
  - developing rapport and responding to patient's emotions.
- Bayer Institute for Health Care Communication E4 model (Keller and Carroll 1994):
  - engaging the patient
  - empathising with the patient.
- The Four Habits Model (Frankel and Stein 1999; Krupat *et al.* 2006):
  - demonstrate empathy.
- The SEGUE Framework for teaching and assessing communication skills (Makoul 2001):
  - understand the patient's perspective.
- The Maastricht Maas Global (van Thiel and van Dalen 1995):
  - emotions
  - flexibility.
- Essential Elements of Communication in Medical Encounters: Kalamazoo Consensus Statement (Participants in the Bayer-Fetzer Conference on Physician–Patient Communication in Medical Education 2001):
  - build a relationship.
- Patient centred medicine (Stewart *et al.* 2003):
  - enhancing the doctor-patient relationship.
- The Model of the Macy Initiative in Health Communication (Kalet *et al.* 2004):
  - build a relationship.
- The Six Function Model (de Haes and Bensing 2009):
  - fostering the relationship
  - responding to emotions.

Skills

Box 5.1   Building the relationship

Using appropriate non-verbal communication
- **Demonstrates appropriate non-verbal behaviour**
  - eye contact, facial expression
  - posture, position, movement
  - vocal cues, e.g. rate, volume, intonation
- **Use of notes:** if reads, writes notes or uses computer, does so in a manner that does not interfere with dialogue or rapport
- **Picks up patient's non-verbal cues** (body language, speech, facial expression, affect); checks them out and acknowledges as appropriate

Developing rapport
- **Acceptance:** accepts legitimacy of patient's views and feelings; is not judgemental
- **Empathy:** uses empathy to communicate understanding and appreciation

of the patient's feelings or predicament; overtly acknowledges patient's views and feelings

- **Support:** expresses concern, understanding, willingness to help; acknowledges coping efforts and appropriate self-care; offers partnership
- **Sensitivity:** deals sensitively with embarrassing and disturbing topics and physical pain, including when associated with physical examination

Involving the patient
- **Sharing of thoughts:** shares thinking with patient to encourage patient's involvement (e.g. *'What I'm thinking now is ...'*)
- **Provides rationale:** explains rationale for questions or parts of physical examination that could appear to be non sequiturs
- **Examination:** during physical examination, explains process, asks permission

'What' to teach and learn about building the relationship: the evidence for the skills

Next we examine in detail the individual skills for building the relationship, listed in Box 5.1, and explore the evidence from theory and research which validates their use in the consultation.

USING APPROPRIATE NON-VERBAL COMMUNICATION

We cannot emphasise enough the importance of non-verbal communication throughout the medical interview. We need to pay as much attention to the effect of our non-verbal interaction with patients as we do to the impact of our words (Friedman 1979; Hall *et al.* 1995; Roter *et al.* 2006). Two intimately related aspects of non-verbal communication require consideration:

1. the non-verbal behaviour of patients
2. the non-verbal behaviour of doctors.

As doctors, we need to recognise patients' non-verbal cues in their speech patterns, facial expression, affect and body posture. But we also need to be aware of our own non-verbal behaviour, how the physician's use of eye contact, body position and posture, movement, facial expression and use of voice can all influence the success of the consultation (MacDonald 2009). Box 5.2 lists the variety of behaviours and cues that contribute to non-verbal communication (Mehrabian 1972; Gazda *et al.* 1995).

Box 5.2   What do we mean by non-verbal communication?

- **Posture:** sitting, standing, erect, relaxed
- **Proximity:** use of space, physical distance between and positioning of communicators
- **Touch:** handshake, pat, physical contact during physical examination
- **Body movements:** hand and arm gestures, fidgeting, nodding, foot and leg movements
- **Facial expression:** raised eyebrows, frown, smiles, crying
- **Eye behaviour:** eye contact, gaze, staring
- **Vocal cues:** pitch, rate, volume, rhythm, silence, pause, intonation, speech errors
- **Use of time:** early, late, on time, overtime, rushed, slow to respond
- **Physical presence:** race, gender, body shape, clothing, grooming
- **Environmental cues:** location, furniture placement, lighting, temperature, colour

---

What is the difference between verbal and non-verbal communication?

What are the differences between verbal and non-verbal communication (Verderber and Verderber 1980)?

- Verbal communication is discrete with clear endpoints – we know when the message has come to an end. In contrast, non-verbal communication is continuous – it goes on for as long as the communicators are in each other's presence. We cannot stop communicating non-verbally (Watzlawick *et al.* 1967) – even when people are together in silence, the atmosphere is filled with messages. The difference between comfortable and uncomfortable silence is mediated by our non-verbal communication.
- Verbal communication occurs in a single mode, either auditory (spoken) or visual (written), whereas non-verbal communication can occur in several modes at once. We can send and receive all the non-verbal cues listed in Box 5.2 simultaneously; all of our senses can be receiving signals at once.
- Verbal communication is mostly under voluntary control whereas non-verbal communication operates at the edge of or beyond our conscious awareness. Non-verbal communication can be amenable to deliberate control: for instance we use non-verbal cues from voice, body, head and eye movement deliberately to help to co-ordinate the taking of turns in conversation. However, non-verbal communication also operates at a less conscious level. Our non-verbal communication may be 'leaking' spontaneous clues to the receiver that we are not even aware of and may be providing a better representation of our true feelings than our more considered verbal comments. DiMatteo *et al.* (1980) have shown that this is particularly true for body posture and movement.
- Verbal messages are more effective in communicating discrete pieces of information and in conveying our intellectual ideas and thoughts. In contrast, non-verbal communication is the channel most responsible for communicating our attitudes, emotions and affect, for conveying the way we present ourselves

and how we relate. Considerably more information about liking, responsiveness and dominance is provided by non-verbal than verbal means. Non-verbal communication plays an increasingly important role when someone is unable or unwilling to explicitly express feelings verbally – for example, when cultural taboos dictate against disagreeing with a superior or where words are inadequate to describe love or grief or pain (Ekman *et al.* 1972; Mehrabian 1972; Argyle 1975).

Why understanding non-verbal communication can make a difference in the consultation

Non-verbal communication can work to accent, qualify, regulate, take the place of or contradict verbal communication. In most circumstances, verbal and non-verbal communication work together to reinforce one another. Non-verbal cues enable verbal messages to be delivered more accurately and efficiently by strengthening the verbal message. For example, after the doctor has summarised and asked, *'Have I got that right?'* the patient says, *'Yes, that's spot on'* and smiles, leans forward and uses an animated voice; or as the patient talks of her fears about her surgery, she looks down, talks more slowly and plays with her fingers.

When we are deprived of accompanying non-verbal confirmation, our verbal conversation is more liable to misunderstanding. We have all encountered problems communicating over the telephone where we are denied so many non-verbal cues.

We can intentionally use non-verbal communication to reduce uncertainty and misunderstanding in our verbal communication. *'Are you happy with that plan?'* accompanied by eye contact, hands opened out and an enquiring facial expression will indicate your genuine interest. Alternatively, the same phrase accompanied by a closure of the notes, hands banged on the table and a quick look at the patient and then away all suggests that you don't want to know if the answer is no.

As we can see from the last example, the two channels can also work to contradict each other. Communication research has shown that when the two are inconsistent or contradictory, non-verbal messages tend to override verbal messages (Koch 1971; McCroskey *et al.* 1971). If the verbal statement is *'Tell me about your problem'* while the non-verbal cues are speaking quickly and looking agitated, the patient will make the correct interpretation that time is at a premium today. If the doctor says there is nothing to worry about but hesitates in her speech as she delivers this verbal message, the patient will assume that perhaps there is some concern and that information is being withheld. However, this generalisation may apply only to normal adults. Young children and emotionally disturbed adults or adolescents tend to believe the verbal message when faced with contradictions or inconsistencies (Reilly and Muzarkara 1978).

A further use of non-verbal behaviour relates to the reinforcement theory of social interaction (Mehrabian and Ksionsky 1974) and to non-verbal synchrony (DeVito 1988). People tend to act in ways that reinforce their general expectations. People also tend to mirror or imitate each other's non-verbal behaviour – to move or talk in synchronisation – as a gesture of affiliation. Doctors can use these concepts to advantage first by anticipating a positive experience and second, by modelling relaxed attentive listening skills. Unconscious mirroring and reinforcement of this behaviour by patients will enable them also to relax and become more attentive. We can affect others positively through our behaviour. On the other hand, if we act disinterested, our non-verbal behaviour will be picked up by the patient and communication can deteriorate.

What is the research evidence that non-verbal communication makes a difference to the consultation?

Harrigan et al. (1985) have demonstrated that doctors who face their patients directly, have more eye contact and maintain open arm postures are regarded as more empathic, interested and warm.

Weinberger et al. (1981) in a study of hospital-based internal medicine out-patients have reported a positive relationship between patient satisfaction and physician non-verbal communication in the form of physician nods and gestures and closer distance between doctor and patient in the information-gathering phase.

Larsen and Smith (1981) have demonstrated in family medicine that non-verbal immediacy, defined in terms of touch, closer distance, leaning forward, body orientation and gaze, is related to patient satisfaction as well as patient understanding.

Hall et al. (1981) used the technique of filtered speech to separate verbal messages from vocal cues. In electronically manipulated recordings, vocal expression could be heard but not the content of words. They showed in a family and community health clinic that patients and doctors reciprocated their emotions in their voice quality. If one party appeared satisfied or angry or anxious, so did the other. This reciprocation was far more apparent in filtered speech than in non-filtered speech or written transcripts. The authors inferred that much of the affective communication actively responded to in the interaction takes place via non-verbal cues. They also demonstrated a difference between verbal and non-verbal channels in relation to patient satisfaction. Verbal messages using words that appeared less anxious and more sympathetic were related to greater patient satisfaction. In contrast, non-verbal messages that were more angry or anxious led to more patient satisfaction. Similar findings were demonstrated in relationship to patient compliance in appointment keeping. The authors suggest that non-verbal cues of anger and anxiety are interpreted by the patient as reflecting concern and seriousness on the part of the physician. Clearly, the verbal and non-verbal channels offer very different information about affect.

Haskard et al. (2008) also used filtered speech and found that affect in physicians' voices was correlated with patients' satisfaction, perceptions of choice/control, medication adherence, mental and physical health, and with physicians' satisfaction.

Hall et al. (1987) demonstrated that doctors in primary care who were high information givers were also rated highly on their voice tone by independent observers – they were more interested, more anxious and less bored. In contrast, physicians who gave less information spent more time in pleasantries but had voices that were perceived as bored or calm. Again the authors conclude that anxiety in the doctor's voice is perceived as anxious regard. This interpretation would fit well with the work of Kaplan et al. (1989), which we discuss in detail in Chapter 6. They found that 'negative affect' expressed by both physician and patient was related to better health outcomes. The authors concluded that this may represent 'healthy friction' or it may be that doctors who are more engaged with their patients appear more anxious or concerned.

DiMatteo *et al.* (1980, 1986) have shown that internal medicine residents and family practice residents who tested highly on objective laboratory tests of their ability to communicate emotion through their faces and voices ('encoding') had patients who were more satisfied with their medical care and, interestingly, more patients on their lists! Physicians who tested highly on their ability to recognise the meanings of patients' non-verbal cues ('decoding') had more satisfied patients with better appointment keeping!

Goldberg *et al.* (1983) demonstrated that family practice residents who established eye contact were more likely to detect emotional distress in their patients.

Bensing (1991) showed that non-verbal affective behaviour had the strongest predictive power in determining the quality of psychosocial care and in predicting patient satisfaction.

Ambady *et al.* (2002a) have shown a relationship between judgements of surgeons' voice tone and their malpractice claims history. Surgeons were audiotaped while speaking to their patients during office visits, and very brief samples of the conversations were rated by coders blind to surgeons' claims status. Two 10-second clips were extracted for each surgeon from the first and last minute of their interactions with two different patients. Controlling for content, ratings of higher dominance and lower concern/anxiety in their voice tones significantly identified surgeons with previous claims compared with those who had no claims. This study underscores the potency of vocal cues in medical interactions.

Ambady *et al.* (2002b) have also linked physical therapists' patterns of non-verbal communication and their therapeutic efficacy. Independent raters' judgements of videotaped samples of therapists' non-verbal behaviour were correlated with clients' physical, cognitive and psychological functioning at admission, discharge and at three-month follow-up. Therapists' distancing behaviours, defined as not smiling and looking away from the client, were strongly correlated with short- and long-term decreases in physical and cognitive functioning. In contrast, facial expressiveness reflected in smiling, nodding and frowning was associated with short- and long-term improvements in functioning.

Griffith *et al.* (2003) examined the association of internal medicine residents' non-verbal communication with standardised patients' satisfaction with the interview. Non-verbal communication skills (facial expressivity, frequency of smiling, eye contact, nodding, body lean, body posture and tone of voice) were found to be an independent predictor of standardised patient satisfaction for three very different patient stations: (1) a straightforward, primarily 'medical' problem (chest pain); (2) a patient with more psychosocial overlay (a depressed patient with a history of sexual abuse); and (3) a counselling encounter (HIV risk factor reduction counselling). The effect sizes were substantial, with non-verbal communication predicting 32% of the variance in patient satisfaction for the chest pain station, 23% of the variance for the depression–sexual abuse station, and 19% of the variance for the HIV counselling station. The authors conclude that better non-verbal communication skills are associated with significantly greater patient satisfaction in a variety of different types of clinical encounters with standardised patients.

Unfortunately, there is still evidence that doctors respond to increased patient participation with non-verbal blocking behaviours (Zandbelt *et al.* 2007).

In a simulation study in a US teaching hospital where patients observed a pre-recorded simulated consultation involving disclosure of error, Hannawa (2012) demonstrated that physicians' non-verbal behaviours had a significant impact above and beyond what physicians *said*. Physicians' non-verbal behaviour affected patients' ratings of trust, closeness, empathy, forgiveness, avoidance, distress, and satisfaction.

Swayden *et al.* (2012) showed that something as simple as sitting rather than standing has a positive impact. In a prospective, randomised, controlled study of inpatients admitted for spinal surgery, Swayden and colleagues found that patients whose providers sat during brief post-operative consultations perceived that the provider was present at the bedside longer than when the provider stood. This was the case even though the actual time the physician spent at the bedside did not change significantly. Patients with whom the physician sat reported a more positive interaction and a better understanding of their condition.

Cocksedge *et al.* (2013) explored qualitatively the use of touch in general practice consultations, both procedural and expressive, and found that patients in general welcomed expressive touch and were less concerned than their doctors about invasion of body space (although it should be noted that this was in a study group with little ethnic diversity).

What then are the lessons for physicians?

Physicians therefore need to be aware of both their patients' and their own non-verbal behaviour.

Reading the non-verbal cues of patients

Being able to 'decode' non-verbal cues is essential if we wish to understand our patients' feelings. The cultural norms of the healthcare setting militate against patients' expressing their feelings verbally – patients are reluctant to express their thoughts or feelings openly, but instead use indirect or tacit messages (*see* p. 177–88, Chapter 6). Non-verbal cues may therefore be one of the few indicators to the physician of a patient's desire to contribute their own concerns about a problem.

However, just because spontaneous cues representing true feelings are being sent does not mean that you can interpret those cues accurately simply by noticing them – there are many sources of possible distortion and misunderstanding inherent in receiving non-verbal messages. To ensure accurate interpretation of such *non-verbal* behaviour, it is important not only to observe carefully but also to verify our perceptions *verbally*. Your interpretations and assumptions may or may not be right – they need to be checked out with the patient. Checking your assumptions encourages patients to talk further about what they are thinking or feeling and has a double payoff – both doctor and patient avoid possible misinterpretation and discover more information.

The skills of picking up non-verbal cues and checking them out verbally ('*You seem upset – would you like to talk about it?*') are described in Chapter 3.

Picking up on non-verbal cues not only helps the doctor to understand the emotional impact of the patient's illness but is also of considerable diagnostic importance in its own right. Reading the non-verbal cues of depression is an essential part of diagnosing the illness itself (Hall *et al.* 1995), while emotional problems only hinted at through non-verbal channels are often the root cause of physical symptoms.

Transmitting your own non-verbal cues

Similarly, without attention to your own non-verbal communication skills and the messages that you are transmitting through the non-verbal channel ('encoding'), many of your other efforts to communicate may be undone. If your verbal and non-verbal signals are contradictory, at the very least you risk confusion or misinterpretation, and at worst your non-verbal message will win out. Non-verbal skills signalled through eye-contact, posture, position, movement, facial expression, timing and voice can assist in demonstrating attentiveness to the patient and facilitate the formation of a helping relationship; ineffective attending behaviour in contrast closes off the interaction and prohibits relationship building (Gazda *et al.* 1995). Again the disparity in power and control between patient and doctor leads patients to be particularly attentive to non-verbal cues regarding doctors' attitudes and meanings. Patients rarely ask for verbal confirmation of cues that they pick up and commonly base their impressions primarily on non-verbal messages.

Use of notes and computers

One of the most important of all non-verbal skills is eye contact. Yet so often doctors lose eye contact when they refer to the patient's written or computer record during the consultation while the patient is speaking. In a qualitative study in general practice in the UK, Heath (1984) examined the consequences of physicians attempting to read the patient's records and listen to the patient at the same time. She demonstrated how instead of increasing efficiency, quite the opposite occurs:

- patients withhold their initial reply to the doctor's solicitation until eye contact is given
- patients pause in mid-utterance when the doctor looks at the notes and resume when eye contact is regained
- patients use body movement to catch the doctor's gaze if he is reading the notes while the patient is talking
- patients' fluency deteriorates as the doctor looks away and recovers on re-establishment of gaze
- doctors frequently miss or forget information given to them while they are reading their notes.

Eye contact allows the patient to infer that the doctor is prepared to participate and listen. In the absence of eye contact, the patient makes non-verbal efforts to encourage the doctor to realign his gaze and there is a reduction in quality and quantity of information provided. This study concludes that using records while the patient is speaking is not an efficient way to conduct the consultation for either patient or doctor. The patient will give their information more slowly and less completely and the doctor may well not 'hear' the information provided. Heath suggests various strategies to overcome the common problem of needing to both hear the patient's story and examine their records:

- deliberately postpone using the records until the patient has completed their opening statement
- wait for opportune moments before looking at the notes

- separate listening from note reading by signposting both your intention to look at the records and when you have finished, so that the patient understands the process.

These findings have been replicated more recently by Robinson (1998) and Ruusuvouri (2001). Ruusuvouri elegantly shows how both body position and eye contact work together to signal whether the doctor is engaged in listening to the patient's story. A base position where the lower body faces the patient rather than the desk is more helpful in allowing the patient to tell their story with fluency. Gaze withdrawal to look at the notes is less damaging if the lower body is still facing the patient than if the whole body now faces towards the desk. Ruusuvouri also showed that gaze withdrawal is more disruptive at critical moments when the patient is describing points of particular importance to them. Eye contact is not necessary throughout the interview (and, indeed, doctors do need to look at their notes at times) but at certain points in the patient's storytelling, eye contact is critical. Gorawara-Bhat and Cook (2011) analysed and subdivided eye contact into sustained and brief episodes and noted that brief episodes involved a greater focus on charts rather than patients.

Perhaps the most important lesson for clinicians to grasp is the skill of structuring the consultation into separate elements, with a deliberate attempt to start the interview by giving full attention to the patient and then explaining to the patient when attention has to be given to the records. In this way, a happy medium can be reached where the doctor has both the skills to communicate well with the patient and is also able to manage the consultation in such a way as to refer to the records when appropriate and record the necessary data.

Increasingly, doctors are using computers during the consultation as an adjunct to handwritten records and in many situations computers have replaced written notes entirely. Even more care with regard to eye contact and body positioning needs to be taken to consult effectively while using a computer (Greatbach *et al.* 1993; Als 1997; Makoul *et al.* 2001; Frankel *et al.* 2005; McGrath *et al.* 2007; Pearce *et al.* 2008; Shachak and Reis 2009; Shachak *et al.* 2009; Silverman and Kinnersley 2010; Noordman *et al.* 2010), although many advantages can also ensue (Mitchell and Sullivan 2001; Booth *et al.* 2002). Communication benefits of using the computer collaboratively in the consultation include:

- sharing information (e.g. a table of cardiovascular risk)
- discussing prompts (*'I see it is time I re-checked your blood pressure – shall we also do that today?'*)
- recording agreed plans and follow-up.

However, Bensing *et al.* (2006) observed that communication between Dutch general practitioners during the period 1986–2002 had become more task oriented, with the doctors less likely to engage in building partnerships with their patients, less likely to express concern for their patients and less likely to provide a structure to the consultation. Bensing and colleagues considered that a likely cause of the deterioration in communication they observed was the increasing use by general practitioners of computers.

Margalit *et al.* (2006) showed that the way in which physicians use computers in the examination room can negatively affect patient-centred practice by diminishing dialogue, particularly in the psychosocial and emotional realm. Screen gaze appeared particularly disruptive to psychosocial inquiry and emotional responsiveness, suggesting that visual attentiveness to the monitor rather than eye contact with the patient may inhibit sensitive or full patient disclosure.

In contrast, and perhaps more hopefully, Chan *et al.* (2008), in a small study from Ireland, found that general practitioners were able to vary their use of the computer depending on the patient's presenting problem. For non-psychological problems the computer was used from 10% to 32% of the time, but if the problem was classified as psychological this time was reduced to 6%–16%.

Duke *et al.* (submitted for publication 2013) have very helpfully reviewed the literature on use of computers within the consulting room. The major strategy that they identified to improve physicians' communication skills while consulting with the electronic health record was dividing the encounter into patient- and computer-focused stages that are clearly demarcated from one another and signalled both verbally and by changes in body language and focus of gaze. Another key strategy was engaging patients by sharing the screen with them or reading out loud while typing. The authors have modified 'ten tips' for physicians on how to incorporate the computer into consultation as originally suggested by Ventres *et al.* (2006) and have also formulated a model to help clinicians, residents, and students improve physician–patient communication while using the electronic health record. This model integrates patient-centred interview skills and aims to empower physicians to remain patient centred while effectively using electronic health records.

DEVELOPING RAPPORT

Acceptance

In Chapter 3, we looked at the importance of understanding the patient's perspective. We examined the need to elicit patients' *thoughts* (their ideas, concerns and expectations) and take note of their *feelings*. But having discovered these thoughts and feelings, what should be our first response? The concept of acceptance as proposed by Briggs and Banahan (1979) is helpful here. It suggests that instead of immediate reassurance, rebuttal or even agreement, our initial response to patients' contributions should be to give an 'accepting response'.

The accepting response

Also called the 'supportive response' or the 'acknowledging response' elsewhere in the literature, the accepting response provides a practical and specific way of:

- accepting non-judgementally what the patient says
- acknowledging the legitimacy of the patient to hold their own views and feelings
- valuing the patient's contributions.

The accepting response acknowledges and accepts both the patient and the patient's emotions or thoughts wherever and whatever they are. Note that acceptance here does not mean that you necessarily agree with the patient but rather that you hear and acknowledge the patient's emotion or point of view. This approach is effective in relationship building because it establishes common ground between doctor and patient through a shared understanding of the patient's perspective. Acceptance is at the root of trust and trust is the bedrock of successful relationships (Briggs and Banahan 1979; Gibb 1961). The accepting response demonstrates empathy.

Accepting patients' ideas and emotions without initial judgement may not be easy – especially if they do not accord with your own perceptions. However, by acknowledging and valuing the patient's point of view rather than countering immediately with your own ideas, you can support your patients and enhance your relationship. The key concept here is acknowledging the patient's rights to hold their own views and feelings. It helps for patients to understand that not only it is reasonable for them to have thoughts and emotions about their illnesses but also it is important to you as a doctor for these to be expressed so that you can be aware of and appreciate the patient's perspective and needs. In their qualitative study done in Finland, Steilhaug *et al.* (2012) showed that recognising a patient's perspectives through skills similar to those of the accepting response may also help to reduce potential conflict and make it easier to tolerate disagreement when, for example, patients have values and perspectives that conflict with the doctor's or with sound medical practice. Based on the work of Schibbye (1993), Stielhaug *et al.* (2012) usefully called these skills and behaviours 'recognising interactions' or a 'recognising attitude'.

Functions of the accepting response

The accepting response has three valuable functions:

1. to respond supportively to the patient's expression of feelings or thoughts
2. to act as a facilitative response to obtain a better understanding of these thoughts and feelings
3. to value the patient and their ideas even when their feelings or concerns seem unjustified or perhaps even wrong.

Skills of the accepting response

The following set of skills can be used in the sequence shown to signal acceptance to the patient. In this example, the patient has expressed his thoughts by saying, *'I think I might have cancer, doctor. I've been getting an awful lot of wind lately'*:

- **acknowledge the patient's thought or feeling by naming, restating or summarising:** *'So, you're worried that the wind might be caused by cancer'*
- **acknowledge the patient's right to feel or think as he does by using legitimising comments:** *'I can understand that you would want to get that checked out'*
- **come to a 'full stop'; use attentive silence and appropriate non-verbal behaviour to make space for the patient to say more:** *'Yes, doctor, you see my mother died of bowel cancer when she was 40, and I remember she had a lot of wind; I'm terrified of getting it too'*
- **avoiding the tendency to counter with *'yes, but …'***

Although not a necessary part of every accepting response, it can also be helpful to:

- **acknowledge the value to the doctor of the patient expressing his views:** *'Thank you for telling me that – it's very helpful to know your concerns.'*

Responding to overt feelings and emotions

In the example just given, we use the accepting response to respond to a patient's belief. Acceptance is equally valuable as our initial response to feelings and emotions. For instance, consider this accepting response to a bereaved patient saying of her dead husband: *'I'm so angry with him, how could he have left me alone like that? He didn't even make a will.'*

Doctor: *'So, you feel angry about being left alone and about the will, I can see that must be upsetting.'*

(Pause – a 'full stop' gives the patient time and space to go on)

Patient: *'Yes, I am, I'm so alone and I get so cross with him for not being with me and then I feel guilty for being angry with him. Am I going mad, doctor?'*

Doctor: *'Those are strong emotions to deal with – I'm glad you mentioned them.'*

(Pause)

Responding to indirectly expressed feelings and emotions

The next two examples demonstrate that the accepting response can be useful when the feeling or thought is indirectly expressed – for instance, through non-verbal behaviour alone. Here we can combine picking up a cue to the patient's feelings (as we discussed in Chapter 3) with the accepting response:

'I sense that you feel uneasy about having to come to see me [the doctor is a hae-matologist], *am I right? … That's OK, many people feel that way when they first come here.'*

(Pause/full stop)

or

'I can see you're delighted with these test results. I'm glad they're so good too.'

(Pause/full stop)

An important part of the accepting response is to come to a *full stop* after giving the initial acknowledgement, to wait briefly and attentively in silence and to avoid saying 'yes, but …', which automatically negates the acceptance. This is almost a knee-jerk reaction for most of us. We are so eager to help that instead of waiting we say 'yes, but …' and go on to give our point of view or correction to erroneous thinking or our reassurance before we give the patient a chance to feel the acceptance or to say anything further. All of this can come later, perhaps considerably later in the interview, *after* the patient has had an opportunity to respond to our statement of acceptance. It is of course imperative that we correct, advise and reassure – the question is when.

What happens if we make a full stop rather than adding the 'but …' clause?

Usually patients will respond with a brief outpouring of whatever thought or feeling has been acknowledged, share the burden or exhilaration, and get it 'back' to a less overwhelming perspective so that they can talk about it further or go on to focus on other matters.

Acceptance is not agreement

It is important to differentiate acceptance from agreement. Acknowledging that a patient would like further surgery is not the same as agreeing to perform it. It is a two-stage process. First, identify and acknowledge a patient's beliefs without immediately countering. This enables you to understand the patient without provoking initial defensiveness. If the patient's thoughts do not fit with your own, later on in the consultation and after due consideration go to the second stage – offer your own perspective and correct misapprehensions.

Consider, for instance, if the patient in the example given earlier were a 20-year-old man. Contrast the following possible replies to his statement *'I think I might have cancer, doctor. I've been getting an awful lot of wind lately'*:

Doctor:	*'Oh, we all get wind, but that's not a sign of cancer at your age. What exactly have you noticed?'*
Patient:	*'Well, I've just felt more blown up after meals and keep passing wind in the evenings.'*
Doctor:	*'That doesn't sound like anything to worry about.'*

This approach devalues the importance of the patient's views and although most probably correct, the reassurance comes too early in the consultation to be accepted by the patient. The patient will not be encouraged to propose his own theories in the future.

Instead, we could follow the plan we proposed earlier:

Doctor:	*'So, you're worried that the wind might be caused by cancer.'*
(Pause)	
Patient:	*'Yes, doctor, you see my mother died of bowel cancer when she was 40 and I remember she had a lot of wind.'*
Doctor:	*'I can understand your concern – we'll check that out carefully. Tell me a bit more about your symptoms and then I'll examine you to see if you're OK.'*

Here, instead of countering the patient's view or giving premature or ineffective reassurance, the importance to you of hearing and explicitly acknowledging the patient's concerns is emphasised. You can explain and correct misconceptions later. In fact, Donovan and Blake (2000) found that the key to reassurance was the doctor's ability to acknowledge the patient's perspectives of their difficulties or concerns – patients who felt their problems were acknowledged felt more reassured.

Acceptance is the second stage in the three-stage process of discovering patients' beliefs that we introduced in Chapter 3.

1. **Identification**: discover and listen to the patient's ideas, concerns and expectations.
2. **Acceptance**: acknowledge the patient's views and their right to hold them, without necessarily agreeing with them; then pause so the patient can say more.
3. **Explanation**: explain your understanding of the problem in relation to the patient's understanding and reach mutually understood common ground.

Acceptance makes it possible for us to remain open to our patients. It precludes judgemental remarks. It reinforces a tentative frame of mind, prevents premature closure or defensive reactions and instead establishes mutually understood common ground. It is this that ultimately allows for change.

The problem of premature reassurance

Acceptance also enables us to avoid the trap of premature or ineffective reassurance. Simple reassurance by itself may not be an effective supportive response (Wasserman *et al.* 1984). Often reassurance is given before adequate information has been obtained, before patients' concerns have been discovered and before rapport has been developed. Unless we obtain sufficient information first, reassurance may sound false or in fact be inappropriately optimistic. Unless we understand our patients' fears, we may be addressing the wrong concern. Unless we have developed rapport with the patient, reassurance may well be interpreted as indifference or as being dismissive. And lastly, unless appropriate and relevant information is provided to back up our reassurance, patients will not understand the basis for our assertions (Kessel 1979). Acceptance prevents premature reassurance – by discovering and accepting the patient's concerns, trust is developed and more information can be obtained about the patient's illness and their concerns before an opinion is offered. Reassurance when it comes can then be appropriately timed, properly explained and matched to the patient's concerns.

Before we have collected further information or ordered tests, we may not be in a position to provide reassurance that there is nothing to worry about. However, we still have much to offer. We can accept the patient's concern and then use reassurance in other more appropriate ways. Instead of reassuring about the disease, we can, for instance, reassure the patient about our intent – we can offer our support by demonstrating that we wish to work with the patient and that we will give careful attention to their concerns.

Empathy

One of the key skills in building the doctor–patient relationship is the use of empathy (Spiro 1992; Garden 2009). In a recent review of the literature, Neumann *et al.* (2009) go much further and suggest that clinical empathy is a fundamental determinant of quality in medical care, enabling the clinician to fulfil key medical tasks more accurately and thereby leading to enhanced health outcomes.

Goleman (2011), whose work focuses on emotional and social intelligence, calls empathy the essential building block for compassion. He describes three interdependent varieties of empathy. The first variety is cognitive empathy, which is the capacity to understand others' perspectives, to see how others think about things and to know cognitively how they are feeling. Clearly, this is an important capacity for physicians to develop. However, Goleman also points out a downside: if I do not care about you and have only this kind of empathy, I can use it to manipulate or take advantage of you. So cognitive empathy alone is insufficient. The second variety is emotional empathy, which is the capacity to sense how the other person is reacting, to feel with the other, to have an emotional connection. As essential as this kind of empathy is, it too has a downside: I can internalise another's emotion to the point that it overwhelms or leads me to emotional exhaustion and burn out. The antidote here is not to stop feeling emotional empathy but to learn what Goleman calls 'emotional self-management skills', which allow you to keep emotional empathy in balance. The third variety is empathic concern. This is the capacity not only to understand the other's predicament and to feel with them but also to spontaneously want to take action to help them.

Of all the skills in the consultation, empathy is the one most often thought by learners to be a matter of personality rather than skill. Certainly, a first step in empathy is the internal motivation and commitment to understand the patient's perspective, and this must be present as well as appropriate communication skills (Norfolk 2007). However, although some of us may naturally be better at demonstrating empathy than others, the skills of empathy can be learned. The challenge is to identify the building blocks of the empathic response and enable learners to integrate the elements of empathy into their natural style so that it appears genuine to both doctor and patient (Bellet and Maloney 1991; Platt and Keller 1994; Gazda *et al.* 1995; Coulehan *et al.* 2001; Buckman 2002; Frankel 2009).

Empathy is a two-stage process:

1. the understanding and sensitive appreciation of another person's predicament or feelings
2. the communication of that understanding back to the patient in a supportive way.

The key to empathy is not only being sensitive but also overtly demonstrating that sensitivity to the patient so that they appreciate your understanding and support. It's not good enough to think empathically – you must show it too. *Demonstrating* empathy in this way overcomes the isolation of the individual in their illness and is strongly therapeutic in its own right. It also acts as a strong facilitative opening, enabling the patient to divulge more of their thoughts and concerns. What then are the building blocks of the empathic response?

Understanding the patient's predicament and feelings

Many of the skills that we discuss throughout this book demonstrate to patients that we are genuinely interested in hearing about their thoughts. Together they provide an atmosphere that facilitates disclosure and enables the first step of empathy – understanding the patient's predicament – to take place:

- welcoming the patient warmly
- clarifying the patient's agenda and expectations
- attentive listening
- facilitation especially via paraphrasing of content and feelings and repetition

- encouraging the expression of feelings and thoughts
- picking up cues, checking out our interpretations or assumptions
- internal summary
- acceptance
- non-judgemental response
- use of silence
- encouraging the patient to contribute as an equal
- offering choices.

Having set up a climate conducive to patient disclosure, the doctor has to pick up patients' verbal and non-verbal cues, become aware of their predicament and consider their feelings and emotions. In a descriptive qualitative study of medical interviews in a variety of settings, Suchman *et al.* (1997) demonstrated that patients seldom verbalised their emotions directly. Instead they offered clues in statements about situations or concerns that might plausibly be associated with an emotion. Doctors needed to pick up these 'potential empathic opportunities' by inviting elaboration (a 'potential empathic opportunity continuer') in order for the patient to directly express their emotional concern. Only then could the doctor respond by communicating empathy. In many instances that they observed, physicians used 'potential empathic opportunity terminators', redirecting the interview with an unrelated biomedical question or comment and thereby preventing the patient's emotion from being voiced. Levinson *et al.* (2000) similarly found that physicians only responded positively to patient cues in 38% of cases in surgery and 21% in primary care and in the remainder missed the opportunity to respond to the patients' cues and acknowledge their feelings. Morse *et al.* (2008), in a study of patients with lung cancer and their thoracic surgeons or oncologists, found that physicians responded empathically to 10% of empathic opportunities and provided little emotional support, often shifting to biomedical questions and statements. When empathy was provided, 50% of these statements occurred in the last one-third of the encounter, whereas patients' concerns were evenly raised throughout the encounter. Considering the value of acknowledgement from the standpoint of relationship building, both the infrequency and delay seem particularly unfortunate.

Communicating empathy to the patient

The skills outlined here do not complete the second step of empathy, which is communicating your understanding back to the patient so that they know that you appreciate and are sensitive to their difficulty. Both non-verbal and verbal skills can help us here.

Empathic non-verbal communication can say more than a thousand words. Facial expression, proximity, touch, tone of voice or use of silence in response to a patient's expression of feelings can clearly signal to the patient that you are sensitive to their predicament. But what are the verbal skills that allow us to demonstrate empathy?

Empathic statements are supportive comments that specifically link the 'I' of the doctor and the 'you' of the patient. They both name and appreciate the patient's affect or predicament (Platt and Keller 1994).

- *'I can see that your husband's memory loss has been very difficult for **you** to cope with.'*
- *'I can appreciate how difficult it is for **you** to talk about this.'*
- *'I can sense how angry **you** have been feeling about your illness.'*
- *'I can see that **you** have been very upset by her behaviour.'*
- *'I can understand that it must be frightening for **you** to know the pain might keep coming back.'*

It is not necessary to have shared an experience to empathise, nor to feel yourself that you would find that experience hard. However, it is necessary to see the problem *from the patient's position* and to communicate your understanding back to the patient. Empathy should not be confused with sympathy, which is a feeling of pity or concern from *outside of the patient's position.*

Poole and Sanson-Fisher (1979) have clearly shown that empathy is a construct that can be learned. They utilised a nine-point evaluation scale developed by Truax and Carkhuff (1967) which ranges from stage 1 ('completely unaware of even the most conspicuous of the client's statements; responses not appropriate to the mood and content of the client's statements') to stage 9 ('unerringly responds to the client's full range of feelings in their exact intensity; recognises each emotional nuance and reflects them in his words and voice; expands the client's hints into a full-blown but tentative elaboration of feeling or experience with unerring sensitive accuracy'). Truax has shown that psychotherapists who score highly on this scale achieve change.

Poole and Sanson-Fisher showed that medical students' ability to empathise did not improve over their medical school training without specific training – both first- and final-year students scored poorly on the evaluation scale (average 2.1). However, after participating in eight two-hour workshops using audiotapes, students' ratings significantly improved to an average level of 4.5 (stage 5: 'accurately responds to all the patients' discernible feelings; any misunderstandings are not disruptive due to their tentative nature'). After training, students also:

- used less jargon
- made clear attempts to understand the unique meaning of events, words and symptoms to patients
- less often blocked off emotion-laden areas
- obtained descriptions of more of their patients' problem areas
- more often matched their voice tone to that of their patients
- did less talking
- responded more in an understanding mode
- offered less advice
- were reported by patients to be understanding and caring.

Bonvicini *et al.* (2009) have more recently demonstrated that communication training with practising physicians made a significant difference in physician empathic expression during patient interactions six months after the training, as demonstrated by outside observer measurements.

Bylund and Makoul (2002) developed a measure of empathic communication in the physician–patient encounter and confirmed that female physicians tend to communicate higher degrees of empathy in response to empathic opportunities created by patients. Interestingly, they demonstrated that patients provide empathic opportunities irrespective of familiarity with the clinician and length of relationship (Bylund and Makoul 2005).

Hojat *et al.* (2009) demonstrated in a four-year US medical school programme that although empathy scores did not change significantly during the first two years of medical school, a significant decline in empathy scores was observed at the end of the third year and this persisted until graduation. Patterns of decline in empathy scores were similar for men and women. The authors call for targeted educational programmes to retain and enhance empathy at the undergraduate, graduate and continuing medical education levels. Newton *et al.* (2008) have also shown that empathy significantly decreased during undergraduate medical education, especially after the first and third years. Students choosing career specialties characterised by continuity of patient care had higher empathy levels.

There has been debate about whether skills-based training and assessment of empathy trivialises the very qualities we are trying to instil by reducing them to surface behaviours, potentially preventing learners from acquiring the habits of mind and sensitivity needed for 'earnest attempts to understand and relate to patients' stories'. Others believe that surface manifestations of behavioural empathy should be assessed and taught because these are essential skills for the compassionate and effective care of patients. A student who is unable to display these basic communication skills is likely to be deficient in the other, deeper, components of empathy as well. Clearly, skills-based training should be complemented by other approaches that enhance students' capacities for compassion and authentic presence and enable students to more readily identify with patients' feelings (Stepien and Baernstein 2006; Steele and Hulsman 2008; Wear and Varley 2008; Teherani *et al.* 2008).

Blatt *et al.* (2010) used the approach of perspective taking, common in the fields of social psychology and neurobiology, to devise a very brief intervention with medical students. Prior to a clinical skills assessment scored on history taking, physical examination and patient communication, an intervention group was given the following additional instructions: 'When you see your patient, imagine what the patient is experiencing as if you were that person, looking at the world through the patient's eyes and walking through the world in the patient's shoes.' Simulated patient satisfaction with the interview increased over control students.

More recently, Salmon *et al.* (2011) have postulated that explicit emotional engagement is not always necessary in every context. In a study of breast surgeons and their patients, despite finding very little emotional talk on observing consultations, later interviews with patients and doctors suggested that they both still felt their relationship was personal and emotional and that this was mediated by 'practitioners' conscientious execution of their role'. Salmon *et al.* postulate that an authentic caring relationship can be developed through the surgeon's expertise and character.

Taking a different approach, Hsu *et al.* (2012) attempted to understand reasons for the repeated finding that providers miss 70%–90% of opportunities to express empathy (Morse *et al.* 2008; Byland and Makoul 2005; Levinson *et al.* 2000). In this study with HIV patients, providers also missed most opportunities to respond empathically to patients' emotion. Instead providers often addressed the problem underlying the emotion – in so doing, providers did attempt to respond to the patient's cues, albeit not with an empathic response. In other words, in response to the patient's cue, the physician provided instrumental support (trying to solve the underlying problem) rather than explicit emotional support (acknowledgement). When the provider's initial response to the patient's cue was problem solving, empathic statements rarely occurred in subsequent dialogue. The study found that providers 'rarely ignore the patient's cue altogether; rather, they recognize and acknowledge the patient's cue but may fail to respond adequately.' The researchers suggest that a better alternative for clinicians would be to recognise the importance of both kinds of support. By offering both problem solving and empathic responses, 'providers may build stronger therapeutic relationships and achieve better health outcomes for their patients in moments of vulnerability'.

Support

Several other supportive approaches contribute to relationship building and rapport formation (Rogers 1980; Egan 1990). They are often used to complete the empathic response:

- concern

> *'I'm concerned that you'll be going home on your own tonight and might not be able to cope with your arm in a cast.'*

- understanding

> *'I can certainly understand how you might feel angry with the hospital for cancelling your operation.'*

- willingness to help

> *'If there is anything else I can do for Jack, please let me know.'*
>
> or
>
> *'Although, as I say, we can't cure the cancer, I can help with any symptoms that it might cause so please tell me right away if anything happens.'*

- partnership

> *'We'll have to work together to get on top of this illness, so let's work through the options that we can choose from.'*

- acknowledging coping efforts and appropriate self-care

> 'You've really done exactly the right things in trying to get his temperature down.'
>
> or
>
> 'I think you've coped really well at home despite some very considerable problems.'

- sensitivity

> 'I'm sorry if this examination is embarrassing for you. I'll try to make it as quick and easy as I can.'

The key point here is that our thoughts and acknowledgements need to be verbalised to be supportive. Communication must be overt to be truly effective and not liable to misinterpretation. Without explicit comment, the patient may well not be fully aware of your support.

Williamson (in Suchman *et al.* 2011) has provided an acronym, PEARLS, to help more readily remember the variety of relationship-building statements available to us:

- partnership
- empathy
- acknowledgment
- respect
- legitimisation
- support.

What is the research evidence that rapport-building skills make a difference to the medical consultation?

Throughout this chapter we have summarised studies demonstrating how relationship matters. Here we sample additional research regarding the impact of rapport-building skills on the consultation and outcomes of care.

Buller and Buller (1987) described two general styles displayed by physicians in medical interviews. The first, affiliation, was composed of behaviours designed to establish and maintain a positive doctor–patient relationship. Many of these behaviours were those discussed in the sections earlier, including friendliness, interest, attentiveness, empathy, non-judgemental attitude and social orientation. The second style included behaviours that established the doctor's power, status, authority and professional distance. Patient satisfaction was found to be significantly higher when doctors in both specialist and family practice adopted the affiliative style.

Bertakis *et al.* (1991), in a study of physicians from both internal medicine and family practice, have demonstrated that patients are most satisfied by interviews that encourage them to talk about psychosocial issues in an atmosphere characterised by an absence of physician dominance and the presence of friendliness and interest.

Hall *et al.* (1988), in a meta-analysis of 41 independent studies, reported that patient satisfaction was related to the amount of information given by doctors, technical and interpersonal competence, more partnership building, more positive talk, more positive non-verbal behaviour and more social conversation. The definitions used to group behaviours together under 'partnership building' and 'positive talk' include many of the rapport-building skills discussed earlier.

Wasserman *et al.* (1984) analysed the effect of supportive statements made to mothers during paediatric visits. They found that empathic statements led to increased satisfaction and reduction in maternal concerns. Encouragement (such as acknowledging coping efforts and appropriate self-care) led to increased satisfaction and higher opinions of clinicians. In contrast, simple reassurance, which was the commonest intervention, led to no improvements in outcome. This confirms the suggestion that reassurance without understanding the patient's concerns or providing adequate information may be of little value. Donovan and Blake (2000) added further confirmation of this suggestion – their study found that patients who felt their problems were acknowledged felt more reassured.

Wissow *et al.* (1994) found that paediatricians' use of supportive statements (compliments, approval, concern, empathy, encouragement and reassurance) was positively associated with parents' disclosure of psychosocial problems.

Spiegel *et al.* (1989) conducted a longitudinal study of women with metastatic carcinoma of the breast, comparing a control group with a second group of women assigned to a year of weekly supportive-expressive group therapy. Women in the experimental group were encouraged to provide mutual support, to express and discuss their feelings and concerns about dying, to develop a life project for their remaining time, to examine their relationships with others, to work through doctor–patient problems and to use self-hypnosis to aid pain control. After four years, all of the control group patients had died and one-third of the experimental group were still alive. Over 10 years, women attending the support group had lived on average 15 months longer than women in the control group. Although this study looked at the effects of supportive group therapy rather than the doctor–patient relationship *per se*, we report this study here because it speaks to the importance of expressing feelings in a supportive climate and the power of relationship in healthcare. It also serves as a reminder that in addition to developing the best relationship possible with their patients, doctors can also point them in the direction of support groups and other professionals who can fulfil additional relationship needs.

Dimoska *et al.* (2008a) have shown that patients seeing an oncologist who was rated as warmer and discussed a greater number of psychosocial issues had better psychological adjustment and reduced anxiety after the consultation.

Levinson *et al.* (2008) examined the content and process of informed decision-making between orthopaedic surgeons and elderly white versus African American patients. Differences in the process of relationship building and in patient satisfaction ratings were clearly present. Overall there were practically no significant differences in the content of informed decision-making elements based on race. However, coder ratings of relationship were higher on responsiveness, respect and listening in visits with white patients compared with African American patients. Patient ratings of communication and overall satisfaction with the visit were significantly higher for white patients.

In a study in which Swiss university students interacted via computer with a virtual physician, Cousin *et al.* (2012) found that a more caring physician communication style led to higher participant satisfaction regardless of participants' attitudes toward high or low caring. However, satisfaction with a physician's high or low sharing communication style was influenced by participants' attitude toward sharing. Taking study limitations into account, the researchers concluded that a physician may adopt a high caring style, confident that all patients will benefit, but adoption of a sharing style must be more carefully aligned to patient attitudes.

Kim *et al.* (2004) demonstrated in Korea that patient-perceived physician empathy significantly influenced patient satisfaction and compliance.

In an audiotape study of 461 discussions of weight, Cox *et al.* (2011) showed that when physicians expressed empathy along with other patient-centred techniques, patients' weight-related attitudes and behaviours improved.

In a randomised controlled trial of 719 patients, Rakel *et al.* (2011) found that positive patient perception of physician empathy had significant effects on reducing the duration and patient-reported severity of the common cold. Their study was also able to correlate these subjective measures with objective findings regarding physical immune changes measured by interleukin-8 and neutrophil counts.

Hojat *et al.* (2011) correlated physician empathy scores on a self-completed empathy scale with HbA_{1C} and low-density lipoprotein cholesterol tests and found a positive relationship between physicians' empathy and patients' clinical outcomes.

In a large retrospective correlational study of 20961 patients performed in an Italian primary care setting, Canale *et al.* (2012) compared physician empathy scores with clinical outcomes for patients with diabetes mellitus. They found that 'patients of physicians with high empathy scores, compared with patients of physicians with moderate and low empathy scores, had a significantly lower rate of metabolic complications.'

Since 2005 when we completed the second edition of this book, the evidence points increasingly to the impact of relationship and relationship building skills on physiological as well as psychological outcomes of care. This influence may, as Street *et al.* (2009) suggest, follow an indirect pathway. The skills that contribute to building relationship may, for instance, enhance accuracy of understanding and trust, which in turn influence patient involvement, clinical reasoning, quality decision making and patient adherence, which then influence health outcomes such as pain control, functional ability, cure or recurrence, and survival. Whether direct or indirect, the influence is unmistakably there. These findings concerning the impact of relationship on health outcomes represent another confirmation of the interdependence of communication content, process and perceptual skills that we discussed in Chapter 1.

INVOLVING THE PATIENT

One of the principles of effective communication that we presented in Chapter 1 was *reducing unnecessary uncertainty*. Unresolved uncertainties can lead to lack of concentration or to anxiety, which in turn can block effective communication. The distractions associated with uncertainty can be particularly evident – for example, during rushed visits where the patient has little opportunity to ask questions, or in contexts such as emergency departments (Slade *et al.* 2008), where interruptions in the physician–patient encounter are common and where the consultation becomes fragmented, where multiple clinicians may be interacting with patients during the same visit, where the patient may have limited understanding and be given little explanation of what is happening. Patients may be uncertain about what to expect during a given interview, about the significance of a line of questioning, about the role of a particular member of the healthcare team, or about the attitudes, intentions or trustworthiness of the other individual. Therefore, one important aspect of building the relationship in the consultation is to employ skills that limit the uncertainty that can so easily block communication.

Sharing of thoughts

Throughout this book, we have espoused a system of medical communication that encourages a collaborative understanding between patient and doctor. We have seen how important it is for patient and doctor to understand each other and the steps that we can take to ensure that communication in the consultation is an interaction rather than a one-way transmission. Techniques such as *the use of internal summary* in information gathering and *checking understanding* in information giving not only ensure accuracy but also act as facilitative openings by encouraging a truly interactive process.

Sharing one's thinking with the patient is another example of encouraging the patient's involvement:

> 'What I'm thinking now is how to sort out whether this arm pain is coming from your shoulder or your neck.'
>
> or
>
> 'Sometimes it's difficult to work out whether abdominal pain is due to a physical illness or is related to stress.'

Sharing one's thought processes in this way not only allows the patient to understand the reasons for your questions but also acts as a facilitative probe:

> 'I think you might be right about stress, doctor. I've had a terrible time with my son just recently and I just don't know how to cope.'

This overt approach allows the patient an insight into the process of the interview, enabling him to understand the drift of your questioning and providing a very open-ended method of eliciting further information. It is often more acceptable than thinking through the dilemma internally and then posing closed questions without explanation:

> *'Are you under any stress at the moment?'*

Closed questions so often feel unsettling to the patient because of uncertainty about what lies behind the doctor's choice of direction:

> *'Does the doctor think I'm just neurotic?'*

Heritage and Stivers (1999) explore the use of 'online commentary', talk that describes what the physician is seeing, feeling or hearing during the physical examination, and hypothesise that online commentary may be associated with successful physician resistance to implicit or explicit patient demands for inappropriate medication.

Peräkylä (2002) also used conversation analysis to explore the effect of doctors explaining overtly their reasoning for a diagnosis. Patients talked about the diagnosis more often and became more involved than after diagnostic statements in which such explication was not done.

Robins *et al.* (2011) explore the concept of transparency, of clear signalling to the patient about the process as well as the content of the interview, so that not only the physician but also the patient understands where the interview is going and why. They clarify how this promotes relationship building, reduces uncertainty for the patient and enables a more collaborative consultation. They particularly comment about the importance of sharing thinking and providing a meta-commentary to the patient about why the physician is exploring a particular pathway. Robins *et al.* demonstrate in their study how physicians spent little time using such process-related transparency.

Providing rationale

Explaining the rationale for questions or parts of the physical examination is another specific example of the principle of reducing uncertainty. Many of our questions and examinations remain a mystery to the patient unless explained. When taking a history from a patient with chest pain, we ask:

> *'How many pillows do you sleep with?'*

This appears to the patient to be a complete non sequitor. Why is the doctor asking him about his bedtime habits? Yet we could so easily have asked:

> *'Do you get breathless when you lie flat at night?'*
>
> followed, if necessary, by
>
> *'Do you have to prop yourself up on several pillows?'*

Similarly, without explaining why we are performing parts of the examination, we leave the patient in confusion and may even lay ourselves open to medico-legal attack. The young female patient who comes in with a sore throat will be surprised if the male doctor starts to examine her groin unless he explains that she might have glandular fever and that he wishes to check for lymphadenopathy. The man with sciatica may be worried by the doctor who starts to test perineal sensation with a pin, unless the doctor explains about the danger of central prolapsed discs. Both these examples have led to formal complaints against doctors. Reducing uncertainty can decrease anxiety for the doctor too!

During physical examination, asking permission to perform each task is not only a matter of common courtesy but demonstrates to the patient that you are sensitive to their potential discomfiture and therefore promotes relationship building.

Summary

In this chapter, we have examined the skills of building the relationship, a task that is central to the success of the consultation. Without attention to both our own and our patients' non-verbal communication, without efforts to develop rapport, without taking pains to involve the patient in the process of the consultation, many problems will arise. Not only will our long-term relationship with the patient suffer but also, even in the short-term, our patients will feel less understood and supported, the other tasks of the interview will become much more difficult to achieve and patient satisfaction and adherence will diminish.

Throughout the interview, the doctor has to pay specific attention to the skills of relationship building while completing the more sequential tasks of the consultation. By keeping in mind the skills outlined in this section of the Calgary–Cambridge Guides, the doctor will be rewarded with a more accurate, efficient and supportive consultation that paves the way for a the development of a trusting and productive long-term relationship.

Chapter 6

Explanation and planning

Introduction

Explanation and planning is the Cinderella subject of communication skills teaching. Most teaching programmes concentrate on the first half of the interview and tend to neglect or underplay this vital next stage in the consultation (Maguire *et al.* 1986b; Sanson-Fisher *et al.* 1991; Elwyn *et al.* 1999b). To some extent this emphasis is understandable, as so many problems in communication arise from the beginning or information-gathering phases of the interview. Also, as we show in this chapter, many of the skills of successful explanation and planning are inextricably linked with the skills of information gathering – effective explanation needs both to be based on information gathered about the disease aspects of a patient's problems and to be framed in terms that take into account the patient's illness framework of ideas, concerns and expectations.

Yet explanation and planning is of utmost importance to a successful consultation. There is little point in being able to discover what the patient wishes to discuss, in taking a good history and in being highly knowledgeable if you cannot make a joint management plan that the patient feels comfortable with, understands and is prepared to adhere to. Prescribing treatment that is not taken wastes all our efforts in assessment and diagnosis.

If the first half of the consultation represents the foundations of medical communication, explanation and planning is the roof. Neglecting this aspect may ruin all of the hard work already expended on understanding the patient's problems.

Problems in communication

Research identifies substantial difficulties in the explanation and planning phase of the interview. In fact, the statistics concerning these problems pose worrying questions about the value of many of our everyday activities! Here we provide just a few examples from a large body of evidence collected over many years.

Are there problems with the amount of information that doctors give?

Many studies show that, in general, physicians give sparse information to their patients.

- Waitzkin (1984) has demonstrated that American internists devoted little more than one minute on average to the task of information giving in interviews lasting 20 minutes and overestimated the amount of time that they spent on this task by a factor of nine.

- Makoul *et al.* (1995) found that doctors in UK general practice overestimated the extent to which they accomplished the following key tasks in explanation and planning: discussing the risks of medication, discussing the patient's ability to follow the treatment plan and eliciting the patient's opinion about medication prescribed.
- Boreham and Gibson (1978), in a study in Australian general practice, showed that despite a lack of basic knowledge prior to the consultation and a strongly expressed desire to gain information concerning their illness, the majority of patients did not obtain even basic information concerning the diagnosis, prognosis, causation or treatment of their condition.
- Svarstad (1974) studied doctors' instructions to patients when prescribing drugs and found no discussion at all in 20% of cases, no information about the name or purpose of the drug in 30%, no mention of the frequency of doses in 80% and no mention of the length of the course in 90% of cases.
- Richard and Lussier (2003) studied the discussion of medications in Canadian general practice. They assessed audiotapes of 40 experienced general practitioners engaging in 462 patient encounters. Several of their findings echo and extend those from earlier research. In instances of the prescription of new medications, instructions were discussed in 75.9% of cases, warnings and side effects were rarely discussed and reasons to re-consult were discussed in only 35.4% of cases. Discussion of compliance issues regarding these new prescriptions occurred in only 5% of cases.
- In a subsequent study of 442 encounters involving 1492 discussions of medications, these researchers again found a generally low level of physician–patient dialogue when discussing medications during primary care consultations (Richard and Lusseier 2007). Patients had little opportunity to discuss their concerns and perspectives. Using the Medicode coding system, Richard and Lussier (2006a) determined that physician initiation and monologues dominated, pointing to a lack of mutuality in exchanges on medications.
- More recently in the UK, Sibley *et al.* (2011) found that nurse prescribers discussed medications with patients in a more dyadic manner than their physician counterparts but still initiated most discussion, asked patients about their concerns and perspectives infrequently, and rarely took on the role of listener, respondent or participant.
- Tarn *et al.* (2006) come to the same conclusions: 'When initiating new medications, physicians often fail to communicate critical elements of medication use.'

Are there problems with the type of information that doctors give?

We also know that patients and doctors disagree over the relative importance of different types of medical information

- Kindelan and Kent (1987), in a study in UK general practice, showed that patients placed the highest value on information about the diagnosis, prognosis and causation of their condition. However, doctors greatly underestimated their patients' desire for information about prognosis and causation and overestimated their desire for information concerning treatment and drug therapy. Patients' individual information needs were not elicited.
- Jenkins *et al.* (2011) discovered that oncologists frequently omitted discussion

of prognosis in discussions about phase 1 trial participation, 'a fundamental and ethical prerequisite for patients' being able to consider how best to use the time left to them'. Interestingly, 50% of doctors reported discussing prognosis in the consultation, but only 12% of patients and 20% of coders agreed that it had been mentioned.

- In a study that combined personal narrative with other evidence, Anderson and Marlett (2004) looked at the nature of the information (rather than the amount of information) that healthcare providers give to stroke patients and their families and how people use that communication to restructure life after stroke. They considered how communication influences stroke outcome, often for the worse because of its emphasis on what will no longer be possible.

Can patients understand the language that doctors use?

Many studies have shown that doctors not only use language that patients do not understand but also appear to use it to control their patients' involvement in the interview.

- Korsch *et al.* (1968) found that paediatricians' use of technical language (e.g. 'oedema') and medical shorthand (e.g. 'history') was a barrier to communication in more than half of the 800 visits studied. Mothers were confused by the terms used by doctors yet rarely asked for clarification of unfamiliar terms.
- Svarstad (1974) suggested that doctors and patients engage in a 'communication conspiracy'. In only 15% of visits where unfamiliar terms were used did the patient admit that they did not understand. Doctors in turn seemed to speak as if their patients understood all that they said. Physicians deliberately used highly technical language to control communication and to limit patient questions – such behaviour occurred twice as often when doctors were under pressure of time.
- McKinlay (1975), in a study of obstetricians and gynaecologists in the UK, showed that physicians were well aware of the difficulties that patients had in understanding doctors in general. Despite this, in their interviews with patients, physicians continued to use terms that they had previously identified as the very ones that they would not expect their patients to understand.
- Castro *et al.* (2007) described physicians' use of jargon with diabetes patients with limited health literacy in the United States and concluded that physicians caring for these patients employed unclarified jargon during key clinical functions such as providing recommendations.
- Koch-Weser *et al.* (2009), in a study of rheumatologists in the United States, showed that doctors did not explain, or use as part of an explanation, 79% of the medical words they introduced, and that patients seldom responded in a way that would indicate whether or not they had correctly interpreted those terms.
- Bagley *et al.* (2011), in the UK, investigated patients' understanding of orthopaedic terms and discovered low levels of understanding of commonly used terms in orthopaedic clinics.

Do patients recall and understand the information that we give?

It is clear that patients do not recall all that we impart, nor do they make sense of difficult messages. As we shall see later, earlier studies showed that only 50%–60% of information given is recalled. Further studies in general practice have suggested that in fact much more is remembered and the real difficulty is that patients do not always understand the meaning of key messages, nor are they necessarily committed to the doctor's view.

- Dunn *et al.* (1993) found that cancer patients in their first interview with an oncologist remembered only 45% of 'key points' as determined by the oncologist.
- Braddock *et al.* (1997) showed, in a study of audiotaped patient encounters with primary care physicians in the United States, that patient understanding was assessed only 2% of the time.
- Murphy *et al.* (2004) demonstrated that 30% of patients undergoing laparoscopy for acute abdominal pain in Ireland were either not given or did not reliably recall basic information regarding the procedure.

Are patients involved in decision making and to the level that they would wish?

- Degner *et al.* (1997) studied women with a confirmed diagnosis of breast cancer attending hospital oncology clinics, and found that 22% wanted to select their own cancer treatment, 44% wanted to select their treatment in collaboration with their doctors, and 34% wanted to delegate this decision making to their doctors. Only 42% of women believed that they had achieved their preferred level of control in decision making.
- Looking at informed consent in cancer clinical trials in Australia, Brown *et al.* (2004) showed that oncologists rarely addressed aspects of shared decision making, and that in almost one-third of consultations, doctors made implicit statements favouring one option over another – either standard or clinical trial treatment.
- Audrey *et al.* (2008) looked at how much oncologists in the UK tell patients about the survival benefit of palliative chemotherapy during consultations in which decisions about treatment are made. Most patients were not given clear information about the survival gain of palliative chemotherapy, preventing them from being fully involved in decision making.

Do patients comply or adhere to the plans that we make?

Here the research is clear-cut and salutary.

- Studies have consistently shown that between 10% and 90% of patients prescribed drugs by their doctors (with an average of 50%) either do not take their medicine at all or take it incorrectly (Haynes *et al.* 1996).
- Many studies have shown that patients do not follow their doctors' recommendations, with 20%–30% non-adherence to medications for acute

illness, 30%–40% for medications for illness prevention, 50% for long-term medications and 72% for diet.

- Yet, surprisingly, doctors have a tendency to ignore non-adherence as a possible cause of poor outcome.
- Non-adherence is enormously expensive. The cost of wasted funds spent on prescription medications used inappropriately or not used in Canada amounts to CAN$5 billion a year, based on an annual expenditure of CAN$10.3 billion and data indicating that 50% of prescription medications are not used as prescribed. Estimates of the further costs of non-adherence (including extra visits to physicians, laboratory tests, additional medications, hospital and nursing home admissions, lost productivity and premature death) were CAN$7–9 billion in Canada (Coambs *et al.* 1995) and US$100 billion plus in the United States (Berg *et al.* 1993).
- Yet, in a more recent meta-analysis of published research, Zolnierek *et al.* (2009) showed that communication in medical care is highly correlated with better patient adherence, and that training physicians to communicate better enhances their patients' adherence.

For further information about non-adherence, the following texts provide excellent reviews of the field: Haynes *et al.* (1979), Meichenbaum and Turk (1987), Ley (1988), Coambs *et al.* (1995), Haynes *et al.* (1996), Butler *et al.* (1996) and DiMatteo (2004).

Are there problems in the teaching and learning of explanation and planning in medical education?

Maguire *et al.* (1986a,b) looked at the information-giving skills of young doctors who five years previously had completed training in interviewing skills at medical school. This training had, however, not included any specific training in information giving *per se*. The results were disturbing. Doctors were weakest in many of the very techniques that have been found to increase patients' satisfaction with and adherence to advice and treatment, namely:

- discovering the patient's views and expectations (70% made no attempt)
- negotiation (90% made no attempt)
- encouraging questions (70% made no attempt)
- repetition of advice (63% made no attempt)
- checking understanding (89% made no attempt)
- categorising information (90% made no attempt).

No difference at all was detected in information-giving skills between those who had completed the course on interviewing skills at medical school and controls. Yet the same students had maintained their superiority over controls in key information-gathering skills. This demonstrates the need for teaching not only in information-gathering skills but also in the specific skills of explanation and planning if we wish doctors to become effective in information transfer in the consultation. Two decades ago, Sanson-Fisher *et al.* (1991) argued that training medical practitioners in information transfer was the new challenge in communication skills teaching. That challenge continues today but, as we shall see, now includes shared decision making and mutual collaboration as well as information transfer.

Campion *et al.* (2002) looked at 2094 candidates' scores on the consulting skills module of the examination for membership of the Royal College of General Practitioners in the UK. For this national high-stakes examination, residents nearing completion of their three-year residency programme submit a videotape of seven actual consultations with their own patients, which the candidate self-selects to represent their best performance – the first five of these were assessed for each candidate. Even in this highly select set of consultations in which candidates were fully aware of the performance criteria, Campion *et al.* found significant deficits in four patient-centred competencies related to explanation and planning:

1. exploring patients' beliefs about the illness was not seen in 14% of the candidates – only 39% met this performance criterion in three or more of their five consultations
2. using beliefs in explanation was not seen in 31% of the candidates – only 17% met this criterion in three or more of the five consultations
3. checking patients' understanding of explanations was not seen in 45% of the candidates – only 9% met this criterion in three or more of the five consultations
4. involving patients in decisions was not seen in 14% of the candidates – only 36% met this criterion in three or more of the five consultations.

Are these problems improving with time?

Unfortunately, these difficulties do not appear to be resolving with the passage of time. Bensing *et al.* (2006) compared communication patterns between general practitioners and patients in 1986 and 2002. Contrary to expectations, patients were less active in 2002, talking less, asking fewer questions and raising fewer concerns or worries. General practitioners provided more medical information but expressed their concern about the patients' conditions less often. In addition, they were less involved in process-oriented behaviour and partnership building. Overall, these results suggest that consultations in 2002 were more task-oriented and businesslike than 16 years earlier, perhaps reflecting the recent emphasis on evidence-based medicine, protocolised care and the effect of computerisation.

How does all of this relate to the growing field of health literacy?

There is increasing and considerable interest and research into the issue of patient health literacy. Low health literacy contributes to possible communication gaps between physicians and patients. Patients with low health literacy may have less familiarity with medical concepts and vocabulary and ask fewer questions. They may also hide their limited understanding from shame or embarrassment. Physicians commonly overestimate patients' literacy levels. Clearly, in all consultations, there is a need to tailor information giving to each individual patient and actively discover what will be helpful to the patient. Interestingly, research into explanation and planning and research into patient health literacy have arrived at the same conclusions as to the skills that physicians can employ to help improve their consultations. Kripalani and Weiss (2006), Sudore and Schillinger (2009) and Coleman (2011) provide very useful reviews of strategies for communication in low health literacy situations that have remarkable similarity to the skills that we promote in this chapter.

Objectives

Our objectives for explanation and planning can be summarised as:

- gauging the correct amount and type of information to give to each individual patient
- providing explanations that the patient can remember and understand
- providing explanations that relate to the patient's perspective
- using an interactive approach to ensure a shared understanding of the problem with the patient
- involving the patient and planning collaboratively to the level that the patient wishes, so as to increase the patient's commitment and adherence to plans made
- continuing to build a relationship and provide a supportive environment.

These objectives encompass many of the tasks and checkpoints mentioned in other well-known guides to the consultation:

- Pendleton *et al.* (1984, 2003):
  - to enable the patient to choose an appropriate action for each problem
  - to achieve a shared understanding of the problems with the patient
  - to involve the patient in the management and encourage them to accept appropriate responsibility.
- Neighbour (1987):
  - handing over – doctors' and patients' agendas; negotiating, influencing and gift-wrapping.
- AAPP Three-Function Model (Cohen-Cole 1991):
  - education, negotiation and motivation
  - developing rapport and responding to patient's emotions.
- Bayer Institute for Health Care Communication E4 model (Keller and Carroll 1994):
  - educating the patient
  - enlisting the patient in his or her own healthcare.
- The SEGUE Framework for teaching and assessing communication skills (Makoul 2001):
  - giving information.
- The Maastricht Maas Global (van Thiel and van Dalen 1995):
  - information sharing
  - diagnosis
  - management.
- Essential Elements of Communication in Medical Encounters: Kalamazoo Consensus Statement (Participants in the Bayer-Fetzer Conference on Physician–Patient Communication in Medical Education 2001):
  - share information
  - reach agreement on problems and plans.

- The Four Habits Model (Frankel and Stein 1999; Krupat *et al.* 2006):
  - invest in the end
    - › deliver diagnostic information
    - › provide education
    - › involve the patient in making decisions.
- Patient-centred medicine (Stewart *et al.* 2003):
  - finding common ground
  - incorporating prevention and health promotion.
- The Model of the Macy Initiative in Health Communication (Kalet *et al.* 2004):
  - patient education
  - negotiate and agree on plan.
- The Six Function Model (de Haes and Bensing 2009):
  - providing information
  - decision making.

The content of explanation and planning

In Chapter 3 we described how the process skills for gathering information as delineated in the Calgary–Cambridge Guides relate to the Calgary–Cambridge content guide. The process skills for explanation and planning also correspond to three specific areas of the content guide. Box 6.1 shows these content guide components.

Box 6.1   The content of explanation and planning

Differential diagnosis – hypotheses
Including both disease and illness issues

Physician's plan of management
Investigations
Treatment alternatives

Explanation and planning with patient
What the patient has been told
Plan of action negotiated

Note that these content components include aspects of the physician's internal thinking and planning as well as the explanation and planning that occurs jointly with the patient. Throughout the rest of this chapter on explanation and planning, it will be useful to keep in mind how process and content skills work together during this important part of the consultation.

The process skills of explanation and planning

Box 6.2   The process skills of explanation and planning

Providing the correct amount and type of information

Aims: to give comprehensive and appropriate information
             to assess each individual patient's information needs
             to neither restrict nor overload

- **Chunks and checks:** gives information in assimilable chunks, checks for understanding; uses patient's response as a guide to how to proceed
- **Assesses patient's starting point:** asks for patient's prior knowledge early on when giving information; ascertains extent of patient's wish for information
- **Asks patients what other information would be helpful,** e.g. aetiology, prognosis
- **Gives explanation at appropriate times:** avoids giving advice, information or reassurance prematurely

Aiding accurate recall and understanding

Aims: to make information easier for the patient to remember and understand

- **Organises explanation:** divides into discrete sections, develops a logical sequence
- **Uses explicit categorisation or signposting** (e.g. *'There are three important things that I would like to discuss. First …' 'Now, shall we move on to …'*)
- **Uses repetition and summarising:** to reinforce information
- **Language:** uses concise, easily understood statements, avoids or explains jargon
- **Uses visual methods of conveying information:** diagrams, models, written information and instructions
- **Checks patient's understanding of information given (or plans made),** e.g. by asking patient to restate in own words; clarifies as necessary

Achieving a shared understanding: incorporating the patient's perspective

Aims: to provide explanations that relate to the patient's perspective of the problem
             to discover the patient's thoughts and feelings about the information given
             to encourage an interaction rather than one-way transmission

- **Relates explanations to patient's perspective:** to previously elicited ideas, concerns and expectations
- **Provides opportunities and encourages patient to contribute:** to ask questions, seek clarification or express doubts; responds appropriately
- **Picks up and responds to verbal and non-verbal cues,** e.g. patient's need to contribute information or ask questions, information overload, distress
- **Elicits patient's beliefs, reactions and feelings:** regarding information given, terms used; acknowledges and addresses where necessary

Planning: shared decision making
Aims: to enhance patients' understanding of the decision making process
       to involve patients in decision making to the level they wish
       to increase patients' commitment to plans made
- **Shares own thinking, as appropriate:** ideas, thought processes and dilemmas
- **Involves the patient:**
  - offers suggestions and choices rather than directives
  - encourages patient to contribute their ideas, suggestions
- **Explores management options**
- **Ascertains level of involvement that patient wishes** in making the decision at hand
- **Negotiates a mutually acceptable plan:**
  - signposts own position of equipoise or preference regarding available options
  - determines patient's preferences
- **Checks with patient:**
  - if accepts plans
  - if concerns have been addressed

Options for explanation and planning
(includes content and process skills)
If offering an opinion and discussing significance of problems
- Offers opinion of what is going on and names if possible
- Reveals rationale for opinion
- Explains causation, seriousness, expected outcome, short- and long-term consequences
- Elicits patient's beliefs, reactions and concerns (e.g. if opinion matches patient's thoughts, acceptability, feelings)

If negotiating a mutual plan of action
- Discusses options – e.g. no action, investigation, medication or surgery, non-drug treatments (physiotherapy, walking aids, fluids, counselling), preventive measures
- Provides information on action or treatment offered:
  - name
  - steps involved, how it works
  - benefits and advantages
  - possible side effects
- Obtains patient's view of need for action, perceived benefits, barriers, motivation
- Accepts patient's views, advocates alternative viewpoint as necessary
- Elicits patient's reactions and concerns about plans and treatments, including acceptability
- Takes patient's lifestyle, beliefs, cultural background and abilities into consideration
- Encourages patient to be involved in implementing plans, to take responsibility and be self-reliant

- Asks about patient support systems; discusses other support available

If discussing investigations and procedures
- Provides clear information on procedures, e.g. what patient might experience, how patient will be informed of results
- Relates procedures to treatment plan – value, purpose
- Encourages questions about and discussion of potential anxieties or negative outcomes

Communication process skills: the evidence

We now explore the individual skills for explanation and planning listed in Box 6.2 and examine the evidence from theory and research that validates their use in the consultation. We have divided the skills of explanation and planning into five sections and will look at each in turn:

1. providing the correct amount and type of information
2. aiding accurate recall and understanding
3. achieving a shared understanding: incorporating the patient's perspective
4. planning: shared decision making
5. options in explanation and planning.

As we progress through these sections, we will illuminate the skills of explanation and planning in the one-to-one situation by considering the skills involved in delivering a lecture. We have all attended many lectures in our lifetime, not all of them of the highest quality. Thinking about the poorly delivered lecture provides us with many insights into the skills required in information giving in the medical interview. Nobody has escaped sitting through lectures in which some or all of the following apply:

- the lecture has no apparent structure, and as a listener you cannot tell where it is going
- the lecturer uses language or jargon you cannot understand
- the lecturer loses you early on and you struggle to keep up from then on
- the information given is either way below or way above your current level of understanding
- you are given too much or too little new information
- the lecturer has made assumptions about your personal needs that are incorrect and the questions you wish to be answered are not addressed
- you are not sure what the key points are at the end.

At its worst, the following scenario ensues. The lecturer speaks for 45 minutes without interruption in a darkened room with poor-quality slides. You concentrate for a while and a question enters your head that needs clarifying in order for you to make sense of what has been said so far. While you are thinking about this, you miss the next few minutes of the speech. You start to drift into a daydream and return to concentrate on the lecture after an unclear amount of time. When you do so, the rest of the lecture does not quite make sense. At the end, the lecturer asks if there are any questions but you are too embarrassed to ask the question you thought of earlier as you do not know if it was answered when you were day-dreaming. You say nothing.

We can apply lessons learned from this scenario not only to how to give a lecture but also to conducting the explanation and planning component of the doctor–patient interview. To optimise information giving in both of these settings, it is useful to revisit two approaches to communication outlined in Chapter 2 of our companion book *Teaching and Learning Communication Skills in Medicine*. Barbour (2000) metaphorically labelled these approaches:

1. the shot-put approach
2. the frisbee approach.

The shot-put approach defines communication simply as *the well-conceived, well-delivered message*. From the classical Greek times of its origins right through to the early twentieth century, formal communication training in the professions has focused almost entirely on the shot-put approach. Effective communication meant content, delivery and persuasion. Formulate your message well, heave it out there and your communication job is done. An early communication model developed by a telephone company reflects the 'shot-put' approach – the sender puts together a clear, well-argued message and transmits it, the receiver picks it up and that is perceived to be the end of the communication.

The traditional lecture in its most basic form exemplifies the shot-put approach. The skills that make for effective lecturing are part of what makes for effective communication in the doctor–patient relationship – we need to know how to deliver a message effectively and how to package and articulate the message we want to get across to the patient so that it can be both remembered and understood. However, the shot-put approach is only part of what is needed.

In the 1940s, our understanding of effective communication began to shift toward a more interactive, give-and-take approach. This new perspective – appropriately dubbed the frisbee approach – finally caught on in the 1960s. In this approach *mutually understood common ground* is perceived to be a necessary foundation for both trust and accuracy, so achieving this common ground is one of the central concepts of the approach. If mutually understood common ground is important to effective communication, then our time-honoured, one-dimensional focus on the well-conceived, well-delivered message falls short. In the interpersonal or frisbee perspective the message is still important, of course, but the emphasis shifts to interaction, feedback and collaboration.

This brings us back to one of the principles of communication that we have outlined earlier: *effective communication ensures an interaction rather than a direct transmission process*. If communication is viewed as direct transmission, the senders of messages assume that their responsibilities as communicators are fulfilled once they have formulated and sent a message. However, if communication is viewed as an interactive process, the interaction is only complete if the sender receives feedback about how the message is interpreted, whether it is understood and what impact it has had on the receiver. Just imparting information is not enough – responding to feedback about the impact of the message becomes crucial and the emphasis moves to the interdependence of sender and receiver in establishing mutually understood common ground (Dance and Larson 1972).

Happily, this frisbee approach has gradually infiltrated lecturing styles. The first step in the modernisation of the lecture was the provision of 10 minutes at the end for questions from the audience. This enables some of the interaction of the frisbee approach but only for a defined part of the proceedings. An increasingly common pattern now is for the lecturer to stop and ask for questions from the audience at several points as the lecture proceeds. And some lecturers now even start by first exploring the audience's needs and expectations – the learner-centred lecture.

In the doctor–patient interview, we need to take an even more interactive approach. As we shall see, we need to take into account each patient's individual and unique requirements, their different capacity to take in information and their different needs and concerns. What does this patient know already, how much information would the patient like, what is the patient most concerned about and how much would the patient like to be involved in decision making? And we have to do all of this without sacrificing the important organisational and linguistic skills that have been learned from the shot-put approach.

PROVIDING THE CORRECT AMOUNT AND TYPE OF INFORMATION

One of the key issues of explanation and planning is how to gauge just what information to share with the patient. How do we negotiate the delicate path between not giving enough information and overloading the patient with too much? How do we ascertain the individual information needs of each patient and tailor our information giving accordingly? How do we discover what information each patient requires to make sense of the situation rather than give a predetermined lecture based on our assumptions of what the patient needs?

Do patients and doctors disagree over the amount of information that should be imparted?

We have already seen that there are problems with the amount of information doctors give to patients. But do patients wish to be better informed?

Doctors frequently misperceive the amount of information that their patients want, with a consistent tendency to underestimate the amount of information required. Waitzkin (1984) showed that in 65% of encounters, internists underestimated their particular patient's desire for information; in only 6% did they overestimate it.

Faden *et al.* (1981) looked at the differences between attitudes of neurologists and their epileptic patients to the disclosure of information. They found that patients preferred to receive detailed disclosure of almost all risks associated with medication, even those that were quite rare. Physicians, however, said that they were likely to disclose only those risks with a high probability of occurrence. Physicians felt that detailed disclosure of information about drugs would decrease adherence, whereas patients felt that disclosure would improve their adherence.

Many studies have shown that, with the best of intentions, physicians choose to withhold information in an attempt to protect patients from worry. Pinder (1990) found that on making a diagnosis of Parkinson's disease, family doctors were most concerned with issues of 'protection': deciding how, when and whom to tell and deciding just how much to share about the diagnosis and prognosis. Patients, on the other hand, were attempting to comprehend and adjust to their illness, with many questions in their minds about the course of the disease and possible treatments, and many fears about the illness and their future prospects. Doctors tended to be positive, over-optimistic and protective. For instance, they avoided detail about drugs, were low-key about side effects and did not explore the problems of long-term use of anti-parkinsonian medication. Patients on average wanted to be given information and not to be protected. Most patients wanted to understand their drugs and be forewarned about side effects.

If the research shows that in general patients want more information (Cassileth *et al.* 1980; Beisecker and Beisecker 1990), why do doctors persist in giving them less? Why is there such a wide gulf between what doctors think patients want and what patients tell us they need? And how can doctors determine just how much information each individual patient would like in each situation? Much of the disparity between the amount of information that doctors give and the amount that patients would prefer to receive has its roots in the traditional view of the doctor–patient relationship. In Chapter 3 we contrasted the traditional method of history taking with the disease–illness model of the University of Western Ontario. We now take a similar approach to explanation and planning by comparing the traditional view of information giving with more modern concepts that mirror changes in society as a whole.

The traditional view of the doctor–patient relationship

An unbridgeable competence gap

The traditional view of the doctor–patient relationship held in the first part of the twentieth century was of an unbridgeable competence gap that made it impossible to achieve any semblance of true patient understanding. Parsons (1951) felt that doctors' vast training and knowledge created such a difference between them and their patients that it was not possible to explain complex issues appropriately. Patients simply acquiesced with their doctors' advice because of their faith in their doctor as a person and in the medical profession as a whole. According to this theory, patients relied on the wisdom of their doctor and were safeguarded by the profession's strong code of ethics, which compelled the physician to act in the patient's best interests.

In this analysis, the medical consultation is somehow different from other situations where experts convey and share information with less expert clients – e.g. the specialist advising the general practitioner, the lawyer advising the house purchaser, the scientist collaborating with the businessman, or the teacher instructing students. In all of these situations, people with different levels of understanding and knowledge have to try to reach a compromise. Sufficient information has to be imparted to allow successful communication and to enable clients to make informed choices or plans without being confused by excessive detail.

The emotional nature of illness

So what is so different in the medical consultation to justify Parson's viewpoint? One argument used is that the highly emotional nature of illness prevents rational communication and understanding. It is suggested that the anxiety and fear induced by being placed in the patient role make patients passive, willing to adopt a dependent 'sick' role, and willing to accept a well-intentioned, paternalistic medical adviser. By adopting the privileges of illness and convalescence, the patient is excused from everyday responsibilities. Following on from this argument is the fear that providing information to patients about the seriousness of their illness might well be harmful to them, and that it is often best for the doctor to protect the patient from the possible emotional consequences of such disclosure.

Professional authority

An opposing view (Freidson 1970) is that the difference between the medical interview and other information-giving circumstances is not due to any emotional difficulty within the consultation, but is more an inevitable result of doctors' desire to retain their high status within society. This analysis suggests a much less altruistic reason for withholding information. If the difference in social standing between doctor and patient is something that the profession desperately wishes to preserve, in part this can be achieved by limiting the provision of information to the lay population. Mystification of the doctor's knowledge and devaluation of the patient's knowledge might be said to be more powerful driving forces than the higher motive of creating informed and autonomous patients. Maintaining clear water between professional and client necessitates a degree of ownership of information by the doctor. The use of Latin terms can be seen as one part of this complicated process of obfuscation – the patient presents a sore throat, the doctor advises that it is acute pharyngitis. Of course, this impressive title is simply a translation of the patient's words into an unshared medical language (Bourhis *et al.* 1989).

The perceived 'competence gap', the emotional difficulties of the doctor–patient relationship and the need to preserve professional authority may then have predisposed physicians to withhold information and patients to remain passive bystanders in the explanation and planning phase of the interview.

Why has modern research been misinterpreted as confirming the traditional stereotype of information giving?

Tuckett *et al.* (1985) have argued that the medical profession has incorrectly interpreted some of the results of research about information giving so as to confirm its own traditional prejudices.

Early studies of recall of information

In earlier studies, patients' recall of information was shown to be poor. Ley (1988) quotes figures of around 60% in hospital settings from various authors, with better recall in repeat rather than new interviews. In general practice, Ley found 50% and 56% recall, respectively. Bertakis (1977) reported 62% recall in first attenders, and Hulka (1979), mainly with repeat consultations, showed higher levels of 67% for diabetics and pregnant mothers and 88% for mothers whose infants were ill.

Ley also demonstrated a relationship between the amount of information presented and the amount of information recalled. His research showed that in laboratory experiments, the more items of information that were given, the greater the proportion that was forgotten. He was able to confirm this finding in the clinical situation of hospital outpatients, although not in general practice.

This research has been widely quoted as evidence that:

- *'patients recall very little of what you tell them'*
- *'the more you tell them, the less they remember'*

and the almost inevitable conclusion

- *'it's therefore not worth telling them very much in the first place.'*

But are these conclusions correct? Even if only 50% of information is remembered, does this mean that it is not worth giving information at all, or does it suggest that we should look at ways of improving that figure?

More recent studies

More recent research suggests that patients actually recall much more than had previously been reported. Tuckett *et al.* (1985), using a different methodology that looked more closely at what was being recalled and specifically analysed key points rather than every piece of information given by the doctor, showed that only 10% of patients in a study in primary care failed to remember all of the key points that they had been told. Interestingly, as predicted, recall may not be as good in those settings where the information provided is more concerning and the patient is potentially more anxious. Dunn *et al.* (1993) found that cancer patients in their first interview with an oncologist remembered only 45% of 'key points' as determined by the oncologist. Jansen *et al.* (2008) looked at the recall of information presented to newly referred patients with cancer and showed that younger and older patients correctly recalled 49.5% and 48.4% of information, respectively. Although age decreased recall of information, this effect was only present when the total amount of information presented was taken into account. Older patients have more trouble remembering information if more information is presented. Again, patients with a poorer prognosis consistently remembered less information than patients with a better prognosis.

Ley, in fact, never meant to imply that we should not strive to give patients information. Commenting on his work on the relationship between the amount of information presented and the amount of information recalled, he makes the following point: 'Note that it is the proportion forgotten that increases, and this is quite compatible with patients given more information about their disease knowing more about their condition than those given less. The finding is not an argument for providing patients with less information.' Although the proportion of the total remembered goes down in Ley's studies, the absolute amount remembered still goes up.

Confirmation of prejudices

Tuckett has written eloquently of how these misconceptions concerning Ley's findings have confirmed the medical profession's traditional views and have been accepted as standard teaching. Those aspects of Ley's work that fit well with the traditional model have reached prominence, and those that do not have been discarded. Students are told that their patients will not remember most of what they are told and that they should keep it simple. They are taught not to be overambitious in information giving and that 'only when the number of statements is limited to two is recall good' (Horder *et al.* 1972). Doctors have seized on Ley's findings to justify their view that there is little scope for more than basic information giving.

Yet, as already mentioned, these were not Ley's own conclusions. His view was that doctors should use strategies to improve the amount of information given to patients, thus increasing the total of that information that their patients can then recall and understand. He wished doctors to give more, clearer and better-ordered information, and for patients to become better informed.

What recent trends in society have influenced medical information giving?

Changes in society

Recent decades have brought many changes in society and the breaking down of a multitude of class and social barriers. Moves towards freedom of speech, sexual and racial equality and freedom of information have changed society irrevocably. As educational standards and personal wealth have increased, expectations have followed suit and demands on many services, including health, have escalated. Changes away from just curative medicine towards prevention of illness and maintenance of health have led to an increased awareness of health issues in the population. The mushrooming of articles and programmes in the written and broadcast media and the explosion of information on the Internet has led to much greater availability of information about health and disease, and the emergence of consumer and patient advocacy groups has changed patient awareness and the influence of the patient on the consultation.

Hay *et al.* (2008) have shown that 87.5% of patients attending their first appointment in rheumatology outpatients looked up their symptoms or suspected condition prior to their first appointment, with 62.5% of all patients seeking that information on the Internet. Only 20% of online information seekers discussed that information with their physicians during the consultation. Bylund *et al.* (2007) looked at patients' experiences talking to their providers about Internet health information. Providers' validation of patients' efforts was associated with higher patient ratings of satisfaction and validation and reduced concern, while providers' disagreement with the information was associated with lower ratings. The provider taking the information seriously was associated with higher patient satisfaction. Bowes *et al.* (2012) showed patients used the Internet to become better informed about their health and hence make best use of the limited time available with their general practitioner and to enable the general practitioner to take their problem more seriously. Patients expected their general practitioner to acknowledge the information; discuss, explain or contextualise it; and offer a professional opinion. Patients tended to prioritise general practitioner opinion over Internet information. However, if the general practitioner appeared disinterested, dismissive or patronising, patients reported damage to the doctor–patient relationship, occasionally to the extent of seeking a second opinion or changing their doctor.

Legislation focusing on patients' rights in healthcare have followed these changes and cemented their influence. Society has not stood still, nor has the doctor–patient relationship – the public routinely questions both the knowledge and the motivation of doctors and no longer demonstrates a blind faith in the profession. Patients do not now accept the concept of an unbridgeable competence gap.

Bracci *et al.* (2008) have shown that in Italy, cultural attitudes towards communication in oncology are changing on the sides of both the physician and the patient. There are still significant geographical differences within the country, but there is a general trend suggesting improved awareness about diagnosis and treatment.

Claramita *et al.* (2011) explored the perceived ideal communication style for doctor–patient consultations and the reality of actual practice in a Southeast Asian context in Indonesia. Patients, doctors and medical students appear to be in favour of a partnership style of communication, which was in sharp contrast to observed communication styles, where a paternalistic style prevailed, irrespective of patients' educational background. Patients were unprepared and hesitant to participate in consultations, despite their preference to do so, and doctors therefore concluded that this style was not required. Also, doctors were not equipped to use a partnership style. Moore (2009) reported similar findings in Nepal.

Mitchison *et al.* (2012) studied the prognostic communication preferences of migrant patients and their relatives in Australia. Differences in the preferred level of information disclosure emerged between migrants and Anglo-Australians. Yet, contrary to previous research, migrant patients and not Anglo-Australian patients reported a desire to be well informed of their disease, often including disclosure of prognosis. On the other hand, the preferences of migrant families differed from migrant patients and tended to reflect the more traditional conceptualisations of non-Western attitudes to communication during cancer care, including non-disclosure of prognosis and the mediatory role of the family between the oncologist and the patient.

Changes in medicine

While some patients may adopt a dependent role with very serious illness and be only too grateful for the doctor to take charge, most consultations in modern Western medical practice are not about life-threatening illness. Furthermore, chronic care and prevention are playing ever-expanding roles. As a result, anxiety levels and consequent blocks to communication are reduced – patients feel that they can cope with being fully informed and involved in their care.

Patient autonomy

Patient autonomy has become a central tenet of medical ethics and the paternalistic relationship between doctor and patient is increasingly viewed as anachronistic. As we shall see later, there is a danger of too large a shift towards a consumerist relationship. A collaborative and mutual approach has been suggested as a more appropriate path forward.

Doctors have seen these changes gradually reflected in their working practices. Patients far more frequently come for information about preventive measures (e.g. calcium supplements for osteoporosis) with the expectation that they themselves will make an informed decision based on the arguments put before them. In the past the doctor would simply have made a recommendation and expected the patient to follow it. Ward rounds less frequently consist of discussions at the end of the bed about patients who are considered to have no thoughts, feelings or involvement in the process of their own medical care. Perhaps the biggest change has been in the area of withholding information about serious illness or bad news. Not long ago it was the norm to withhold news of conditions such as cancer from patients on the basis that the information might harm them. Physicians shielded their patients from information that they might not be able to cope with. It was the physician's responsibility to decide whether to favour discretion and complicity with relatives over the duty to tell the truth. Now the pendulum in the West has swung to the patients' right to information, for physicians to provide opportunities to inform patients sensitively about their disease and to withhold that information only if patients give out signals that they would prefer not to know (Buckman 1994). Important cultural differences still exist in various countries concerning the balance between individual autonomy and the importance of the family in decision making. In Japan, for instance, physicians were recently still giving patients optimistic accounts of prognosis and families pessimistic accounts (Akabayashi *et al.* 1999; Elwyn *et al.* 2002).

What is the research evidence to suggest that giving more information is helpful?

Patients wish to receive more information than they are routinely given. But can we demonstrate that this provision of information actually affects the outcome of their healthcare?

There is much evidence to confirm the value of information giving. In a meta-analysis of the influence of the various 'provider behaviours' that might make a difference in medical encounters, Hall *et al.* (1988) searched the literature from 1966 to 1985 and discovered 41 independent studies where communication variables by the health professional were related to improvements in satisfaction, recall or compliance. Having grouped the possible variables into six overall categories, they concluded that, of all of the categories, the amount of information imparted by physicians was the most dramatic predictor of patient satisfaction, compliance, recall and understanding. This positive relationship between patient satisfaction and the amount of information given has been a highly consistent finding in the communication literature (e.g. Bertakis 1977; Stiles *et al.* 1979; Deyo and Diehl 1986).

Many studies link the provision of information to substantial benefits in health outcomes such as symptom reduction and physiological status (e.g. Kaplan *et al.* 1989; Stewart 1995). Egbert *et al.* (1964) showed that preoperative education from an anaesthetist about postoperative pain control led not only to less use of analgesia but to shorter hospital stays. Mumford *et al.* (1982) reviewed many similar findings of information giving or psychological intervention speeding recovery and improving outcome in patients post surgery or post myocardial infarction.

Do all patients want more information?

But do all patients want more information and, if not, how can we individualise our information giving to match our patients' needs and preferences?

In Pinder's (1990) study of information giving to patients with Parkinson's disease, doctors adopted a set style with all patients despite individual patients varying greatly in the amount of information that they wished to be given. Most patients were keen to hear more information about their illness and medication, but not all. Jenkins *et al.* (2001), in a large study of 2331 patients with cancer, showed that 87% of patients wanted as much information as possible, while 13% preferred to leave disclosure of details to the doctor. Many other studies have shown that patients can be divided into seekers (around 80%) and avoiders (around 20%)

with regard to information, with seekers coping better with more information and avoiders coping better with less (Miller and Mangan 1983; Deber 1994). Steptoe *et al.* (1991) showed that information avoiders report a better understanding and satisfaction with doctor–patient communication than seekers but paradoxically they have a worse understanding. Seekers, on the other hand, are less satisfied with communication and would like even more information, despite having already gained a better understanding. Tuckett *et al.* (1985) found that 19% of patients did not ask questions of their doctors because they were not interested in knowing about medical matters. Broyles *et al.* (1992) showed that only half of mothers of newborn babies at risk of respiratory failure, when presented with brief information about mechanical ventilation and then asked if they wished to have further detailed information, requested more.

While most patients do want their doctors to provide more information, a minority would like less. But it is not at all easy to predict which patient is in which group. For instance, as Waitzkin (1985) has said, 'research has clearly shown that the commonly expressed assumption that working-class patients do not want a full explanation of their illness seems to derive from the hesitancy of patients to ask questions rather than from any actual disinterest in information'. Barsevich and Johnson (1990) showed that there was only a moderate relationship between the information wishes of women undergoing colposcopy and their information-seeking behaviour. Repeated studies have also shown that the assumption that elderly patients do not wish to receive information about their illness is unfounded. Although slightly more elderly than younger patients prefer to receive less information, by far the majority of older patients want to be kept very well informed about their illness (Davis *et al.* 1999; Stewart *et al.* 2000b).

Hagerty *et al.* (2004) showed that most metastatic cancer patients want detailed prognostic information but prefer to negotiate the extent, format and timing of the information they receive from their oncologists. More than 95% of patients wanted information about side effects, symptoms and treatment options, and 85% wanted to know longest survival time with treatment, 80% wanted to know five-year survival rates and 81% wanted to know average survival time.

In a study of 60 mixed-ethnicity older adults who were presented with hypothetical scenarios and asked about their preference for discussing prognosis, 65% wanted to discuss prognosis if their doctor estimated they would have less than five years left to live and 75% if less than one year (Ahalt *et al.* 2012). A significant proportion said they would not want to discuss prognosis at any time. Though differences emerged between ethnic groups, nearly all participants said doctors should not make assumptions based on ethnicity.

What skills can learners use to help gauge the correct amount and type of information to give to each individual patient?

We have seen that doctors in the past have underestimated patients' information needs in general and also that a substantial minority of patients would prefer not to be given as much information. Therefore, a key challenge in information giving is to find out how much information a patient wants in a given situation, rather than making assumptions about it, and then to tailor the amount of information to the needs of the individual patient. In the past, we have tended to withhold information from all in order to protect the few who would rather not know. The challenge now is how to inform the majority while being sensitive to the needs of the minority. And we also have to consider tailoring not just *how much* but also *what* information to tell patients. How do we take into account patients' pre-existing knowledge and discover the questions that they would like us to answer?

Returning to the comparison with lecturing, how could you personalise a lecture to the needs of the audience rather than give a predetermined speech based on your assumptions about the audience's requirements? First, you could start on the path that you had planned, but break the lecture up into discrete sections and ask the audience for questions about what you have said within each section. This would allow you to answer questions as you go and, equally as important, to gauge the learners' level of understanding and their further requirements. Second, you could deliberately ask the audience early on what they already know about the topic, what problems they have in this area and what specific questions they would like to have answered. And you could repeat the process as the lecture proceeds, constantly asking what further information would be helpful. In other words, you could increase the interactivity and thereby move from the shot-put to the frisbee approach. This is exactly what is helpful in the context of the medical interview.

Chunking and checking

Chunking and checking is a vital skill throughout the explanation and planning phase of the interview, not only for gauging the correct amount of information to give but also as an aid to *accurate recall* and to *achieving a shared understanding*.

In chunking and checking, the doctor gives information in small pieces, pausing and checking for understanding before proceeding and being guided by the patient's reactions to see what information is required next. This technique is a vital if indirect component of assessing the patient's overall information needs. If you give information in small chunks and give patients ample opportunity to contribute, they will respond with clear signals about both the amount and type of information they still require.

Doctor:	*'So really, given the symptoms you have described and the very typical way that you wheeze more after exercise and at night, I feel reasonably confident that what you are describing is asthma and that we should consider giving you some treatment for it.'* (Pause) *'Does that make sense so far?'*
Patient:	*'Yes – I think so, but I'm not sure I really understand what asthma is. Is it something that runs in families?'*

Assessing the patient's starting point

One key interactive approach to giving information to patients involves *assessing the patient's prior knowledge*. How can you determine at what level to pitch information unless you take active steps to find out the patient's starting point? How can you assess the degree to which your view of the problem differs from that of the patient and the approach that you will need to take to achieve mutual understanding unless you discover early on the patient's understanding of his or her problem?

Explaining a new diagnosis of diabetes to either a university lecturer or a manual labourer is apparently not the same task, with potentially very different levels of understanding and different capabilities of processing information. However, making this assumption without directly asking for the patient's prior knowledge is dangerous. The lecturer in astronomy may have a poor understanding of diabetes and know it only as a possibly disastrous cause of blindness and a threat to his vocation. The labourer may have grown up with parents with diabetes and have a high level of understanding of the condition. It would therefore be helpful before proceeding too far into a detailed explanation to ask:

Doctor:	*'I don't know how much you know about diabetes already?'*
Patient:	*'Well, I know a little about it – my best friend at college had it.'*
Doctor:	*'It would be helpful for me to understand a little of what you already know so that I can try to fill in any gaps for you.'*

Similarly, it is important to *ascertain each individual patient's overall desire for information*. As we have already seen, while most patients wish their doctors to provide more information, a significant minority would prefer less. How can we discover whether a particular patient is a seeker or an avoider of information? Chunking and checking and asking for the patient's questions are indirect approaches to assessing the patient's overall information needs. A more direct approach is to ask the patient early on in the process:

Doctor:	*'There's a lot more information that I'd be happy to share with you about Parkinson's disease and the drugs we use to treat it. Some patients like to know a lot about these things and some prefer to keep it to a minimum. How much information would you yourself like?'*
Patient:	*'Well, I'm not sure I can take a lot in today doctor. Perhaps we could just organise some treatment and I could come back with my wife in a few weeks' time.'*

Remember that a patient's preference and need for information may change over time and from one situation to another. For instance, a terminally ill patient may move from a position of avoidance and denial towards acceptance and more open discussion as he comes to terms with his illness. We need to be aware of this possibility and not assume that the answer to the doctor's question regarding preference and need for information will remain constant for any one individual.

Asking patients what other information would be helpful

As we have seen, doctors often misconstrue the types of information that the patient requires. They often do not address the 'what has happened, why has it happened, why to me, why now, what would happen if nothing was done about it?' questions that patients would like to have answered in preference to information about treatment (Helman 1978). It is difficult to guess each patient's individual needs, and asking directly is an obvious way to prevent the omission of important information.

> Doctor: *'Are there any other questions you'd like me to answer or any points I haven't covered?'*
> Patient: *'Do you think I could pass this on? I mean, is it infectious?'*

Giving explanation at appropriate times

A common difficulty in consultations arises from giving advice, information or reassurance prematurely. For example, during the information-gathering phase, a mother of an asthmatic child may ask the following:

> Patient's mother: *'Sophie's quite unwell with this cold – could she have some antibiotics?'*
> Doctor: *'I'm sure the answer isn't antibiotics – her cold will have triggered her asthma – it's not that she has infection on her chest – what we really need to do is treat the asthma.'*
>
> You deliver your standard lecture. You then take more history, and find that Sophie has been hot and sick in the night. Examination reveals unilateral signs. You start backtracking and feel you have lost the mother's confidence.
>
> Doctor: *'Ah, despite what I said, there is a problem here that needs antibiotics.'*

Instead, you could simply acknowledge the mother's question and deal with it later after you have all the facts at your disposal:

> Doctor: *'That's a very good question. Would you mind if I put that on hold just for a second and come back to it after I've examined Sophie? Then I'll be able to give you a much better answer.'*
>
> Then, after you have explained your findings:
>
> Doctor: *'Coming back to your question, there clearly is a problem with her chest today that needs antibiotics. Are you happy gauging when it is the asthma itself that's worse and when she might have a chest infection?'*
> Patient's mother: *'Yes, I think so, but it's not always easy.'*
> Doctor: *'Well, on most occasions, it's just that a cold triggers asthma without the infection going on to the chest ...'*

AIDING ACCURATE RECALL AND UNDERSTANDING

Another important area in explanation and planning is how to give information that can be more easily remembered and understood. In the previous section on providing the correct amount and type of information, we explored the need to move towards a highly interactive, 'frisbee' approach to information giving in order to tailor our message to the needs of the patient. However, that does not mean that we abandon the lessons learned from the shot-put approach. The way in which we give information can lead to excellent recall and understanding or to an extremely unsatisfactory learning experience.

So how do you achieve the *well-conceived, well-delivered message*? How do you give information so that people can understand and remember what you say? The old adage from lecturing, 'Say what you are going to say, say it and then say what you have said', identifies some of the organisational and structuring tools that can make information giving effective. To these we need to add the appropriate use of language and visual aids as well as the skills involved in checking for understanding. These are the very skills we shall now explore in the setting of medical interviews.

Ley's research into patient recall

In the 1970s and 1980s, Ley (1988) undertook comprehensive research to establish which communication skills could improve patients' recall of information. His work was initially based on experiments in the psychology laboratory. He later transposed his research into clinical settings – doctors in both hospital and general practice were taught various techniques to see if earlier laboratory findings could be reproduced in the consulting room. The following is our interpretation of Ley's findings.

Categorisation: an example of signposting

In this technique, the clinician forewarns the patient about which categories of information are to be provided and then presents the information category by category:

> 'There are three important things I want to explain. First I want to tell you what I think is wrong; second, what tests we should do; and third, what the treatment might be. First, I think you have ...'

Ley demonstrated that the level of recall was higher using this method in both laboratory and clinical experiments, with typical increases in recall rates from 50% to 64%.

There are two processes at work here. The first is the organisation of information giving. Categorisation allows the information to be divided into discrete sections and enables a logical sequence to be followed. The second is making that categorisation explicit to the patient. This is a further example of signposting, a technique that we introduced in Chapter 3. Signposting is the process of explaining to the patient where the interview might go next and why. Providing an overt structure to the consultation reduces uncertainty and anxiety that can otherwise block effective communication and reduce recall and understanding. This is similar to effective lecturers having a plan that they make explicit to their audience at the beginning of the lecture.

Labelling important information: another example of signposting

In his writings, Ley places much emphasis on the primacy effect – that people remember best what they are told first. He demonstrated in laboratory experiments that medical facts given to volunteers early in a sequence of information were recalled more than those given later. He then proceeded to a clinical setting. In a previous study he had shown that patients recalled information about diagnosis better than information about instructions and advice, since patients considered information about diagnosis to be more important than information about treatment. People recall better what they think is most important. To see whether recall of instructions and advice could be improved, he used the outpatient setting to give information in varying orders. Patients who were given information about treatment first remembered 86% of this information, compared with 50% in patients who were given the information later. Interestingly, there was no improvement in the amount of information retained overall – as recall of instructions and advice increased, so recall of diagnosis declined.

Although the primacy effect is clearly of importance in information giving, we do have some reservations about Ley's conclusion that we should present 'important' information first. Ley suggests that to increase compliance we should give information about treatment and advice before diagnosis and rationale. This view is based on the premise that patients remember treatment issues less well, and that compliance with treatment plans will suffer if recall is not maximised. However, total recall remains unchanged and recall of diagnosis and rationale diminishes. Although remembering treatment plans is a necessary condition for compliance, will this approach actually achieve increased adherence to plans in practice or are there other factors involved? Ley has already said that patients view diagnostic statements as more important than instruction and advice, so does it not seem likely that reducing patients' understanding about their diagnosis will have deleterious effects on their compliance? What if the patient remembers exactly what the doctor said about treatment but has no intention of complying because he has little understanding of his condition or commitment to the doctor's views?

> *'He told me to take this steroid inhaler twice a day all the time, but I'm fine now so I don't need to take anything.'*

Clearly, recall is not everything. And who is to say what is the most 'important' information? What the patient and doctor consider to be important might be completely different. Ley's approach here is doctor-centred in that it is the doctor who decides what is the most important information for the patient to understand. This runs contrary to the work of Tuckett *et al.* (1985), presented in the next section, where the importance of discovering and addressing each patient's very individual information needs is emphasised.

One further message of value here is Ley's finding that it might help if the physician labels certain pieces of information as important to raise the patient's awareness of the physician's point of view. This is another example of signposting:

> *'It is very important that you remember this ...'*

Chunking and checking

We would argue that the key issue here is not so much about ordering information in terms of importance but about avoiding giving a large amount of information all at once. A long monologue will produce a strong primacy effect – the patient is still thinking about the first point as the next three are being presented, and is distracted from listening to later pieces of information. If the aim is to increase recall, understanding and commitment to plans, we suggest reducing the likelihood of a primacy effect occurring in the first place.

This can be achieved by chunking and checking – that is, giving information in small pieces, pausing and checking for understanding before proceeding, and being guided by the patient's reactions to see what information is required next. Only then is it likely that patients will both recall and understand. As they assimilate each section of information, they will become ready for the next one. This technique is also a vital component of assessment of the patient's overall information needs. If the doctor gives information in small chunks and gives the patient ample opportunity to contribute, the doctor will receive clear signals about the amount and type of information the patient still requires.

Repetition

There are two elements to repetition that can make a considerable difference to patient recall:

1. repetition of important points by the doctor
2. restatement of information by the patient.

Repetition by the doctor of important points has been shown to be of value in assisting recall in laboratory conditions (Ley) and in the consulting room (Kupst *et al.* 1975). Kupst showed the rate of immediate recall to be 76% for single presentation and 90% after physician repetition.

> Doctor: *'So just to recap, we have decided to treat this as a fungal infection with a cream that you put on twice a day for two weeks, and if it is not better by then, you are going to come back to see me.'*

Patient restatement is also a highly effective technique. Here the doctor checks the patient's understanding of information given by asking the patient to restate, in the patient's own words, what they have understood. The doctor then clarifies as necessary. In Kupst's work, patient restatement achieved an immediate recall rate of 91%, which matched physician repetition. However, for recall at one month, patient restatement with feedback was shown to be the most effective method. Patient restatement has the added benefit of giving you and the patient early insight into what the patient understands.

Bertakis (1977) undertook a study to evaluate the usefulness of patient restatement and physician clarification. When family practice residents were trained in this technique, patients were more satisfied and showed an increase in retention of information from 61% to 83 %.

The difficulty of requesting patient restatement is all in the phrasing and tone of voice. It is so easy to sound patronising by implying that the patient has limited capacity to understand what the clever doctor has said! Practising phrases that work for you as an individual is all-important:

Doctor: *'I know I've given you a lot of information today and I'm concerned that I might not have made it very clear – it would help me if you repeated back to me what we have agreed on so far, so I can make sure we are on the same track.'*

Kemp *et al.* (2008) looked at which approaches to assessing patients' understanding were preferred and perceived to be most effective by a panel of patients observing pre-prepared videotapes of physician behaviours. Three options were presented:

1. Yes–no: *I've given you a lot of information. Do you understand?*
2. Tell back–collaborative: *I imagine you're really worried about this clot. I've given you a lot of information. It would be helpful to me to hear your understanding about your clot and its treatment.*
3. Tell back–directive: *It's really important that you do this exactly the way I explained. What do you understand?*

The 'Tell back–collaborative' inquiry, involving both patient restatement and a patient-centred approach, was significantly preferred over the other two approaches.

In an observational study of primary care doctors, Bravo *et al.* (2010) demonstrated again that patients leaving the consultation remembered more of the recommendations if they had been asked by the physician to restate these during the consultation.

Fink *et al.* (2010) explored the value of restatement in discussions regarding informed consent for surgery. In a randomised controlled study, restatement implemented within an electronic informed consent system significantly improved patient understanding.

Language

We have seen that the use of jargon is a major problem in communication and that patients rarely ask for clarification for fear of appearing ignorant. It is not just technical language that is the problem (Hadlow and Pitts 1991), as even simple everyday words in a medical context can be ambiguous. Mazzullo *et al.* (1974) showed that 52% of people thought that a tablet prescribed *'for* fluid retention' would *cause* fluid retention. Ley therefore recommends simplification of information to aid recall and understanding. This can be achieved by:

- reducing the use of jargon
- explaining jargon when used
- using shorter words
- using shorter sentences.

Recent work demonstrates again the need for clarity and simplicity in information giving, irrespective of health literacy, and that the most valued method of transmission of information from health professionals continues to be face-to-face consultations (Shaw *et al.* 2009).

Making explanations or advice specific enough for the patient to understand or act upon

Ley quotes Bradshaw *et al.* (1975) to demonstrate that specific statements are more easily recalled than general statements. Obese women given dietary advice remembered 16% of general and 51% of specific statements.

Making advice more specific clearly makes sense in certain situations, such as explaining to patients how to take pills. However, we have reservations about promulgating this method in all circumstances of information giving; there is a danger that giving specific advice can become confused with being inappropriately dogmatic.

As we shall see later, there is much evidence to favour a collaborative model of explanation and planning where patients are involved in choices and doctors offer options and suggestions rather than directives. Adherence to plans has been shown to be improved when doctors actively seek patients' reactions to suggestions and engage in appropriate negotiations. Ley suggests that telling a patient to lose 30 pounds will lead to better recall than just telling the patient to lose weight. But will this produce better compliance? What if all the patient remembers is:

> *'30 pounds!! I've never been that weight in my life – no way!'*

There is a third approach. Make suggestions, elicit reactions and negotiate. Then, at the end of that process, clarify *specifically* what the agreed upon plan involves. How to 'be specific' therefore depends upon the complexity of the task. In simple instructions, being specific is relatively easy. But in complex areas such as health promotion or preventive medicine, it is pointless engineering excellent recall without motivation. Being specific needs to be balanced by the skills of negotiation and motivational interviewing.

Using visual methods of conveying information

Many studies have shown that the use of diagrams, models, written information and instructions can improve patient knowledge and adherence. There is a considerable literature on the effective design of printed material to improve patient use, understanding and recall, which is well summarised in Ley (1988). Recent work, such as De Morgan *et al.* (2011) with patients with ductal carcinoma in situ, has concentrated on the provision of written consultation aids that enable a highly personalised approach to be taken by clinicians in discussing diagnosis, prognosis, treatment and support.

Tattersall *et al.* (1997), McConnell *et al.* (1999), Sowden *et al.* (2001), Scott *et al.* (2001) and Minhas (2007) provide reviews of more modern approaches to providing patients with tailored information about their illness. These include the provision of audio- or videotapes of the actual interview and writing to patients after their consultation, both of which have been shown to increase patient satisfaction, recall and understanding, and patient activity. In contrast, general audiotapes about a condition do not increase and may actually decrease patient recall and satisfaction with a specific interview. Tattersall *et al.* (1994) showed that patients ranked audiotapes more highly than the provision of letters or talks with the oncology nurse specialist. Hack *et al.* (2007) showed that audiotapes are rated highly by men with prostate cancer, and these audiotapes help to enhance their perception of having been provided with critical disease and treatment-related information.

Van der Meulen *et al.* (2008) undertook a systematic review of interventions to improve recall of medical information in cancer patients. They concluded that an audiotape of the patient's own consultation has added value compared with oral information only, but that providing patients with a general audiotape does not improve recall of information and might even inhibit patients' recall.

A few cautionary notes are in order with respect to the use of visual materials or tapes:

- Written or taped material does not work well as a stand-alone or substitute for interaction with the physician. To optimise its use, health professionals need to:
  – introduce, follow up and personalise the material for the individual patient
  – set up opportunities for patients to ask questions after they have looked at the material.
- The material may be inappropriate when the patient is not fluent in the language in which the materials are presented (Brown *et al.* 2007).
- Written material (including written instructions and diagrams) is inappropriate when the patient is functionally illiterate. Even in countries where education is widespread, the percentages of functionally illiterate people are much higher than many healthcare professionals realise.

A summary of the skills that can help patients to remember and understand doctors' explanations is given in Box 6.2 (*see* pages 157–9).

ACHIEVING A SHARED UNDERSTANDING – INCORPORATING THE PATIENT'S PERSPECTIVE

In the earlier analysis, we have looked in detail at the skills that can be employed to improve patients' recall of information. This approach is concerned primarily with the recall of information that doctors consider to be important. However, as we have already seen from the work of Kindelan and Kent (1987) and, indeed, from Ley's own analysis, what the patient and doctor think is important is not always the same. So just looking at what doctors think their patients should be told and discovering the best ways to give that information is only half the story. What about the information needs from the patient's perspective (Grol *et al.* 1991)?

Asking this question does not negate the findings of Ley and others, who present important skills that doctors can use to make information giving clearer and that can lead to better patient recall. However, a further analysis is needed of how to match information giving to patients' perceived needs. How do you provide explanations that relate to the patient's perspective of the problem? How do you ascertain the patient's thoughts about the information that you have given? How do you achieve a shared understanding with your patient?

Tuckett and colleagues' research into patient understanding

Described in their book *Meetings Between Experts: An Approach to Sharing Ideas in the Medical Consultation* (Tuckett *et al.* 1985), Tuckett *et al.*'s research is central to our understanding of a shared approach to information giving. Their findings and use of a different methodological approach greatly extended our understanding and challenged previous perceptions.

The methodology of Tuckett and colleagues

Tuckett *et al.* studied 1302 consultations conducted by 16 doctors in general practice in the UK in considerable depth, setting out with the following three principles in mind.

1. **Not all information is of equal importance.** Previous work had assessed information giving by counting how many of the total number of statements made by the doctor were remembered by the patient. But perhaps some information is more important than other information. Does it matter that patients forget a certain proportion of information given if they remember the most important points? Does it help if patients remember more statements if this isn't the information they really need to understand their problem? We need to consider what information has been imparted rather than simply how much. Tuckett's team therefore devised a method for deciding what were the 'key' points made by the doctor. This enabled the subsequent analysis of patient recall to be examined in relation not to all possible statements made by the doctor but only to those statements necessary for the patient to make sense of their illness and treatment.
2. **Recall does not necessarily imply understanding or commitment.** Just improving recall will not necessarily lead to better health outcomes. What if the patient can recall what the doctor said but it appears to make no sense? We have to look beyond recall to understanding – although recall is important, it is not by itself a satisfactory endpoint in information-giving research. Tuckett *et al.* therefore looked at the following three outcome measures:
    *   patient recall
    *   patient understanding – did the patient make correct sense of what they were told?
    *   patient commitment – did the patient agree with the doctor's key ideas, and were these ideas in conflict with the patient's own explanatory models?
3. **Information giving needs to be looked at from the patient's perspective as well as that of the doctor.** The problem of information giving is not simply about how doctors can give information that they wish to impart. It is also about how patients can discover the information they themselves would like and how doctors can assist in that process. Tuckett *et al.* therefore examined two approaches to information giving. First, they examined Ley's concept of clarity in information giving. What influence did doctors' abilities to use Ley's suggestions (explicit categorisation, grammatical statements, coherence of phraseology, avoidance of jargon, avoidance of unexplained assumptions, pace and

audibility) have on patient recall, understanding and commitment? Second, they looked at a totally different perspective, mutual sharing by exchange of views, which was based on the work of social anthropologists such as Helman (1978). This perspective is very similar to the disease–illness model that we explored in Chapter 3 and moves toward the all-important concept of mutually understood common ground. Does understanding the patient's belief systems and taking into account the patient's own perspective of their illness help information giving? Responding to this question, the Tuckett team looked at doctors' efforts to encourage patients to volunteer and elaborate on their ideas, doctors' responses to any evidence of a patient having ideas, the extent to which doctors' reasoning was directly related to patients' ideas, and the extent to which doctors checked for patient understanding.

What does the research of Tuckett and colleagues show about the information given by doctors?

- As expected, doctors' information giving placed far more emphasis on diagnostic-significance and treatment action than preventive action or implications.
- On only a small percentage of occasions were doctors' views presented clearly.
- On only 50% of occasions were rationales included to substantiate doctors' views.
- Even when rationales were given, they were mostly parsimonious in content and lacking in clarity.
- Doctors almost never related their explanations to patients' view or beliefs. In only 12 out of 405 consultations were doctors' explanations related to their patients' beliefs at all.
- In only 6% of consultations were patients' ideas and explanatory beliefs elicited in the first place.
- Even when patients volunteered their ideas either as hinted cues or as spontaneous outright statements, doctors still only asked patients to elaborate on their ideas in 7% of consultations.
- Not only were patients not asked to elaborate on their ideas but also doctors often evaded them, interrupted them or deliberately inhibited their expression.
- In only 7% of consultations did doctors in any way check their patients' understanding of what had been said.

In summary, the research of Tuckett *et al.* showed that doctors rarely exhibited the organisational and other communication skills to make their efforts clear to patients. They also showed little interest in their patients' theories, hypotheses or understanding. More recent research, such as that of Campion *et al.* (2002), suggests that this is unfortunately still the case. Therefore, in relation to both models of 'how' to give information – Ley's and the disease–illness model – doctors would not be expected to be particularly effective in their efforts at information giving!

What does the research of Tuckett and his colleagues show about the influence patients can have on their doctors' information giving?

Do patients attempt to influence their doctors' information giving and do they do it overtly or covertly? To assess how often patients tried to play an active role in this part of the consultation, Tuckett *et al.* examined the following strategies that could be used by patients to influence the information obtained from their doctors:

- indicating their own explanatory models
- seeking clarification of a doctor's views and instructions
- asking for a doctor's reasons and rationales
- expressing doubts.

They could do this

- overtly
- covertly.

A remarkably high level of participation was demonstrated. In fact, 85% of patients engaged in at least one of the four activities. However, this participation was mostly performed in a covert way, utilising hints and vague questions, rather than overtly, with clear statements or questions. This fits in well with other work showing that the proportion of patients asking overt questions is small (Svarstad 1974; Roter 1977; Stimson and Webb 1975; Beisecker and Beisecker 1990) and that patients' indirect attempts to make their views and questions heard are important (Levinson *et al.* 2000). Hudak *et al.* (2008) showed that patients raised only 53% of their concerns with orthopaedic surgeons. Orthopaedic surgeons responded positively to 66% of the concerns raised by the patients. Only two concerns were raised in response to direct surgeon inquiry.

What effect does patients' participation have on doctors' information giving? When patients did contribute overtly, they were more likely to receive more information. Covert participation led to a much smaller effect. Svarstad (1974), Boreham and Gibson (1978) and Roter (1977) have also shown that when patients ask questions overtly, doctors provide answers and patients obtain more detailed explanations.

Thus patients can exert considerable control over how their physicians behave and are wise to ask questions openly rather then covertly if they wish to receive more information. However, there is a potentially less desirable outcome. Where doctors did not respond positively to patients asking them for their rationale or expressing doubts, patients were more likely to experience a consultation characterised by evasive attitudes and behaviour from the doctor and an increase in tension. Roter (1977) and Kaplan *et al.* (1989) also found that more question asking by the patient led to increased doctor anxiety and anger, although this was interpreted as an indication of being engaged rather than as a negative finding.

Do patients feel they would like to ask their doctors questions and if so, why don't they do so overtly? In Tuckett *et al.*'s research, 76% of the patients said afterwards that they had specific doubts or questions during the interview that they did not mention to the doctor. Why do patients hold back from asking questions? And why when they do pluck up courage do they often ask questions covertly and provide only indirect cues to their information needs? Patients in the study gave the following reasons for their behaviour.

- It was not up to them to ask questions, express doubts or behave as if their view was important (36%).
- They were afraid of being less well thought of by the doctor (22%).

- They were frightened of a negative reaction from the doctor (14%).
- They were too flustered or hurried to ask coherently (27%).
- They doubted that the doctor could tell them any more at the moment (22%).
- They forgot or were waiting until next time to ask, when they would be more certain of what they thought was reasonable to ask (36%).
- They feared the truth (9%).

Only 19% of patients who exhibited gaps in their knowledge said that they did not ask questions because they were not interested in the answer.

In an Australian study of communication in a large emergency department that combined observation with analysis of audiotapes and transcripts, Slade *et al.* (2008) showed that overwhelmingly doctors asked questions and patients answered. This pattern of doctors' questions dominating occurred not only during history taking but throughout the encounter. With little opportunity to deviate from the question/answer structure, patients and their families rarely asked any questions suggesting that they did not think it appropriate for them to ask questions or felt too intimidated by the context to do so.

What are the combined effects of patients' and doctors' approaches to patient involvement in information giving?

Tying together the results of Tuckett *et al.* for both patients' and doctors' behaviour in the consultation leads to some depressing conclusions. Both parties appeared to adopt the roles predicted by the traditional view of the doctor–patient relationship. Patients felt that it was not relevant for them to understand or up to them to ask questions. They were afraid of the doctor's reactions to questions that they might ask. In total, 85% of patients attempted to contribute their ideas, ask questions or express doubts, but the majority used hints and vague questions rather than overt questions. Doctors were poor at picking up on such cues or covert messages, did not encourage and even actively discouraged patients from expressing their ideas, and often responded with increased tension when ideas were ventured or questions were asked. Therefore, doctors' behaviour and patients' perceptions together act to confirm a passive role for the patient in which shared understanding is unlikely to occur.

The tradition of the doctor controlling information appears to be very strong – patients adopt a passive role and are assumed to be disinterested by doctors who take the initiative. Unfortunately, doctors' and patients' behaviour are self-perpetuating – past experiences of patients and physicians reinforce the attitudes of authority and deference that overshadow the doctor–patient relationship.

Can doctors and patients more positively influence each other towards a shared understanding in information giving?

We have already seen that the more active patients are in the consultation, the more likely they are to obtain the information that they would like. There is also no doubt that doctors, if they wish, can influence patients and enable them to take a more active role. Svarstad (1974) showed that doctors who avoided certain inhibiting behaviours enabled their patients to ask more questions. Inhibiting conditions included clock-watching, use of jargon, mumbling incomprehensibly, interrupting, ignoring patients' comments, unfriendliness and ending consultations precipitately.

Doctors appeared to be able to vary their behaviour according to circumstances, and utilised communication-limiting strategies much more when they were under pressure of time. Thus both doctors and patients can influence the degree of sharing that occurs in the consultation.

Does the research of Tuckett et al. about recall fit in with previous work?

One very important finding of Tuckett et al.'s work is that patients recalled far more information than previous studies had intimated. Tuckett et al. found that only 10% of information was forgotten, as opposed to 30%–50% in studies such as those of Ley. As doctors had in the past used patients' poor recall to justify giving them only limited information, this new finding is of extreme importance. What could be the reason for this significant difference?

Although it is possible that differences in the settings in which the interviews studied took place may have been responsible, by far the most likely cause is the different methodology for assessing recall used by Tuckett's team. First, they assessed only whether patients remembered the 'key' points made by the doctor. This is very different from seeing how many statements were remembered of all the things said by the doctor. Second, while previous work had used the method of free recall, whereby interviewers asked a general question such as 'What did the doctor say to you about the reasons for seeing him?' and were then not allowed to probe any further, Tuckett et al. used the approach of probed recall, in which interviewers used a standardised interview but were allowed to discover the patient's meaning and clarify answers.

Was correct sense made of the explanations?

Around 90% of the key points of information provided by their doctors were remembered. But was it understood? Tuckett and his colleagues compared patients' understanding of the information that they had received with their doctors' actual meaning as judged by third-party assessment. Again relatively high levels of comprehension were found – 73% of patients made correct sense of the key points that they had been told.

Tuckett et al. then looked at the effect that the two different concepts of 'how' to give information (i.e. clarity and mutual sharing by exchange of views) had on patient understanding. Surprisingly, no relationship was found at all between the clarity of explanation given by the doctor and whether correct sense was made of the doctor's comments by the patient!

Attempts to correlate the value of mutual sharing to patient understanding did however produce evidence of a relationship. Consultations in which the doctor inhibited or evaded their patients' ideas were more likely to result in a failure of recall and understanding than those in which doctors did not inhibit or evade. Understanding dropped from 40% to 29%. This suggests that paying attention to the patient's explanatory framework does increase understanding. It was not possible to assess other aspects of mutual sharing because doctors so rarely demonstrated the appropriate skills required. Patients' understanding was so rarely checked and clarified by the doctor, patients' ideas and beliefs were so infrequently actively discovered, and the rationales given were so rarely related to patients' explanatory beliefs that their effect on understanding could not be ascertained!

To try to discover further information about the importance of a mutual exchange of views, Tuckett et al. undertook a qualitative analysis of a small sample of the consultations. Further examination of the recorded consultations and post-consultation interviews showed that patients had particular problems with recall and making sense of information presented by the doctor when there was a mismatch with the patient's own explanatory framework. The key to the problem of understanding appeared to be the detailed ideas that the patient brought to bear on the explanation of the doctor – if there was a match with the doctor's explanation, good understanding ensued, even if the explanation by the doctor had been unclear or sparse. However, if there was a mis-match in the doctor's and the patient's explanatory frameworks, understanding was likely to suffer. Not surprisingly it is more difficult to assimilate information which is unfamiliar, unexpected or threatening. Then the ambiguous and disorganised information giving of doctors is likely to be particularly unhelpful.

Poor information giving clearly leads to considerable scope for misunderstanding. If the doctor and patient's views are divergent, the patient could arrive at a very different version of what the doctor was trying to say without either party realising. As the doctor has not discovered the patients' views, nor conveyed explicitly that his views differ, nor checked the patient's understanding after giving the information, the patients may well misinterpret information or even assume incorrectly that the doctor is confirming their views. In contrast, if views are very close, doctors are more likely to escape the consequences of disorganisation and ambiguity as there is already a congruity of view and much less likelihood of misunderstanding.

Were patients committed to the doctor's view?

The overwhelming majority (75%) of patients who had remembered and made sense of information that they were given were also committed to the doctor's views. Again consultations in which the doctor inhibited or evaded their patient's ideas were more likely to result in lack of commitment to the doctor's views than consultations in which doctors did not evade or inhibit patients' ideas.

The qualitative analysis showed a major difference between those patients who were committed to a doctor's view and those who were not. Those who were committed usually expected what they heard and already agreed with it. However, if the patient started out with views divergent from the doctor, the consultations appeared to do little to change them. Patients rejected their doctor's views in favour of their own. As doctors rarely paid attention to patients' ideas, they remained uninformed about their patients' thinking and could not direct their explanations precisely to it. Tuckett *et al.* firmly believe that without establishing what ideas the patient has, there is no possibility of a mutual exchange of views and without this there is little likelihood of increasing commitment.

As we have said, many patients expressed doubts or asked the doctor for further explanations of their rationale. Tuckett *et al.* showed that patients showing evidence of questioning their doctor in these ways were more likely not to be committed to the doctor's view by the end of the consultation. Patients, it seems, are keen to warn us of the need to take their views and thinking seriously, yet by and large we ignore their efforts to engineer a mutual exploration of ideas.

What are the main conclusions of Tuckett and colleagues?

Tuckett *et al.* conclude that there is a need for two concerted approaches to encourage success in our goals of patient recall, understanding and commitment.

1. Clarity – so that the patient can understand what is said and comprehend whether there is a difference between the doctor's and their own beliefs.
2. Exploration of the patient's beliefs and ideas together with checking the patient's interpretation and reaction to information given. The doctor needs to be willing to explore the differences in viewpoint and negotiate a shared explanatory model.

Tuckett *et al.* suggest that we need to change our approach to explanation and planning to enable a 'meeting of experts' – an explicit sharing of our explanatory models between two parties with different expertise, one of the medical world and one of the unique experience of the individual.

Although it is clear from their work that differences in explanatory framework lead to poorer understanding and commitment, they could not produce direct evidence to prove the efficacy of the measures that they proposed. So few consultations demonstrated an active search for patients' ideas or included explanations that were related to the patients' explanatory frameworks that a statistical analysis proved impossible. We are still left with the partially unanswered question: if we do elicit our patients' conflicting ideas, take them into account and explain our findings in relation to them, will we improve our patients' understanding and commitment? Fortunately, a number of other studies not only confirm the work of Tuckett *et al.* but also add further insight into these issues.

Other work to support shared understanding

Tuckett and colleagues' concept of an 'explicit sharing of explanatory models' fits very well with the disease–illness model and the concept of mutually understood common ground as discussed in Chapter 3. There we advocated a three-stage plan for discovering patients' beliefs and other perspectives:

1. identification,
2. acceptance
3. explanation

in which integrating the doctor's and the patient's understanding of problems and reaching mutually understood common ground is the final aim. Keeping Tuckett's conclusions about clarity and shared explanatory modes in mind, what other evidence supports this approach?

Eisenthal and Lazare (1976) (*see* Chapter 3) demonstrated that if physicians in a psychiatric walk-in clinic discovered patients' expectations, patients were more likely to feel satisfied and to adhere to plans, whether their requests was granted or not. In other words, we do not discover expectations just so that we can give patients what they want, but so that we can base our negotiation on an open understanding of our respective positions. Eliciting expectations allows the physician to consider the relevance of the patient's position and to produce evidence for and against different approaches. It is not finding out whether the patient wants a CT scan and going along with their wishes that is important but finding out the patient's expectations, explaining the doctor's position in relation to the patient's views and reaching a negotiated plan acceptable to both parties.

Arborelius and Bremberg (1992) in a study in general practice showed that in those consultations where both doctor and patient rated the interview positively, increased efforts were made to establish the patient's ideas and concerns and more time was spent on the tasks of shared understanding and involving the patient in their own management.

Maynard (1990) used a qualitative approach to investigate the importance of discovering patients' prior knowledge and feelings in the arena of giving information to parents about their children's developmental disabilities. In this 'breaking bad news' scenario, Maynard identified that 'interactional alignment' was a critical factor in determining how parents accepted the diagnosis of developmental delay. If the news was given without discovering the parent's knowledge and feelings about their child's condition, there was a high likelihood of outright rejection of the diagnosis. When the clinician discovered the parent's understanding first, there was a much greater chance that the news could be delivered in such a way as to allow the parents to accept the diagnosis. Maynard therefore recommends an interactional style of giving difficult information, where the doctor aligns him- or herself with the patient and can anticipate problems before they arise. Once rejection of information has occurred, it is very difficult to redress the balance.

Maynard's work may go some way towards helping doctors to overcome the problems that have been identified by others' research. A consistent finding in the literature (Bass and Cohen 1982; Starfield *et al.* 1981) is that lack of agreement at the end of the consultation about the nature of the problem or the need for follow-up leads to a reduction in improvement in patient symptoms. One way of improving the situation would perhaps be to adopt Maynard's approach of 'interactional alignment'.

Inui *et al.* (1976) looked at the effect of a single training session on compliance-aiding interviewing skills given to physicians working with patients with known hypertension in hospital outpatient clinics. Physicians were given one tutorial lasting up to two hours that demonstrated that:

- non-compliance was widespread in their patients
- there was a high probability that poor blood pressure control was indicative of poor compliance (90% relationship)
- physicians should discuss their patients' knowledge, attitudes and beliefs about their hypertension and its treatment, rather than just search for complications of hypertension
- physicians should switch from being purely diagnosticians to being patient educators; they should link their patients' beliefs, attitudes and understanding to their explanations as doctors, share their rationale and help patients to overcome their barriers to adherence.

The results of this study showed not only that trained doctors spent more time in considering their patients' ideas and in patient education than did control physicians, that patients' understanding of their condition improved and that compliance increased, but also that there was better control of hypertension even six months after the tutorial! Here then is good physiological outcome evidence for the concept of shared understanding.

Similar increases in compliance following a single training session on compliance-aiding interviewing skills have since also been obtained in the context of patients with otitis media attending paediatric outpatients (Maiman *et al.* 1988).

For further insight into the rationale and means for establishing the common ground of shared understanding with patients, consider again the Headache Study Group of the University of Western Ontario's (1986) study that we referred to in Chapter 3. In that one-year prospective study, the best predictor for resolution of headache problems was not diagnosis, intervention, referral or prescription. It was patients' perception that they had had the opportunity to tell their story and discuss their concerns about the headache fully with their physician during the first visit. Apparently even the perception of shared understanding – of achieving the common ground that is possible when patients have the opportunity to share their story and their concerns – is a potent variable affecting outcomes of care.

In another outcome study that we describe in more detail in the next section of this chapter, Kaplan *et al.* (1989) coached patients to voice their questions and concerns in the medical interview. They found that the subsequent change in patient behaviour not only produced a dramatic difference to what happened in the interview itself but also led to improved physiological outcomes in both diabetes and hypertension.

Smith *et al.* (2011) carefully teased apart cognitive and emotional aspects of shared decision making between oncologists and breast cancer patients. By rating consultations both with the OPTION rating scale for shared decision making and the Respond to Emotional Cues and Concerns coding system, they found that cognitive and emotional aspects of shared decision making have different effects on patient outcomes. Whereas the OPTION scale predicted satisfaction with doctor shared decision-making skills and treatment decisions, emotional blocking predicted decisional conflict while empathy and cue emission predicted post-consultation anxiety. This study demonstrates the importance of both shared decision making and emotional relating in consultations with cancer patients.

What skills can we recommend to help learners achieve a shared understanding with their patients?

How do we make the lessons that we have learned from the research described come alive? How do we put these lessons into practice in the consultation? Again the analogy of the lecture is helpful. The most interactive approach to lecturing is the 'learner-centred lecture'. Here, as well as:

- tailoring the presentation to the learners' needs by chunking and checking and assessing the learners' starting point (frisbee approach)
- paying attention to structure and organisation, language and visual aids (shot-put approach)

the lecturer also deliberately encourages the audience to brainstorm their doubts, concerns and expectations early on in the proceedings. Then as the lecture continues, the lecturer repeatedly:

- refers to the learners' doubts as he proceeds
- checks the response to what he is saying by reading the verbal and non-verbal cues of the audience
- deliberately asks for the audience's reactions to what he is saying.

Note that the lecturer has to be much more flexible here to accommodate the audience's needs and has to be very careful to use structuring and organisational tools at appropriate times to prevent the lecture from becoming too random and disorganised. In other words, we have to be wary that we do not lose all the lessons of the shot-put approach in our desire to be highly interactive.

So far so good. However, the frisbee approach at its most powerful occurs not in the large group context of a lecturer talking with an entire audience but in the interpersonal context of two or three individuals communicating with one another as partners and collaborators. The frisbee approach, then, connotes even greater possibilities for interaction and relationship. In the context of the medical interview, it is not just about what the doctor says but also, equally, about what the patient says. All of the lessons learned from the learner-centred lecture analogy continue to apply but we have even greater opportunity for flexibility and interaction, for doctor and the patient hearing each other, responding to each other and achieving a more shared understanding, and for clearly establishing mutually understood common ground.

Relating explanations to the patient's perspective

In Chapter 3 we discussed gathering information and saw how discovering the patient's perspective was an essential component of the effective medical interview. We saw that the advantages of discovering the patient's ideas, concerns, expectations and feelings include not only being more supportive and understanding but also being of help in making a correct diagnosis and producing a more effective and efficient interview.

However, perhaps the most important benefit of discovering the patient's illness framework is the effect that this has on explanation and planning, as we have seen in the research already quoted. Recall, understanding, satisfaction and compliance are all likely to suffer when an explanation does not address the patient's individual ideas, expectations and concerns.

So early on in this phase of the interview, we need to start to relate our explanations to the patient's illness framework that we have previously elicited when gathering information:

> '*You mentioned earlier that you were concerned that you might have angina … I can see why you might have thought that, but in fact I think it's more likely to be a muscular pain … let me explain why.*'

Providing opportunities and encouraging the patient to contribute

If the first stage of achieving a shared understanding is to provide explanations that relate to the patient's perspective that you have previously elicited, the second stage is to discover and address the patient's thoughts and feelings about the information that you are now in the process of giving. An essential element of this is providing opportunities for the patient to ask questions, seek clarification or express doubts. Doctors have to be very explicit here – many patients, as we have seen, are reluctant to express what is on the tip of their tongue and are extremely hesitant to ask the doctor questions. Unless positively invited to do so, they may well leave the consultation with their questions unanswered and a reduced understanding and commitment to plans:

> *'What questions does that leave you with? Is there something I haven't covered or explained?'*

Then of course the doctor must respond appropriately – without validation and interest from the doctor, the patient will not be encouraged to think that their own views are important to the doctor, and will revert to a more passive role:

> *'Yes that is an important question. I'm glad you asked that – I'll try to answer it for you ...'*

Picking up verbal and non-verbal cues

Another means of discovering the patient's thoughts and feelings is to try to pick up the patient's cues, both verbal and non-verbal. Remember that most patients utilise indirect or oblique hints to express their doubts or questions, rather than overt statements or questions. The physician must therefore search for more subtle cues that the patient may wish to contribute information or ask questions, that they may be getting near to being flooded with information or that they are becoming distressed:

> *'You look unhappy – is it about the possibility of having surgery?'*

Eliciting the patient's beliefs, reactions and concerns

In addition to picking up cues, it is important to actively seek out the patient's reactions to the discussion that you have had by asking explicitly for their feelings and concerns and acknowledging and addressing these as necessary:

> *'I'm not sure how that news has left you feeling ...'*
>
> or
>
> *'Does that leave you with any concerns or doubts?'*

PLANNING – SHARED DECISION MAKING

Following on from explanation comes planning. Not only have there been major advances in concepts of information giving but also there have been considerable moves to change the medical profession's approach to planning and decision making. Medical researchers, educators, ethicists and patient groups have increasingly advocated shared decision-making models incorporating partnership, negotiation and mutual collaboration (Coulter 1999). What is the theoretical and research evidence behind these claims?

Theoretical concepts behind shared decision making

Many writers over the last nearly 40 years have provided theoretical support for the concept of a collaborative approach to planning. Becker's *health belief model* (Becker 1974) explores how adherence to a treatment regimen or to a change in health behaviour is influenced by the balance between patients' understanding and appraisal of the potential benefits that might accrue and the costs of and personal or social barriers to carrying out proposed suggestions. According to this model, the physician should not only educate the patient about the nature and effectiveness of treatments but also discover the patient's perceptions of costs and barriers so that these can be addressed. Only if there is a readiness to embrace a negotiating approach to the consultation can this process be achieved. Slack (1977) argues that patients should be encouraged to make their own decisions with the aid of their physician rather than have the physician choose for them. Doctors would then be freed from feeling responsible for all that occurs to their patients, from the liability that accompanies medical paternalism. Brody (1980) suggests four steps necessary to encourage the patient's role in decision making. These suggestions bring together many of the ideas that are advocated throughout this book:

1. establishing an atmosphere conducive to participation where contributions are welcomed and where the patient's ideas and questions are actively sought
2. ascertaining the patient's reasons for seeing the doctor, and their goals and expectations
3. giving appropriate information about the nature of the problem, including the doctor's rationale, possible alternatives, their advantages and disadvantages, and suggested recommendations (rather than directives)
4. eliciting the patient's informed suggestions and preferences and negotiating any disagreements.

Quill (1983) discusses the role of negotiating and contracting in a consensual relationship. Herman (1985) stresses the importance of sharing possibilities and eliciting patient preferences so that the patient understands their physician's rationale, is involved in decision making and shares control with the physician. Deber (1994) suggests that choosing the optimal treatment is often a marginal decision – the 'correct' decision is greatly influenced by the values that a particular patient attaches to different outcomes and to their perception of particular procedures. Only through knowledge of the patient's unique perspective of these issues can the patient and the doctor together make an informed and appropriate choice. Stewart *et al.* (1997) support mutuality, collaboration, and partnership in their model of patient-centred medicine; so, too, does the Pew-Fetzer Task Force document (Tresolini and the Pew-Fetzer Task Force 1994) on relationship-centred care.

The mutuality model

Roter and Hall (1992), in their book *Doctors Talking with Patients / Patients Talking with Doctors*, describe four possible models of the doctor–patient relationship: paternalism, consumerism, default and mutuality.

The *paternalistic model* is characterised by high doctor/low patient control. The doctor makes decisions that he considers to be in the best interest of the patient; the patient co-operates with the advice and does as he is told. At certain times, the patient welcomes this style of relationship – for instance, by those who are seriously ill, vulnerable and unable to take part in a more equal relationship. It is also the preference of certain patients, possibly more so among some elderly or less educated patients (Haug and Lavin 1983). However, there are questions about the appropriateness of this type of relationship, even when both patient and physician appear to agree with it. Patients and doctors are often on an unequal footing and few patients really have an effective role in shaping the relationship. A passive role may be the natural consequence of many years of deference without a full understanding of the alternatives (Deber 1994). Explicit discussions of the different decision-making stances available to the patient are unlikely to occur in paternalistic approaches. It has been suggested that part of the doctor's role should be education and encouragement of patients to take part in adult–adult relationships with their physicians.

Consumerism is the other extreme. Here, there is low doctor / high patient control. A younger or better-informed patient may take a more assertive role; the doctor may simply co-operate by acceding to the patient's requests for, say, investigation or medication. There are problems here too – for example, if the patient's requests are outside normal practice, if they are not in the patient's best interests or if they are a waste of precious healthcare resources. In a healthcare system in which patients as consumers can exert their choice to change doctors until they find one who will accommodate their requests, and in which the doctor's income is dependent on attracting more patients and performing more tasks, good medical practice can be sacrificed on the altar of consumerism and financial incentive. In this model, trust between doctor and patient is eroded and the doctor's expertise is diminished just as the patient's is in the paternalistic model.

Default or *laissez faire* describes a model in which no one takes responsibility, where both doctor and patient have low control and the relationship becomes aimless and unproductive for both parties.

In *mutuality*, there is both high doctor and high patient control. Patients' preferences are actively sought and compared explicitly with doctors' thoughts – doctors explain their reasoning in relation to patients' ideas. Open negotiation leads to a meeting of minds between two more equal parties, and to the production of a mutually agreed upon collaborative plan. Patients can openly explain which option they might prefer or why they might not be able to follow a particular course of action. Similarly, doctors can openly discuss their own dilemmas, explain why a patient's suggestion is not to the patient's advantage and why the doctor may not feel able to fulfil it. Often, both doctor and patient perspectives can be accommodated with minor adjustment; potential disagreements are discovered within the consultation and can be addressed then and there. In a more doctor-centred approach to planning, such doubts may not surface during the interview but appear later on, when the patient has left the room, to initiate the insidious process of non-adherence.

The shared decision-making model

Charles *et al.* (1997, 1999a, 1999b) advocated a shared decision-making model. Here they contrasted three possible positions:

1. paternalistic
2. informed choice
3. shared decision making.

The *paternalistic approach* is as already described. Interestingly, the authors point out that even in a paternalistic relationship, it is still possible for the doctor to discover the patient's preferences and build them into the decision-making process. This has been described as the physician acting as perfect agent for the patient – the doctor tries to make the same decision as the patient would *were the patient to be party to the same clinical expertise as the doctor* (Gafni *et al.* 1998). Although the doctor may feel that this has been a collaborative approach to decision making, the doctor still makes the final decision on behalf of the patient and is in command of the decision-making process. So by definition a true doctor–patient partnership in planning does not exist.

In *informed choice*, such a partnership does exist but is based on a strict division of labour. Here the doctor's role is information giving only. The doctor goes first and provides information on all relevant treatment options, their benefits and their risks. Sufficient information must be transferred for the patient to make an informed choice. Now it is the patient's turn. At this point the patient has both the information necessary and the personal preferences required for decision making. The patient deliberates alone and makes a choice. The doctor has no responsibility or claim to be involved here and should not influence the patient for fear of denying the patient their control over the decision-making process – the doctor should neither advocate nor advise (Eddy 1990). A potential problem here is that the patient may feel increased anxiety and even abandonment as they face a difficult decision alone and without the physician's support. It also removes physicians from having any input into the decision-making process and may force them into actions that they do not consider are acceptable either to themselves or to society overall. The patient is fully empowered but at considerable potential cost to all parties (Quill and Brody 1996).

In contrast, the *shared decision-making model* is more interactional in nature, in that the doctor and the patient share all stages in the decision-making process. It recognises that the effective transfer of all information from a well-informed doctor to a highly capable and independent patient is a flawed model for many consultations. Deficiencies in doctors' communication skills and knowledge, the effect of patients' emotions and varying levels of scientific understanding on comprehension all mitigate against patients being always able to come to a well-informed decision by themselves. In the shared decision model, there is instead a two-way exchange of information (including the technical information that *both* doctor *and* patient bring to the interview and the patient's ideas, concerns and expectations). Both parties reveal their treatment preferences and both agree on a decision to be implemented. Doctor and patient alike have a legitimate investment in decisions and work towards consensus. As in the informed-choice approach, the full sharing of information is essential but now leads on to a further stage of shared decision making – these are separate components of the explanation and planning phase of the interview, requiring separate skills.

In the shared decision-making model, it is perfectly acceptable for the doctor to have a preference as long as he clearly signposts that the patient's position is equally as important as the doctor's and a shared decision is genuinely reached together. However, it is equally possible that the physician is in a position of 'equipoise' (Elwyn *et al.* 2000), and genuinely does not have a preference for which of several treatments the patient might choose. Yet whether in a position of equipoise or of preference, the practitioner should not *disapprove* of the decision the patient eventually makes – it is the discussion that is all-important.

This shared decision-making approach is now widely advocated (Elwyn *et al.* 1999a, 2001a; Coulter *et al.* 1999; Schofield *et al.* 2003; Holmes-Rovner *et al.* 2000). A number of broadly synonymous terms are also in widespread use, which can be confusing – for instance, evidence-based patient choice (Hope 1996; Edwards and Elwyn 2001a; Ford *et al.* 2003), informed shared decision making (Towle and Godolphin 1999, Godolphin *et al.* 2001), informed decision making (Braddock *et al.* 1997; Price *et al.* 2012), integrated decision making (Trevena and Barratt 2003) and participatory decision making (Epstein *et al.* 2004). Makoul and Clayman (2006) have attempted to provide an integrated definition of shared decision making to help bring clarity to research and teaching. They have divided the components of shared decision making into essential and ideal elements.

- *Essential elements* – patients and providers should together:
  - define/explain problem
  - present options
  - discuss pros/cons (benefits, risks, costs)
  - explore patient values/preferences
  - discuss patient ability/self-efficacy
  - discuss doctor knowledge/recommendations
  - check/clarify each other's understanding
  - make or explicitly defer decision
  - arrange follow-up.
- *Ideal elements*:
  - unbiased information
  - define roles (desire for involvement)
  - present evidence
  - mutual agreement.

But do doctors routinely use these approaches? Sadly, the evidence suggests that current practice has not embraced the concept of shared decision making (Makoul *et al.* 1995; Stevenson *et al.* 2000; Elwyn *et al.* 2003b; Campion *et al.* 2002; Richard and Lussier 2003; Cohen and Britten 2003; Ford *et al.* 2006; Edwards *et al.* 2005; Young *et al.* 2008; Hanson 2008; Karnielli-Miller and Eisikovits 2009; Coulter 2009; Godolphin 2009; Sonntag *et al.* 2012) or that despite appropriate intentions to embrace the concept, clinicians in some instances unintentionally communicate in ways that are counterproductive. For example, based on a thematic literature review and their own clinical and educational experience, Wiener and Roth (2006) point out that during discussions with patients and their families regarding goals of care near the end of life, some unintended but common physician communication behaviours may inadvertently impair shared decision making.

Further approaches to encouraging patient participation and involvement have concentrated on the patient's rather than the doctor's role and have utilised methods of enabling patients to prepare for or participate in the interview (Tuckett *et al.* 1985; Kaplan *et al.* 1989; Middleton 1995; Health Canada 1996; Korsch and

Harding 1997; Bayer Institute for Health Care Communication 1999; Fleissig *et al.* 2000; Cegala 2003; Dimoska *et al.* 2008b) by, for instance:

- asking them to prepare lists of issues to discuss before the interview
- providing prompt cards or reminders of useful questions
- providing information about how to get the best out of the visit to the doctor.

From compliance to concordance

Closely allied to shared decision making is the concept of concordance (Marinker *et al.* 1997; Marinker and Shaw 2003; Britten 2003; Stevenson and Scambler 2005). In effect, concordance is shared decision making looked at in the context of medicine taking (Elwyn *et al.* 2003a). Marinker *et al.* (1997) have defined it as:

> *An agreement between a patient and a health care professional that respects the beliefs and wishes of the patient in determining whether, when and how medicines are to be taken. Although reciprocal, this is an alliance in which the health care professionals recognise the primacy of the patient's decisions about taking the recommended medications.*

This definition accepts the obvious truth that, at the end of the day, it is the patient in their own home who decides how or if their medicine is taken. We know that 50% of long-term medications are not taken or taken inappropriately (Haynes *et al.* 1996). This vast non-compliance has serious health and cost issues. Coambs *et al.* (1995), in their review of the literature on non-compliance conclude that of the models that have evolved to explain non-compliance, only those which incorporate patients' attitudes, health beliefs and intentions to comply, rather than patients' biological or social traits, have been successful in predicting non-compliance. They also conclude that 'when the patient–physician relationship is a negotiated process, in which there is increased understanding of and agreement upon a proposed treatment, higher levels of compliance with the therapeutic regime and improved health status can be achieved.'

Increasingly, health professionals are moving away from the use of the word 'compliance' at all with its overtones of passivity, obedience and 'following doctor's orders'. The word 'compliance' does not fit with modern approaches to shared decision making. The compliance literature would suggest that medicine has a rationality whereas patient non-compliance is irrational. Doctors are seen to be the principal contributors to decision making with regard to medication taking. Patients are seen as being passive, obedient, unquestioning recipients of advice. Non-compliers are somehow 'naughty' and the blame for non-compliance lies primarily with the patient.

In reality, of course, patients make their own decisions based on their beliefs, experiences and the information available to them at the time. They have their own rational discourse, which can be different and more wide ranging than the narrower perspective of medical rationality. And prescribing is, of course, not an exact or neutral science – doctors disagree among themselves, there are many commercial and other pressures on prescribers from healthcare systems and pharmaceutical companies, and doctors' personal experience may unduly influence their prescribing (Donovan 1995).

The move to concordance attempts to redress this balance. A patient can be non-compliant, but only an interview or discussion can be non-concordant (Britten 2003). Concordance refers to a relationship between two parties – as doctors we need to know the patient's decision-making quandaries and preferences and openly discuss these, rather than determining a best course of action based on medical imperatives alone. Concordance implies that doctors move from only considering the best possible control of the disease (seizures, say) to looking at the best outcome from the viewpoint of the patient (which may be a balance between seizure control and minimisation of drug side effects). Health outcome in terms of disease needs to take second place to the patient's perceived overall quality of life. The aim of concordance is to make these differences and difficulties overt rather than covert – they will occur anyway, yet in the traditional approach doctors simply do not know that their patients are non-compliant.

Concordance therefore refers to the creation of an agreement with regard to medications that respects the beliefs and wishes of the patient, and not to compliance (the following of instructions) (Britten 1994; Dowell *et al.* 2002). As Marinker and Shaw (2003) have so cogently said:

> *Doctors and patients may not always agree. The implication of concordance is that when this happens the patient's views take precedence. This poses challenging questions about choice and responsibility. If the only treatment to which the patient will agree falls substantially short of what modern medicine can achieve the doctor may be left with a burden of responsibility that is hard to manage emotionally, ethically, and legally. The difficulty for health professionals lies in acknowledging that it is the patients' agendas and not their own that determine whether patients take medicines. Patients have their own beliefs about their medicines and medicines in general. They have their own priorities and their own rational discourse in relation to health and care, risk and benefit. These may differ from and sometimes contradict those of the doctors. They are, however, no less cogent, coherent, or important.*

What would happen if all doctors were to apply the concordance model? What influence would it have on health outcomes for individuals and for whole populations? We do not know as yet. One outcome might be that the amount of money paid out for drugs goes down as we openly take our patients' views into account and do not prescribe medication they would not otherwise take. Will that improve the health of the population? The answer is not necessarily – here we see possible friction between public health medicine (what is 'good' for the population as a whole) and individuals' autonomy.

The research evidence to support shared decision making

What research evidence do we have to demonstrate that a collaborative approach can improve patient outcomes?

Further to their work on the relationship between eliciting patient expectations and subsequent patient satisfaction, Eisenthal *et al.* (1979) demonstrated that higher levels of negotiation and patient participation in the decision-making process are associated with both increased adherence and greater satisfaction. By a 'negotiated approach', the authors meant eliciting patients' expectations and requests for care, actively negotiating treatment plans and checking negotiated plans to see whether the patient agreed with them.

Schulman (1979) found that hypertensive patients who were more actively involved in treatment programmes had higher rates of adherence and more favourable treatment outcomes. 'Active involvement' was defined as viewing themselves as collaborative partners, being involved in two-way communication and joint decision making, being informed of treatment rationales and being encouraged to voice opinions and report side effects. 'Active' hypertensive patients demonstrated a better understanding of their illness, fewer side effects, better adherence, greater adoption of health-promoting behaviour and, most important, better blood pressure control.

Brody *et al.* (1989) showed that patients reporting an active role in their medical visit were more satisfied with their doctors, had lower levels of illness concern and had a greater sense of control over their illness than passive patients.

Kaplan *et al.* (1989, 1996), in studies of chronic diseases (hypertension, insulin-dependent diabetes and rheumatoid arthritis) in both primary care and specialist settings, showed that patients whose physicians were less controlling and more participatory developed better functional status and better physiological outcomes. Patients of doctors who demonstrated a more participatory style were more satisfied and changed their doctors less frequently. Kaplan *et al.* also demonstrated that patients who were more active in the consultation reported fewer health problems and functional limitations due to their illness, and rated their health more favourably. Active patients also achieved better control of their hypertension and diabetes. But were these findings due to intrinsic differences in patients' personalities? Or was patient activity itself the key to these physiological improvements, and, if so, can such involvement in the consultation be improved by education?

To answer these questions, Kaplan *et al.* (1996) conducted a series of randomly controlled trials that separately looked at patients with hypertension, diabetes, breast cancer and ulcer disease. They investigated the effect of coaching patients in behavioural strategies to make them more active participants in the consultation. Patients were coached in how to improve their question asking, provided with techniques in negotiation and shown methods to decrease their embarrassment and fear of feeling foolish. They were also shown their own records and provided with algorithms to understand their treatment. These teaching interventions lead to marked differences in the interview and its consequences. Patients were more active in the interview, made more contributions to the discussion, obtained more information from their physicians and, most important, achieved both better self-reported health and better physiological control of their illnesses (including lower diastolic blood pressure readings and lower HbA_1 results). This improvement in physiological outcome confirms Rost *et al.*'s (1991) earlier work in diabetes. That these results have been obtained in a variety of chronic illnesses lends credence to this being a more generally applicable finding.

One interesting additional result was that more negative affect expressed by both physician and patient was related to better health outcomes. Negative affect in this context was defined as a broad spectrum of behaviours, including tension, anxiety, nervous laughter and self-consciousness as well as outright impatience or anger. This may well represent increased role tension induced by a change in the parties' normal relationship or, as Kaplan has called it, 'healthy friction'. Or it may be that doctors who are more engaged with their patients appear more anxious or concerned. Whatever, patients afterwards expressed a significantly stronger preference for active involvement in medical decision making. Hall *et al.* (1981) also showed that increased physician negative affect is associated with increased patient satisfaction.

These findings confirm the results of an earlier study by Roter (1977), who found that a simple ten-minute intervention prior to patients' consultations in primary care in which patients were helped to ask questions of their physicians led to a doubling of questions asked, a feeling of increased patient control and responsibility for their own health, and less drop-out from follow-up. Butow *et al.* (1994) showed that a question prompt sheet handed to patients 10 minutes before an oncology appointment increased patient question asking about prognosis but not overall numbers of questions. Brown *et al.* (2001) investigated the combined effect of the provision of a question prompt sheet prior to their initial consultation with an oncologist and the active endorsement and systematic review of the question prompt sheet by the oncologist. Patients provided with a question prompt sheet asked more questions about prognosis and oncologists gave significantly more prognostic information. Provision of the question prompt sheet prolonged consultations and increased patient anxiety; however, when oncologists specifically addressed the prompt sheet, anxiety levels were reduced, consultation duration was decreased and recall was improved. The same team found similar findings in terminally ill cancer patients discussing end of life issues (Clayton *et al.* 2007). They also discovered that physician endorsement of question asking itself without a prompt list did not increase question asking in the palliative care situation. Dimoska *et al.* (2008b) reviewed the evidence for the use of prompt sheets: a key finding in this review was that the prompt lists increased the likelihood that a patient would ask at least 1 question about prognosis, a topic that is typically avoided by both cancer patients and physicians during consultation. Later, the same team demonstrated the acceptability of prompt lists to both cancer patients and physicians during routine consultations (Dimoska *et al.* 2012).

Little *et al.* (2004) demonstrated the impact of leaflets encouraging patients to raise concerns and discuss symptoms in the consultation in British general practice. In a randomised controlled trial, a general leaflet encouraging patients to list issues they wanted to raise increased satisfaction particularly with shorter consultations although with some increase in numbers of investigations.

Shepherd *et al.* (2011) tested the effect of a set of three simple questions asked by unannounced simulated patients to general practitioners in a presentation of mild/moderate depression. These questions were:

1. *'What are my options?'*
2. *'What are the possible benefits and harms of those options?'*
3. *'How likely are the benefits and harms of each option to occur?'*

They demonstrated that asking these three questions improved information given by family physicians and increased physician facilitation of patient involvement without any increase in time.

Svarstad (1974) and Tuckett *et al.* (1985) have also shown that patients' willingness to ask questions or exhibit doubts leads to more information giving by doctors by alerting doctors to their patients' needs.

Fallowfield *et al.* (1990) found that women with breast cancer who were seen by surgeons who favoured offering patients a choice between mastectomy and lumpectomy suffered less anxiety and less depression than patients seen by surgeons who favoured either mastectomy or lumpectomy. This at first sight is strong support to the principle of enabling patients to share in decision making by allowing them choice. However, technical considerations prevented surgeons who favoured offering a choice from actually offering such a choice to 50% of their patients. Despite this, these patients still showed the same reduction in anxiety and depression as patients who were actually allowed to make a real choice. As Stewart (1995) comments, 'I would suggest that it is not just the decision making power of the patient that was effective but rather the provision of a caring, respectful and empowering context in which a woman was enabled to make an important decision with both support and comfort.' This conclusion remains conjecture but certainly some aspect of the surgeon's ability to relate and communicate with the patient is making a considerable difference to psychological outcome. Perhaps the willingness to share decision making is a reflection of these surgeons' shift towards a mutual rather than a paternalistic model.

Stewart *et al.* (1997) have shown that interviews in which patients perceived that the doctor and patient found common ground in the decision-making process (involving a mutual discussion of treatment options and goals and roles in management, checking for feedback, etc.) were associated with significantly fewer referrals and investigations over the two months following the interview. This suggests that a collaborative approach can reduce demands on the healthcare system.

While much of the research on patient involvement has been done in primary care contexts, findings in a study of preoperative interviews (Cegala *et al.* 2012) suggest that surgeons also may provide more detailed information to patients who are active participants. In a study assessing audio-recordings of consultations at a large tertiary care centre, Langseth *et al.* (2012) showed that where the shared decision making was of higher quality, patients referred for invasive treatment of cardiac electrical disease were more likely to change to a less invasive treatment option. These consultations often changed expected management.

In a review of evidence on patient–doctor communication, Stewart *et al.* (1999) found that the following aspects of communication about the management plan significantly influenced health outcomes:

- patient being encouraged to ask questions
- provision of clear information
- willingness of doctor to share decision making
- agreement between patient and doctor about the problem and the plan.

Heisler *et al.* (2007) showed that in older adults with diabetes, both their provider's provision of information and their provider's efforts to actively involve them in treatment decision making were associated with better overall diabetes self-management.

These positive associations between doctor–patient communication in this phase of the interview with health-related outcomes need to be tempered by the evidence from systematic reviews. Griffin *et al.* (2004) warned about the lack of rigorous trials of well-specified interventions to inform best practice. Although they found that principal outcomes favoured the interventions in almost three-quarters of the studies, often results failed to reach statistical significance. They did, however, find that there was a greater positive effect of interventions directed to patients than to practitioners, possibly related to the difficulty of consistently altering practitioner behaviour. Harrington *et al.* (2004) reviewed only interventions aimed directly at patients. Although they again found variable results, studies generally demonstrated success in increasing patient participation and control over health. Longer-term outcomes were rarely examined although the results were encouraging. Kinnersley *et al.* (2008) concluded that interventions for patients before consultations produce only small benefits for patients, and that, in general, interventions led to increases in question asking but little other benefit.

In a more recent selective review of the literature regarding patient engagement, including shared decision making, Coulter (2012) described 24 interventions that have been shown to support shared decision making and identified the evidence base behind those interventions. Based on her review of the literature she concluded that 'a) contrary to popular belief, there is a great deal of published evidence on the likely effectiveness of patient engagement strategies and b) there is a compelling case for adapting … healthcare delivery and practice styles to enable active engagement of patients in planning and shaping their health care.'

Do all patients want to be involved in shared decision making?

As with information giving, a proportion of patients will not wish active involvement and will prefer to leave decisions to their physicians. It is a mistake to assume that all patients wish to be involved in a collaborative approach to planning (Cassileth *et al.* 1980; Strull *et al.* 1984; Blanchard *et al.* 1988; Ende *et al.* 1989; Sutherland *et al.* 1989; Beisecker and Beisecker 1990; Hack *et al.* 1994; Guadagnoli and Ward 1998; Levinson *et al.* 2005). For instance, in the study by Strull *et al.* (1984) of hypertensive outpatients, only 53% of patients wished to take an active part in decision making. In a study by Blanchard *et al.* (1988) of cancer patients, 92% wanted information but only 69% wanted to participate in decision making: 25% of those wanting full information still wished the doctor to make the decisions.

Deber *et al.* (1996) questioned the results of previous studies that have shown a low desire of patients to participate in decision making. In their opinion, these studies failed to differentiate between the tasks of problem solving (requiring expertise and necessitating physician input) and decision making (where true choices involving trade-offs of advantages and disadvantages were available to the patient). In their own study, patients did not wish involvement in the former but mostly wished to be involved in the latter.

In a study by Degner *et al.* (1997) of 1012 women with a confirmed diagnosis of breast cancer attending hospital oncology clinics, 22% wanted to select their own cancer treatment, 44% wanted to select their treatment collaboratively with their doctors, and 34% wanted to delegate this decision making to their doctors. Only 42% of women believed they had achieved their preferred level of control in decision making. The substantial difference between women's preferred and attained level of involvement in decision making suggests that we need to look more carefully at how we are dealing with this important aspect of communication and care.

In a study by Gattellari *et al.* (2001) of cancer patients, mismatch between patients' preferred roles in decision making and what they perceived actually happened led to increased patient anxiety. However, whatever the preference of the patient prior to the interview, satisfaction with the consultation and the amount of information and emotional support received was significantly greater in those who reported a shared role. This gives support to the concept that as well as respecting individual differences in patient preference, part of the doctor's role might include gentle encouragement of patients over time to take part in shared decision making. Patients may not understand the benefits they stand to gain from articulating their preferences to their clinician. We know that doctors are not adept at eliciting their patients' preferences for treatment, and that many patients will not have experienced this sort of relationship in the past (Coulter *et al.* 1994; Robinson and Thomson 2001; Kiesler and Auerbach 2006; Burton *et al.* 2010).

Beach *et al.* (2007) looked further at the relationship between shared decision making and patient outcomes in patients with HIV. They found that patients who preferred to share decisions with their HIV provider had better outcomes than both those who wanted their HIV provider to make decisions and those who wanted to make decisions alone. Patients who preferred to make decisions alone were significantly less likely to receive highly active antiretroviral therapy or to have undetectable HIV RNA. They suggest that practising clinicians ought to encourage patients toward a shared decision-making role, not just activating patients who are disengaged but also building trust and rapport with patients who are highly independent.

In their systematic review of 115 studies on patient preferences for shared decisions, Chewning *et al.* (2012) demonstrated that the number of patients who prefer participation in decision making has increased over the past three decades – patients preferred a role in decision making in 50% of studies before 2000, compared with 71% from 2000 and later. This trend is particularly strong for cancer studies, where the majority of patients preferred to participate in decisions in 85% of the 27 cancer studies published in or after 2000 versus 62.5% of studies before 2000. All of the studies in the review also identified a subset of patients who want to delegate decisions. However, the majority of patients still want to discuss options and receive information from their physician even though they may not wish to make the final decision.

Based on focus group discussions and survey interviews with 1068 patients in the United States, Novelli *et al.* (2012) found that nine out of ten patients agreed overall that they want to know all their options; nearly half strongly agreed that they wanted to discuss the option of doing nothing. However, far fewer people said that they were offered options than wanted to discuss them. Patients reported a better experience when they were actively engaged.

The approach that we advocate here is not to make assumptions but to openly ask about patients' preferences for involvement in the process of shared decision making. Even if the patient does not wish to be involved in decision making at the moment, such a discussion will alert the patient to the fact that this is an option that they can return to in the future without criticism from the doctor. The question that we need to address is *how* to discover each patient's individual wishes rather than make assumptions. Although older patients, less educated patients and those with more serious illnesses have in past studies been more likely to prefer a non-participatory role (Degner and Sloan 1992; Belcher *et al.* 2006), many of them will choose to be informed and involved. In a qualitative study in 11 European countries, Bastiaens *et al.* (2007) demonstrated that older patients do want to be involved in their care but their definition of involvement is more focused on the 'caring relationship', 'person-centred approach' and 'receiving information' than on 'active participation in decision making'. Older patients considered involvement as 'taking time to elicit their preferences and needs and enabling them to take an active role in caring for their health accordingly'. However, the authors also comment that older patients' wish for involvement in decision making is highly heterogeneous, so an individual approach for each patient in the ageing population is needed. Similar findings were reported by Ekdahl *et al.* (2010). In their focus group study looking at older adults' views on informed decision making, Price *et al.* (2012) found that participants overwhelmingly endorsed existing criteria for shared decision-making and identified two additional elements: inviting the involvement of trusted others and exploring the impact of decisions in the context of the patient's life.

Strull *et al.* (1984) and Ende *at al.* (1989) have demonstrated how difficult it is to guess each patient's desire for involvement in making decisions without enquiring directly. Rather than guess or force all patients to adopt a collaborative role, it is the doctor's task to ascertain individual patients' preferences for participation and to tailor their approach accordingly.

Muller-Engelmann *et al.* (2011) explored the situational factors involved in whether patients wish to be involved in shared decision making. In severe illness, chronic conditions, more than one therapeutic option, end-of-life decisions and prevention, shared decision making was preferred whereas in emergency situations, a more paternalistic approach was suggested. In a large self-report survey in the Netherlands, van den Brink-Muinen *et al.* (2012) found that chronic care and disabled patients' preferences for shared decision making varied according to the type of care issue involved and that patients' actual involvement also varied, sometimes in the opposite direction of their stated preference. The study suggests that in chronic care contexts, healthcare providers need to pay close attention to their patients' varying preferences for shared decision making each time a new care issue requires decisions.

Since a patient's preferences for participation and information may vary depending on the nature or stage of the illness (Beaver *et al.* 1996; Chewning *et al.* 2012), preferences need to be discussed periodically over time and from situation to situation. Thus, discovering a patient's preference for participation in decision making should be conceptualised as an ongoing task rather than a one-off assessment made at a single meeting.

A monograph by Mulley *et al.* (2012) called 'Stop the Silent Misdiagnosis: Patients' Preferences Matter' summarises the evidence for the importance of patient preferences in decision making.

Ziebland *et al.* (2006) warn of the need for careful support of patients when involving them in choice about their treatments. In a set of qualitative interviews of women with ovarian cancer, they documented how the way in which options were offered to women sometimes lead to confusion and concern, especially if women felt the doctor was unwilling to express his or her own preference. They recommend that clinicians carefully explain about clinical uncertainty and how individual preferences may relate to treatment decisions. They asked clinicians to consider that patients may be left surprised or even shocked.

Politi *et al.* (2007, 2011b) have explored the inherent difficulties for patients in the communication of uncertainty of harms and benefits of medical interventions. In a study of female patients facing breast cancer treatment decisions, communicating uncertainty was negatively related to decision satisfaction. The authors conclude that this outcome could be a natural outcome of the decision-making process and that involving patients in decisions may make them able to tolerate uncertainty better.

Interestingly, Gordon *et al.* (2000) reported the opposite finding, that overt expression of uncertainty by physicians in the consultation was associated with greater patient satisfaction.

What skills can we recommend to learners to help them achieve shared decision making in planning?

A collaborative approach to planning requires the use of many skills through-out the consultation (Towle and Godolphin 1999; Elwyn *et al.* 2003b; Fallowfield 2008). A key challenge for doctors is to create an environment in which the patient feels comfortable to engage in this collaborative process in the first place. The skills of relationship building and development of a partnership, as discussed in Chapter 5, are therefore all important here. But what additional specific skills can we use in this part of the consultation to enable the theory and research on shared decision making to be translated into clinical practice?

Sharing own thinking as appropriate: ideas, thought processes and dilemmas

One specific skill that contributes to a more collaborative approach to planning is for the doctor to share her own thought processes, ideas and dilemmas as appropriate. This offers advantages to doctor and patient alike.

- Uncertainty is reduced and mutually understood common ground established. The patient begins to understand the rationale behind the doctor's suggestions and what the dilemmas in a particular situation are. The patient is not left guessing why you are proceeding along a certain path.
- It encourages patients to contribute their views. After your dilemmas have been made apparent, the patient often contributes a statement that establishes their preference or gives further information helpful to your decision making. Sharing your ideas is a signal that you might be interested in hearing your patient's views, thus encouraging more open communication.
- It forces you to order your information giving. Doctors often skip over diagnosis, aetiology and prognosis and go straight to treatment – the sharing approach helps to prevent the omission of logical steps or information that patients need if they are to participate effectively in decision making.

'There are two possibilities here that might explain your symptoms, either an ulcer or gallstones. It's not clear from just examining you which it is. I'm trying to decide between two ways forward – we can either just treat it as if it is an ulcer or we could do some tests first to get a more definite diagnosis ...'

Involving the patient

Offering suggestions and choices rather than directives

In order to involve the patient in the decision-making process, the physician needs to outline the possible management options that she thinks are available, rather than propose one particular course of action:

> *'Given what you have said, I think there are two choices available that we ought to consider together – first, starting hormone replacement therapy now, and second, simply soldiering on for the moment and seeing what happens to your symptoms over the next few months.'*

Encouraging the patient to contribute their ideas and suggestions

The physician can actively encourage the patient to contribute their ideas and suggestions too. The patient may well have other options in mind that the doctor has not considered. Remember that many patients are reluctant to express their views directly to the doctor and need to be asked overtly if they are to overcome their hesitation. If the doctor signposts a clear interest in the patient's comments, in future the patient may be more confident in coming forth spontaneously with suggestions:

> *'You have probably thought about this a lot, too. Are those the choices as you see it?, What are your own thoughts?'*
>
> *'Well, really I'm most concerned about osteoporosis, so I was also wondering about not taking hormone replacement therapy at all. My friend is on something called a biphosphonate – would that be suitable?'*

Exploring management options with the patient

Next, it is important for the physician to explore the options available to the patient in more depth, and provide information about the risks and benefits of each, including the option of no treatment or action.

> *'So to recap, we have agreed there are three approaches you could take here. The first would be to consider taking hormone replacement therapy, the second would be to see how you go without medication for the time being and revisit the issue at a later date, and the third would be to look at using biphosphonates. Would it help if I ran through the risks and benefits of each courses of action now?'*

The frequency with which patients are provided options varies considerably. Fowler Jr *et al.* (2012) discovered that prostate patients reported more involvement in decision making than elective coronary artery stent patients: 64% of prostate patients were given at least one option, compared with only 10% of stent patients;

63% of prostate patients said their doctors discussed cons, compared with 19% of stent patients.

Two extremely important areas in exploring options with patients have been the subject of considerable research in the last decade. The first is the issue of explaining risks in a truly objective fashion that patients can understand and use in their decision making. The second is the use of written information and decision aids to help patients understand the options available to them and choose between them. It is beyond the scope of this book to explore these complex areas in depth and we merely highlight the issues here.

Risk communication

In the communication of risk (Gigerenzer 2002; Edwards *et al.* 2000; Mazur 2000; Edwards *et al.* 2002; Gigerenzer and Edwards 2003; Halvorsen *et al.* 2007; Apter *et al.* 2008; Gaissmaier and Gigerenzer 2008; Longman *et al.* 2012), great care needs to be taken in the use of the following:

- **the statistical presentation of risk**: use of absolute and relative risk, numbers needed to treat and natural frequencies
- **framing effects**: framing is defined as presenting logically equivalent information in different ways – for example, 'a 98% chance of surviving an operation' as opposed to 'a 2% chance of dying'.

The most accessible way of presenting risk information to patients is by using natural frequencies rather than percentages. An example would be: 'if 100 people just like yourself took no action, at the end of 10 years 6 of those 100 people would have a heart attack or stroke. If those same 100 people took blood pressure medication for 10 years, 4 people would have a heart attack or stroke' (Gigerenzer 2002).

There is great potential to provide biased information of risk by the selective use of statistics and the way that information is presented (the framing effect). An example of this is explored by Hudak *et al.* (2011), who looked at orthopaedic surgeons' consultations in Canada. Although surgeons skilfully adapted their recommendations to the views and expectations of their patients, these efforts were counterbalanced by an overarching institutional bias favouring surgery over other treatment options. This bias shaped not only how recommendations for and against surgery were communicated in the first place, but also extended to differences in the methods surgeons used to counter patient resistance when it arose.

Such bias can be unintentional or deliberate. This issue is particularly important when looking at risk communication in the context of shared decision making (Edwards and Elwyn 2001b). Often in the past the outcome of risk communication was measured by the uptake of screening programmes or the adoption of treatments felt to be most beneficial by doctors. Statistics could easily be quoted that, although true, magnified the benefits and minimised the risks to any one individual of adopting a particular course. In such circumstances, relative risk has often been used to magnify and absolute risk to minimise effects. While this might be justified from the population viewpoint of public health with an eye to the well-being of a whole nation, from an individual's perspective the only acceptable outcome measure for risk communication is the provision of unbiased information leading to an increase in the patient's ability to come to an informed decision (Thornton *et al.* 2003). Otherwise we are back in the area of compliance rather than concordance, and in the province of influence rather than shared decison making.

The way in which risk statistics are represented also needs to be taken into account:

- words vs. numerical representation
- visual and graphic display formats.

A particular problem here is that individuals vary greatly in the way that they prefer to receive complex information, and it is therefore difficult to design formats that will suit everyone. Here again we underscore the value of developing a repertoire of skills and approaches so that you can be more flexible when interacting with each individual (Edwards 2004).

This is not simply a problem of explaining difficult concepts to patients. As Thornton (2009) argues, both doctors and patients need to understand numbers if meaningful dialogues are to occur and there is considerable evidence of statistical illiteracy in the medical profession as well. Collins and Street (2009) describe a shared dialogue approach about risk perceptions between physician and patient to enable quality decisions to be made. A study by Janssen *et al.* (2009) highlights the balance required between the overall finding that patients in general wish to be informed about possible low-risk complications of a procedure and the reaffirmation that patients have different information preference styles. The authors recommend a stepwise approach, where physicians initially tell patients, in broad terms, what the more likely complications of an intervention might be. In a second step, they should try to ascertain to what extent the patient wants to be informed. Based on the patient's information preferences, a tailored approach to discussing risks can be chosen.

Longman *et al.* (2012) raise an additional concern regarding how risk estimates are presented. In a study of university students, they demonstrated that communicating uncertainty in risk estimates has the potential to negatively affect understanding, increase perceptions of risk and decrease perceived credibility.

Decision aids

The field of decision aids is concerned with how to improve the quality of patient's decision making by supplementing existing communication between professionals and patients (O'Connor and Edwards 2001; Robinson and Thomson 2001; Sepucha and Mulley 2003; O'Brien *et al.* 2009; Bunge *et al.* 2010; Elwyn 2011; Myers *et al.* 2011). Some decision aids are designed to be used by patients on their own, as a platform for discussions in further consultations, and some are for use during consultations. Decision aids provide information about possible choices and probabilities of different outcomes, but they go further than simple information leaflets to help clarify patients' values and provide guidance as to how to come to a decision, although there is debate about how far this is possible (Nelson *et al.* 2007; Kaner *et al.* 2007). They help patients balance known benefit/harm ratios as provided by evidence-based medicine, scientific uncertainty and personal values and preferences. Decision aids have been shown to:

- improve patients' knowledge of problems, options and outcomes
- reduce the number of patients who are uncertain what to do
- create more realistic expectations of outcomes

- reduce decisional conflict (uncertainty)
- stimulate patients to be more active in decision making without increasing their anxiety.

Yet decision aids seem to have little effect on patient satisfaction and a variable effect on what decisions are eventually made. However, it is noteworthy that in major surgical decisions, decision aids reduce the preference for surgery by over 20% (O'Connor *et al.* 1999, 2001, 2003). The words of caution that we included earlier regarding written information and patients who are functionally illiterate or whose eyesight is compromised apply here again.

Establishing the level of involvement the patient wishes

One of the key aims of this part of the consultation should be to involve patients in decision making to the level that they wish. We have already seen that the large majority of patients wish to be involved in making choices but that a significant minority would prefer to leave decisions to their doctor. Therefore it is important for the doctors to ascertain each individual patient's preferences for participation in making choices and to tailor their approach accordingly rather than make assumptions without checking. We have also seen that this preference can change over time for each individual patient, so it is necessary to repeat this process periodically.

There are two ways that this can be achieved. Where genuine choice exists (and it often does), the doctor can gently encourage the patient to become involved:

> *'So, here are several things we might try here, each, as I've said, with their own advantages and disadvantages ... have you any clear preference?'*

The patient may respond with either:

> *'Well, overall I'm not a tablet-taking person and, given what you have said, I think I would rather soldier on with the sore throat and let nature take its course.'*

or

> *'I'm not sure – what would you recommend, doctor?'*

Here the patient may be indirectly expressing whether they have a desire to be involved in decision making. A more direct way of discovering the patient's preference in making choices about their care is to ask explicitly:

> Doctor: *'There are several options in the treatment of Parkinson's disease – when to start therapy, which of the drugs we use to treat it, whether you see a specialist. Some patients like to be involved in these decisions and I welcome that. Some prefer for the doctor to take the lead. How would you like to play this yourself at the moment?'*
>
> Patient: *'Well, I'd really like to know what options I have and then discuss the best choice with you.'*

Negotiating a mutually acceptable plan

Next, the doctor and the patient need to come to a decision that both can agree upon.

Signposting position of equipoise or own preferences

As we have said, in the shared decision-making model it is perfectly acceptable for the doctor, having explored the possibilities, to state a preference, as long as he clearly signposts this and also indicates that the patient's position is just as important as that of the doctor. It is equally possible that the physician is in a position of 'equipoise' and genuinely does not have a preference for which of several treatments the patient might choose:

> *'In this particular instance and from a purely medical standpoint, I personally would come down on one side here. I think given the very strong history of ischaemic heart disease in your family and the effect that has on your risk equation, that you would be best to take medication to reduce your blood pressure. But we need to take your views into account here – it is still a balancing of the risks and benefits.'*
>
> or
>
> *'Overall, I think the position is finely balanced and I don't have a strong feeling either way whether you should take blood pressure medication yet. I think it comes down to the relative importance you place on the various things we have discussed.'*

Establishing the patient's preferences

Note that there is a hierarchy of ways of making plans with patients, from paternalistic directives and orders ('You must do the following …') to consumerist handing over of all decision making to the patient ('I'll do whatever you want'). In the shared decision-making model that this chapter espouses, both the doctor's and patient's views can be expressed to good effect, but the doctor is careful both to offer ideas as suggestions for consideration by the patient and to listen carefully to the patient's own ideas and responses:

> *'What do you think overall? What would be your preference?'*

Epstein and Peters (2009) have written eloquently about the difficulties of establishing patients' preferences and have explored the cognitive, emotional and relationship factors that affect how patients' preferences are constructed, especially when patients are faced with complex and unfamiliar situations. When patients confront highly difficult situations, cognitive and emotional elements in decision making are both highly important. The authors suggest that through communication, physicians can more effectively engage patients in constructing preferences in the face of uncertainty, informed by understanding how patients and clinicians think in the complex, unforeseen and sometimes terrifying situations that patients face. Results of Weiner and Roth's (2006) thematic literature review on goals of care discussions with patients and families near the end of life also underscore the importance of including not only cognitive but also integral emotional and social elements of these difficult discussions.

Negotiating differences

The doctor can make it clear to the patient that he wishes to share the decision making, resolve differences and negotiate a mutually acceptable plan:

> *'What I've suggested makes sense to me ... but if it isn't right for you, we'll need to think again ... tell me what you feel about it.'*
>
> or
>
> *'I do have some reservations about taking the approach you suggest. Can I explain them to you and then perhaps we can try to find a solution that works for both of us?'*

Checking with the patient

As a final check at the end of planning, it is good practice to confirm if the patient is happy with the decisions that have been made, if the patient accepts the plans and if her concerns have been addressed:

> *'Now, can I just check that you are happy with the plan?'*

OPTIONS IN EXPLANATION AND PLANNING

The four sections already discussed are common to all consultations featuring explanation and planning. We now discuss three optional elements that may or may not be applicable to any one interview:

1. if offering opinion and discussing significance of problems
2. if negotiating mutual plan of action
3. if discussing investigations and procedures.

We include both process and content items as we look at the skills associated with each option.

If offering opinion and discussing significance of problems

We have already discussed the evidence that doctors tend to discuss treatment and drug therapy while patients are more interested in diagnosis, prognosis and causation of their illness (Kindelan and Kent 1987; Helman 1981) and that patients often come away from the medical interview without even basic information about their illness (Boreham and Gibson 1978; Svarstad 1974). Tuckett *et al.* (1985) have shown that patients' understanding and commitment to management plans is often poor because doctors seldom explain their rationale in any detail or provide explanations related to the patient's illness framework.

So what specific skills can we recommend to help us explain our opinion about a problem? The following are four key skills that help in this section of the interview:

1. offering opinion of what is going on and naming if possible
2. revealing rationale for opinion
3. explaining causation, seriousness, expected outcome, short- and long-term consequences
4. eliciting patient's beliefs, reactions and concerns (e.g. if opinion matches patient's thoughts, acceptability, feelings).

A common example demonstrates these skills in action:

> *'You've told me a lot about this pain in your elbow. I think the problem is tennis elbow ... and the reason why I think that this is the diagnosis is because ... Does that fit in with what you were thinking? All right, I think the reason why it might have come on now is because ... and it may give you discomfort for several months, I'm afraid. I don't think it's serious, and from what you've told me you are not concerned that it might be arthritis. How does that strike you?'*

If negotiating a mutual plan of action

The specific skills that we can use here are as follows.

- Discussing options – for example, no action, investigation, medication or surgery, non-drug treatments (physiotherapy, walking aids, fluids, counselling), preventive measures.
- Providing information on action or treatment offered:
  - name
  - steps involved, how it works
  - benefits and advantages
  - possible side effects or disadvantages.
- Obtaining patient's view of need for action, perceived benefits, barriers, motivation.
- Accepting patient's views, advocates alternative viewpoint as necessary.
- Eliciting patient's reactions and concerns about plans and treatments, including acceptability.

- Taking patient's lifestyle, beliefs, cultural background and abilities into consideration.
- Encouraging patient to be involved in implementing plans, to take responsibility and to be self-reliant.
- Asking about patient support systems, discussing other support available.

Discussing and offering options in management and treatment

Offering options is the first step in enabling patient choice. How can a patient with back pain choose whether to try physiotherapy, osteopathy, pain relief, rest or no treatment without having the possible options clearly explained first?

Providing information on action or treatment offered

Providing information about a proposed management or treatment is a highly skilled task. Consider, for example, the scenario of a man seeking advice about changing his drug therapy for mildly raised blood pressure. Not only does the doctor have to give a clear explanation of how the treatment works and tailor his explanation to the patient's understanding and needs, but also he must describe the risks and benefits of the treatments accurately, taking into account the patient's concerns. The doctor must describe and discuss the potential side effects of the treatments, explain the different preparations available and explain how to take the preparation if the patient chooses to take one.

Obtaining the patient's view of need for action, perceived benefits, barriers and motivation

Balanced against the information that the doctor brings to the consultation are the knowledge, attitudes, values, priorities and beliefs of the patient. These are equally important and valid in reaching a decision about the most appropriate way forward. The patient's views about perceived benefits, barriers and motivations need to be elicited if a shared decision is to be reached.

This is true for any decision in medicine. However, considering barriers and motivation has been particularly emphasised in the field of health promotion. Prevention and health promotion are increasingly important parts of the doctor's domain. Health workers in the fields of drug and alcohol addiction, smoking cessation and weight loss work with a number of useful psychological and communication models that enable them to maximise change in their clients' health-related behaviour.

Greene and Hibbard (2012) provide evidence linking patient activation (i.e. knowledge, skills, beliefs and confidence for managing health and healthcare) with health outcomes. In a cross-sectional study of 25 047 patients undertaken in a Minnesota health service, the authors found that more activated patients were more likely to have received preventive care, less likely to smoke or have a high body mass index and had better clinical indicators. They were less likely to have been hospitalised or to have used the emergency department. The study found no evidence that socio-economic status affected the relationship between patient activation and 10 out of 12 outcomes.

Priest and Speller (1991) cite three sets of skills in which a practitioner needs to be effective to help a patient change to a healthier lifestyle:

1. knowledge about risk factors
2. awareness and understanding about the patient's attitude to the problem affecting his health
3. knowledge and application of the skills involved in helping people to change.

Motivational interviewing

Motivational interviewing (Miller and Rollnick 1991) utilises these three sets of skills to foster the individual's desire to make behaviour changes. In motivational interviewing, the practitioner's immediate task is to discover first the patient's health beliefs and second the patient's readiness for change. Only then can the practitioner determine how best to act to help each patient.

Motivational interviewing is based on the 'stages of change' model (*see* Figure 6.1), originally designed by Prochaska and DiClemente (1986) and further developed in practice by Miller (1983) and van Bilson and van Emst (1989). The model describes a natural series of stages that people work through when considering change. It recognises that at each of these stages people have different frames of mind and that professional intervention is more likely to be successful if

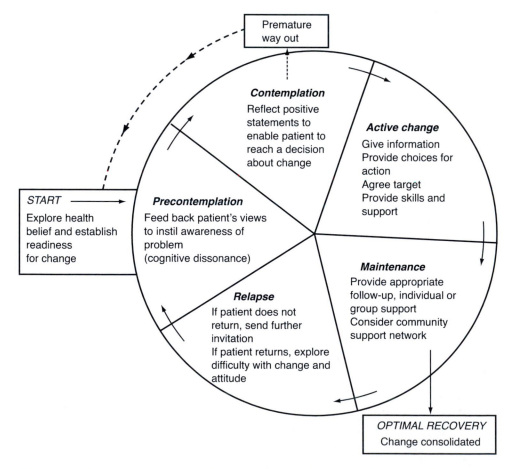

Figure 6.1 Intervention process using the stages of change model. Adapted from the work of Prochaska and DiClemente (1986).

tailored closely to whichever stage the individual is in at present. The practitioner's role is to discover where the patient is in the process of self-motivation and encourage and support their efforts. Patients' levels of confidence (in their ability to make the change) and conviction (regarding how convinced they are that the change is important) will influence their success (Keller and Kemp-White 2001; Rollnick *et al.* 1997). Motivational interviewing attempts to empower patients to take responsibility for their own decisions by increasing their self-esteem and self-efficacy, by respecting their views and concerns and by negotiating suitable targets.

Note that motivational interviewing uses many of the core skills already discussed in this book: listening, exploring patient's beliefs, the use of open questions, reflection, summarising, providing choices, negotiation, acceptance and support. Useful texts that deal with motivational interviewing and the locus of control are Miller and Rollnick (2002), Dye and DiMatteo (1995) and Butler *et al.* (1996).

In contrast to most other models for behaviour change, which are complex and based on the 50-minute counselling session, Keller and Kemp-White (2001) created a model for influencing patient behaviour that enables clinicians to have an impact on patient behaviour in a brief office visit.

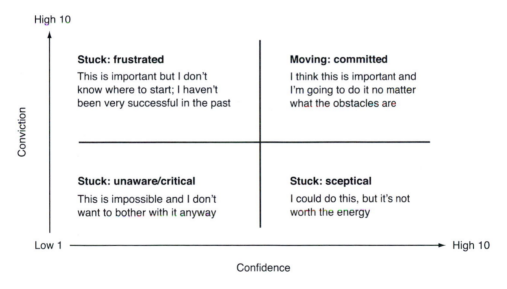

Figure 6.2 Confidence and conviction grid (Keller and Kemp-White 2001).

In this model, the clinician assesses the patient's readiness for change within two dimensions – namely, conviction ('Do I believe that making this change will enhance my well-being?') and confidence ('Do I believe that I can make this change?'). An intervention to increase the patient's confidence, conviction, or both can then be applied to help the patient move into a position of high conviction and high confidence. Specific strategies are suggested for working with patients who are low in both dimensions or high in one and low in the other. The model is applicable to a wide variety of patient health behaviours from following medication regimens to exploring risky behaviour such as smoking or obesity.

Rollnick *et al.* (1999, 2010) offer another approach called 'health behaviour change' that attempts to bring together the lessons from patient-centred method and motivational interviewing while at the same time enlarging the scope of motivational interviewing from addiction and health promotion to many more common clinical encounters. This development helps to deflect one criticism of motivational and behavioural change interviewing – namely, that implicit within a method that attempts to help people to change in a particular way must be an element of 'doctor knows best', of influencing and manipulation, and of attempting to achieve a predetermined outcome dominated by the professional's agenda of what is 'right'. In other words, it sounds suspiciously like attempting to get patients to comply with doctors' advice. This is not surprising, given that motivational interviewing was born from work with patients with severe addictions where the 'right' outcome was clear to see. In this approach to health behaviour change, Rollnick and colleagues more clearly established that the patient must first be allowed to decide what he would like to do with the help of patient-centred interviewing and shared decision making. The practitioner's role is therefore to help people to make decisions within their own frame of reference and only then, once the patient has identified an outcome he would like to achieve, does the practitioner try to enable the patient to assess the importance of the issue, the patient's confidence level in achieving what he would like to do and the patient's readiness to move.

Accepting patient's views and advocating an alternative viewpoint as necessary

In Chapter 5 we discussed the key concept of initially accepting and acknowledging the legitimacy of patients' ideas without necessarily agreeing with them. Non-judgemental acceptance allows us later to offer our own perspective of the problem in light of the patient's beliefs, discuss misperceptions, advocate a different approach if necessary and negotiate an agreed plan. But what if we feel that patients' attitudes are seriously affecting their health yet they brush aside our suggestions? How can we challenge a firmly held belief without denigrating the patient?

Challenging and confronting patients

Being honest in the medical interview can present difficulties for the doctor, particularly when faced with patients who appear not to be confronting an important problem. Conflict with patients is usually unproductive and can leave the patient feeling both angry and unsupported.

Contrast:

> *'You must stop smoking at once. You are a fool not to stop. I can't be responsible for what happens if you don't.'*

with:

> *'I know that it is difficult for you to stop smoking at the moment … you are going through a difficult patch … but your chest has gotten a lot worse in the last year and I'm concerned that you will continue to deteriorate this winter if you don't stop. What could we do to help you?'*

Honesty and the ability to challenge beliefs in a constructive manner are important parts of enabling patients to change

If discussing investigations and procedures

During the medical interview we often need to give information about investigations or procedures. Remember that what may seem to be trivial to the doctor may be highly alarming to the patient. A simple blood test may be terrifying. A two-week wait for the result of a mammogram for a patient who fears breast cancer can seem like a lifetime. Listening, empathy and achieving a shared understanding are all important. There are three key skills in this area of the consultation.

1. Providing clear information on procedures including what the patient might experience and how the patient will be informed of results.
2. Relating procedures to the treatment plan – value and purpose.
3. Encouraging questions about and discussion of potential anxieties or negative outcomes.

Summary: explanation and planning is an interactive process

In much of this chapter we have advocated an interactive approach to explanation and planning – just giving information and dictating plans is clearly not enough. In Chapter 3 we discussed the limitations of direct transmission. If communication is viewed as a direct transmission process, the senders of messages assume that their responsibilities as communicators are fulfilled once they have formulated and sent a message. However, if communication is viewed as an interactive process, the interaction is complete only if the sender receives feedback about how the message is interpreted, whether it is understood and what impact it has on the receiver (Dance and Larson 1972).

We demonstrated that summarising and checking are the key skills that enable this interactive approach to be put into practice in the information-gathering phase of the interview by providing feedback to the patient about what we think we have heard and understood. Now we have seen how further skills are required in the explanation and planning phase to ensure a similar degree of interaction. And we have seen again the significant role that relationship building plays. Shared decision making and other interactive processes in the explanation and planning stages of the consultation are enhanced when a relationship conducive to collaboration and partnership between patient and doctor has already been developed earlier in the interview.

In the explanation and planning phase, we do not give a one-sided speech. To give information accurately, we need to check repeatedly whether we have made ourselves clear and whether the patient understands our thoughts before proceeding to the next chunk of information. We have seen how:

- a two-way interaction enables us to discover what information we have not yet provided

- asking the patient to restate the information they have just been told dramatically increases retention and understanding
- we need to give the patient encouragement to ask questions, express doubts and seek clarification if we are to achieve a shared understanding and prevent non-adherence
- we need to understand our patients' ideas if we want to align our explanations to our patients' needs
- we need to involve the patient in planning by allowing them to be part of the decision-making process and to voice their preferences.

We hope this chapter has convinced you to continue the trend away from merely 'giving' information to patients and towards 'sharing' understanding and decision making. This shift promises not only more satisfying consultations for both patients and doctors but also better long-term health outcomes. The trend toward sharing understanding and decision making is likely to be even more important as populations increase and age in the next 25 years.

Chapter 7

Closing the session

Introduction

Communication problems at the end of the consultation often relate to time issues. Just as you think that you have satisfactorily completed the interview and are drawing the session to an end, the patient introduces another major item. Just as you begin to organise follow-up arrangements, the patient asks a question that makes it clear that he has not understood any of your explanations so far. The doctor wants to close things down and push on to the next appointment – the patient seems keen to open things up again. These unmatched agendas easily lead to conflict and frustration.

What skills can we recommend to help with these problems? Difficulties in closure often emanate from communication issues occurring much earlier in the consultation. They can be avoided by attention to our use of communication skills during the beginning, information-gathering, and explanation and planning phases of the interview. Once these have been addressed, problems in this part of the consultation tend to evaporate.

However, there are specific communication skills in the closing phase, too. Summarising and clarifying plans that have been made and the next steps for both parties, establishing what the patient should do if things do not go according to plan, checking that the patient is comfortable with the follow-up arrangements, continuing to build the doctor–patient relationship – these are all essential elements of the consultation and contribute to improved adherence, satisfaction and health outcomes.

In this chapter we explore two separate but related questions.

1. What are the skills used throughout the rest of the consultation that can help closure to be more efficient?
2. What are the skills during closure itself that will help to bring the consultation to a satisfactory end?

Objectives

Our objectives for this part of the interview may be summarised as follows:

- confirming the established plan of care
- clarifying the next steps for both doctor and patient
- establishing contingency plans
- maximising patient adherence and health outcomes
- making efficient use of time in the consultation

- continuing to encourage the patient to feel part of a collaborative process and to build the doctor–patient relationship for the future.

Again these objectives encompass some of the tasks and checkpoints mentioned in other well-known guides to the consultation.

- Pendleton *et al.* (1984, 2003):
  - to use time and resources appropriately.
- Neighbour (1987):
  - safety-netting: 'what if?' – consider what the doctor might do in each case.
- AAPP Three-Function Model (Cohen-Cole 1991):
  - education, negotiation and motivation
  - developing rapport and responding to the patient's emotions.
- Bayer Institute for Health Care Communication E4 model (Keller and Carroll 1994):
  - educating the patient
  - enlisting the patient in his or her own healthcare.
- The Four Habits Model (Frankel and Stein 1999; Krupat *et al.* 2006):
  - investing in the end.
- The SEGUE Framework for teaching and assessing communication skills (Makoul 2001):
  - ending the encounter.
- The Maastricht Maas Global (van Thiel and van Dalen 1995):
  - management – determining who will do what and when.
- Essential Elements of Communication in Medical Encounters: Kalamazoo Consensus Statement (Participants in the Bayer-Fetzer Conference on Physician–Patient Communication in Medical Education 2001):
  - provide closure.
- Patient-centred medicine (Stewart *et al.* 2003):
  - time and timing.
- The Model of the Macy Initiative in Health Communication (Kalet *et al.* 2004):
  - close.

The process skills for closing the session

The following skills work together to help us to achieve the objectives for this part of the consultation.

Box 7.1 Skills for closing the session

Forward planning
- **Contracting**: contracts with patient regarding next steps for patient and physician
- **Safety-netting**: safety-nets appropriately – explains possible unexpected outcomes, what to do if plan is not working, when and how to seek help

---

> **Ensuring appropriate point of closure**
> - **End summary**: summarises session briefly and clarifies plan of care
> - **Final checking**: checks that patient agrees and is comfortable with plan and asks if any corrections, questions or other issues

'What' to teach and learn about endings: the evidence for the skills

Before looking at the specific skills that contribute to effective endings, it is worth considering some of the issues that commonly arise at this point in the interview and looking at some of the behaviours and skills from *earlier* in the interview that help prevent problems and aid effectiveness.

What actually happens in the closing section of the interview?

White *et al.* (1994) have looked specifically at closure and have attempted to separate this element of the consultation from the explanation and planning phase. Listening to audiotapes of primary care physicians in Oregon, they identified closure by looking for sentences that demonstrated a transition from the educational to the ending phase – for example, *'OK, let's see you back in 5 months'* or *'We'll just see how it goes in the future'*. Their results were as follows:

- length of visits: average 16.8 minutes
- length of closure: average 1.6 minutes (range 1–9 minutes)
- closure initiated by physician: in 86% of consultations
- new problems discussed that were not mentioned earlier in the visit: in 21% of closures
- physician behaviours in closure:
  - clarifying the plan (75%)
  - orienting the patient to next steps (56%)
  - providing information about the condition or therapy (53%)
  - checking for understanding (34%)
  - asking whether the patient has more questions (25%).

Bronshtein *et al.* (2006) showed in a study of Israeli specialists and family physicians, with consultation lengths averaging 9 minutes, that the patient never initiated termination in any of the 320 encounters observed.

Rhodes *et al.* (2004) in a study in an academic medical centre emergency department in the United States showed that discharge instructions averaged 76 seconds. Information on diagnosis, expected course of illness, self-care, use of medications, time-specified follow-up and symptoms that should prompt return to the emergency department were each discussed less than 65% of the time. Only 16% of patients were asked whether they had questions, and there were no instances in which the provider confirmed patient understanding of the information.

What behaviours earlier in the visit prevent new problems from arising during closure?

White *et al.* (1994) found the following behaviours earlier in the visit tended to prevent new problems from arising during closure:

- physicians using signposting to orient patients to the flow of the visit (*'Now I'm going to examine you and then we will have some time to discuss what's going on'*)
- physicians giving more information about the therapeutic regimen
- patients talking more about their therapy
- physicians asking for patients' beliefs and being more responsive to patients.

Barsky (1981) used the term 'hidden agendas' to describe problems that only surface in the closing moments of the interview. These are often emotionally charged or psychosocial issues, and he surmised that such late presentations of problems may well relate to the failure of the physician to facilitate disclosure earlier. Patients wait for the 'right' moment to present their 'real' problem – if it is not deliberately provided earlier on, the opportunity may not present itself until the very end of the interview.

In Chapter 2 we have already described the key research of Beckman and Frankel (1984) on how our use of words and questions can easily and inadvertently direct the patient away from telling us their real reasons for coming to see us. Premature physician interruption and failure to screen for problems early on in the interview lead to an increase in late-arising complaints.

In a study of third-year family physician residents, Ruiz Moral *et al.* (2006) showed that patients mentioned new problems at closure (*'Oh, by the way ...'*) more frequently when physicians redirected the focus of the interview before patients had completed an initial statement of concerns in the early moments of the visit. More than half of the trainees directed the focus of the interview before the patient had completed an initial statement of concerns. Early redirection did not save overall consultation time but instead made closures longer and more dysfunctional by patients raising new problems at this phase of the interview.

What communication skills can we recommend in the earlier sections of the consultation that will aid efficient and satisfactory closure of the session?

Box 7.2

Beginnings
- Attentive listening
- Screening
- Agenda setting

Information gathering
- Signposting
- Exploring the patient's ideas and concerns
- Addressing the patient's feelings, thoughts and emotions
- Discussing psychosocial issues

Explanation and planning
- Information giving
- Involving patients in explanation and planning
- Checking for the patient's understanding
- Asking for the patient's questions

What behaviours during closure are associated with inefficient endings?

White *et al.* (1994) discovered that the following behaviours during closure were associated with longer endings:

- physicians asking open questions
- physicians laughing or showing emotions, concern or responsiveness to patients
- patients engaging in psychosocial discussion, being friendly, dominant, responsive or in distress.

But are we trying to achieve a shorter closure? There is clearly a tension here between efficiency and completeness. If the doctor wishes to end the consultation more efficiently, one option would be to behave in a more closed fashion. However, if the patient has further questions or hidden problems to discuss, closing them down will not maximise the full potential of the interview (Robinson JD 2001). It may instead add time both to the immediate interview and in the long term.

We should not abandon behaving in an open, collaborative and patient-centred way during closure. Our previous behaviour in the consultation will hopefully allow the patient at this stage to say, 'No, I think you have answered all my questions' or 'No, I haven't any other problems'. Yet, however well the consultation has proceeded, there will still be patients who leave their most embarrassing or worrying concern until the very end, until they have plucked up courage to broach it. We must not shut them out simply for the sake of short-term efficiency.

In a further qualitative study, White *et al.* (1997) clarified this area further. They showed that 36% of closures were interrupted, with new problems surfacing in 23% of visits. Interruptions occurred even with open-ended beginnings and early physician requests for all of the patient's concerns. They surmised that interrupted closures that produce new agenda items might be less effective than others, increasing frustration for doctors and reducing patients' satisfaction with care. While recognising that the medical visit is complicated and that doctors and patients can inadvertently forget things until the end, or that doctors may empathise with patients late in the visit, the authors made three observations about interrupted closures that may improve physician efficiency.

1. Only when both patient and doctor are ready to close the visit will they be able to do so successfully – listening and exploring patients' beliefs and concerns earlier in the visit will prepare the way for smooth closure later
2. Doctors should beware of asking, *'Is there anything else?'* or *'Do you have some other concerns you want to discuss?'* so late in the interview that they are not expecting a positive reply. Doctors should ask for any final concerns *before* they start the process of closure rather than at the very end, so that late-arising concerns can be meaningfully addressed. This screening for uncompleted business should therefore precede the move to closure.
3. Clear signposting of the stages of the interview helps the patient to understand the process of the interview and what is happening at each stage – the optimal time for providing unstated concerns may then be more apparent to all. In our view, this would occur throughout the interview and include signalling that you are moving to closure – for example, by saying, *'I think we're just about finished … is there anything else you'd hoped to discuss?'*

Tai-Seale *et al.* (2007) explored the importance of investing in the end of the clinical encounter to ensure patients understand decisions. They discovered that the amount of time a patient spoke was a significant determinant of topics ending with explicit decisions. They recommended strengthening the patient's voice, a clear statement of decisions and written 'exit prescriptions' of plans made.

What are the specific elements of closure itself (see Box 7.1)?

Forward planning

Contracting

Contracting with the patient about the next steps for both patient and physician allows each party to identify their mutual roles and responsibilities (Stewart *et al.* 1997). The doctor may need to state explicitly how he will inform the patient of their results and what the patient should do in the meantime. The patient may need to confirm their willingness to adhere to the agreed treatment plan.

> *'So, I'll dictate a letter to the specialist explaining the problem and fax it later today. If there is anything unusual on the blood tests, I'll phone you before your appointment. Would you call me after your appointment and tell me what Dr Jones has said?'*

Safety-netting

Establishing contingency plans is a key step in closure. Explaining what the patient should do if things do not go according to plan, how they should contact you and what certain developments might mean provides important back-up. As Neighbour (1987) described, explaining possible unexpected outcomes and when and how to seek help are important steps not only in safe medical practice but also in relationship building. If you are told that your sore throat is tonsillitis and will get better with penicillin and it doesn't, you may well return later to another doctor in the practice who diagnoses glandular fever. You may then feel unhappy about the first partner's clinical acumen. However, if the first doctor had mentioned the possibility of glandular fever and that you should return for a blood test if the penicillin had not helped by the end of the course, your regard for the doctor may well have gone up as he correctly predicted the future.

Ensuring appropriate point of closure

End summary

We have looked at the value of internal summary for information gathering and structuring the interview in Chapters 3, 4, and 6. Summary is an essential tool in this part of the consultation too. Summarising the session briefly and clarifying the plan of care not only gives the physician and patient the chance to confirm their deliberations but can also act as a highly valuable facilitative tool allowing the patient to question or amend the physician's perceptions. Summarising is an important aid to accuracy and hence to adherence. Remember to always leave space for the patient to make corrections or additions.

Doctor:	*'So, just to recap, I think your diabetes has crept out of control a little over the last year, probably because of the weight that you have put on, but hopefully we'll be able to get your sugar back to a satisfactory level if you can get your weight down to where it was before. I'll find you the diet sheet that I mentioned, and then we'll see you in two months and see how well you're managing. Is that a reasonable summary of what we've agreed?'*
Patient:	*'Fine, doctor, although, as I said, I think it's the lack of exercise since my husband's heart attack that has been my downfall, and now he's a little better perhaps I'll be able to get out walking more.'*

Final checking

As described earlier, it is important to check finally that the patient agrees and is comfortable with the plans that have been made, and to ask if they have any corrections or questions (Robinson JD 2001). Hopefully the answer will be:

> *'No, that's just fine. Thanks so much for helping me – you've answered all my questions.'*

Summary

In this chapter we have looked at the skills involved in closing the consultation. We have seen how the effectiveness of closure is related both to the appropriate use of communication skills in earlier sections of the consultation and to the use of specific skills identified in this section of the Calgary–Cambridge Guide. Summarising, contracting, safety-netting and final checking all help to round off the interview safely, to establish mutually understood common ground, to reduce uncertainty for doctor and patient about both about what has happened and about what is expected in the future, and to complete the process of sharing, collaboration and partnership that we have promoted throughout this book.

The skills of closure enable patients to feel comfortable with a mutually agreed plan, to be clear about what will happen next and to move on with more confidence. The same skills enable doctors to complete the consultation more effectively and to start the next interview with less unfinished business or anxiety to undermine their concentration. We have already mentioned that the beginning of the consultation is often the root cause of many of the problems of closure. Here we see that, without care and attention, closure can be the root cause of difficulties at the beginning of the next consultation. Putting aside the last patient is an important prerequisite for focusing attention on the next.

Chapter 8

Relating specific issues to core communication skills

Introduction

In this final chapter, we look at specific communication issues in the medical inter-view. Doctors and patients face a number of issues and communication challenges during their interactions with each other. These range from death and dying to relating to people of different ages and cultures, dealing with anger and aggression and difficulties with communication over the telephone. Here, we would like to discuss a selection of these important issues and, in particular, explore examples of how some of the communication process skills from the Calgary–Cambridge Guides are applied in these very different communication contexts.

Many books on communication in medicine devote the majority of their content to specific communication issues and give correspondingly less attention to core communication skills. In this book, we have reversed the balance. Why have we concentrated primarily on core skills that doctors can use in all consultations? We do this because almost all of the skills needed to deal with specific communication issues and challenges are contained in the set of skills that we have already pre-sented in Chapters 2–7. Learning and teaching about individual communication issues is highly important but not because different skills are required in each cir-cumstance. The skills of the Calgary–Cambridge Guides remain the essential toolkit to be selectively, skilfully and deliberately applied in different contexts.

The key concept to bear in mind here is that in each of these highly individual circumstances:

- the context of the interaction changes
- the content of the communication varies
- *but* the process skills themselves remain the same.

Of course, the content of what you are communicating changes in each of these special situations. What you need to say when you are giving someone bad news is clearly different than when you are telling them they have a flu-like illness. Context also changes – for example, in breaking bad news, the level of emotion and the impact of what you are saying on both the patient and family members changes the context of the interview substantially.

However, the process skills that are required in all of these circumstances do not change. There is no need to invent a new set of skills for each issue. Instead, we need to be aware that although most of the skills in the guides are still likely to pertain, depending on the content and particular circumstances, some skills will need to be used with greater intention, intensity and awareness. We need to deepen our understanding of these skills and the level of mastery with which we apply them. For example, in breaking bad news, we need to be particularly skilful and intentional in our use of silence and other non-verbal behaviours and in the use of the acknowledging response.

A sports analogy is helpful here. If you learn to ski in perfect conditions and then suddenly find yourself on ice, the new context will make it seem as though you need a totally new set of skills. In fact, what you have to do is to deepen the level of mastery of the skills that you have already learned and apply some of these skills, like edging, with greater intensity and focus.

In this chapter we have chosen a set of specific issues to demonstrate how to use the skills of the Calgary–Cambridge Guides in more demanding situations.

We explain the first two issues – *breaking bad news* and *cultural diversity* – in some depth. *Age-related issues (older patients and communicating with children and parents), the telephone consultation, mental health issues (psychosis and hidden depression) and medically unexplained symptoms* are then discussed more briefly. At the end of this chapter, we list a number of other communication issues and challenges and include useful sources where these issues are discussed in more depth. In our companion volume on teaching and curriculum building, *Teaching and Learning Communication Skills in Medicine*, we discuss how to incorporate the teaching of specific issues into a primarily skills-based curriculum.

Specific issues

Breaking bad news

The structure and skills of the Calgary–Cambridge Guides provide a secure platform for breaking bad news. Almost all of the process skills needed to deal with this difficult task are included in the guides. For example, the approach to explanation and planning that we have espoused in this book involves building supportive and trusting relationships with the patient and significant others who are present, tailoring information giving to the patient's needs, attempting to understand the patient's perspective and working in a collaborative partnership. All are skills important to breaking bad news. The work of Tuckett *et al.* (1985) demonstrates that finely tuned information giving skills are most required when there is a divergence between the doctor's and the patient's perspective. Breaking bad news is the ultimate example of such a situation. Here the patient's hopes on entering the room are focused on the possibility – however faint – of receiving good news and the doctor has to gradually move the patient's attention towards the worrying facts that he must now begin to communicate.

Breaking bad news is the one communication issue that most doctors appreciate to be a problem and find difficult. The psychological sequelae of breaking bad news in an abrupt and insensitive way can be devastating and long-lasting (Finlay and Dallimore 1991) and over the years there have been numerous articles in the lay and medical press on both sides of the Atlantic that illustrate doctors' deficiencies in this area. In a recent study from the UK (Brown *et al.* 2011), 60% of the patients who had a diagnosis of cancer given to them were satisfied with the way it was given. Although the content of the dialogue was rated as most important, patients were dissatisfied if the doctor was not thought to be warm and empathetic and patients found doctors' pessimism difficult to cope with. Most patients wanted a collaborative role in decision making and some idea of their prognosis. The authors noted the difficulty for physicians in meeting individual information needs – for instance, giving hope, but not giving unrealistic expectations. In a recent study Vail *et al.* (2011) asked 46 experienced hospital consultants in the UK from a wide range of specialties to deliver bad news concerning a presentation of either newly diagnosed or recurrent cancer to simulated patients. They found that the specialists focused mainly on providing biomedical information and did not frequently discuss lifestyle and psychosocial issues.

In a qualitative study concerning recurrent cancer Back *et al.* (2011) concluded

> that oncologists giving news of cancer recurrence could think of the communication as going back and forth between recognition and guidance and could ask themselves: 'Have I demonstrated that I recognise the patient's experience hearing the news?' and 'Have I provided guidance to the next steps?'

In Australia, Shaw *et al.* (2012) suggests that even small differences can be important when breaking bad news. Their study was undertaken to identify and describe the delivery styles doctors typically use when breaking bad news of an unexpected sudden death to a patient's relative. Junior and senior doctors were video-recorded as they conducted the same two simulated scenarios. Analysis of the video recordings revealed three approaches that were consistent across scenarios for a given doctor: (1) a blunt style, in which doctors delivered news within the first 30 seconds of the interaction; (2) forecasting, characterised by a staged delivery of the news within the first 30–120 seconds; and (3) a stalling approach, in which doctors provided very detailed, technically based information describing the events leading up to the bad news but delayed actually delivering the news or avoided explicitly stating the nature of the bad news for more than two minutes. The delivery styles had consequences. Both blunt and forecasting styles appeared to anticipate and elicit (or permit) a spontaneous emotional response from the news recipient and both approaches resulted in clear understanding, although forecasting provided more information. In contrast, the stalling approach resulted in verbal and non-verbal expressions of confusion, anxiety and distress on the part of recipients.

It is encouraging that papers on breaking bad news are now being published not just in the cancer field but also in neurology (Storstein 2011) and dementia (Zaleta and Carpenter 2010) fields, where treatment is often lacking or the prognosis poor.

Despite the attention given to this issue, particularly at undergraduate level, established doctors, residents and medical students still perceive considerable difficulties when delivering bad news to patients and their families (Makoul 1998; Dosanjh *et al.* 2001). Hearteningly, Field (1995) found that between 1983 and 1994, the amount and variety of teaching about death and dying in UK medical schools had grown considerably. The same is true in Australia, North America and other parts of Europe. An increasing number of articles on teaching about breaking bad news have continued to appear in mainstream medical education, which reflects the importance of this issue to both learners and teachers (Garg *et al.* 1997; Vetto *et al.* 1999; Baile *et al.* 1999, 2000; Colletti *et al.* 2001; Elwyn *et al.* 2001b; Orlander *et al.* 2002). A recent literature review of the teaching of breaking bad news showed that considerable attention is being given to this subject at undergraduate level now with good outcomes in terms of satisfaction and skill acquisition. There still seem to be some areas that are not covered well (Harrison and Walling 2010). A UK telephone study of pre-registration house officers has shown that junior doctors are frequently

involved in breaking bad news, and pleasingly they report that their undergraduate teaching on this subject had prepared them for this difficult task (Schildmann
et al. 2005). An interesting study of medical students from the United States suggests that intrapersonal difficulties and lack of self-awareness has a negative direct
effect on the manner and capacity to deliver difficult news (Meitar *et al.* 2009).

In both hospital and family practice, doctors may well have to tell patients that
they have a serious or terminal condition – for example, that a patient has cancer, has a positive HIV test or that a mother has a high risk of carrying a baby with
Down's syndrome. More frequently, doctors have to impart news that the practitioner may not consider to be particularly important or 'bad' but which the patient
perceives to be serious or concerning. Examples include giving the diagnosis of
rheumatoid arthritis or hypothyroidism; telling the patient that they are anaemic;
giving the result of a mildly abnormal cervical smear or even telling a patient who
wishes to go on holiday the next day that they have an influenza-like illness and
are unlikely to be well in time to travel. So often we are unaware of the importance
of our information giving to an individual patient and its likely effect.

Are there cultural differences in the way that patients from different parts of the
world best like to hear difficult or bad news? A study from China (Tse *et al.* 2003)
suggests that many families object to truth-telling to the actual patient, but patients
themselves may have strong views on autonomy and some may disagree with information being withheld. The authors recommend that truth-telling should depend
on what the patient wants to know, rather than on family need. Two papers from
Italy come to similar conclusions. As countries become more developed and people are better educated their desire for information increases. For example, there
seems to be increased awareness from the rural south of Italy about diagnosis and
treatment in cancer care and patients prefer information to be clear and comprehensive and to receive more detail about prognosis (Bracci *et al.* 2008; Mauri *et al.*
2009). A study from Saudi Arabia also supports these conclusions (Aljubran 2010).

Box 8.1 provides a summary of suggestions for 'breaking bad news' – this is
based on a number of people's work (Brod *et al.* 1986; Maguire and Faulkner
1988a; Sanson-Fisher 1992; Buckman 1994; Cushing and Jones 1995). Not surprisingly, these suggestions share considerable common ground with the skills in the
Calgary–Cambridge Guides. Other useful sources include a straightforward guide
produced by the National Council for Hospice and Specialist Palliative Care Services
HS UK (2003), Fallowfield and Lipkin (1995), Maguire *et al.* (1996b), Ptacek and
Eberhardt (1996), Kuhl (2002) and Shaw *et al.* (2012).

Box 8.1 Summary of suggestions for breaking bad news

Preparation
- Set up an appointment as soon as possible.
- Allow enough uninterrupted time; ensure that there are no interruptions.
- Use a comfortable, familiar environment.
- Encourage the patient to invite spouse, relative or friend as appropriate.
- Be adequately prepared with regard to clinical situation, records and
  patient's background.

- Put aside your own 'baggage' and personal feelings wherever possible.

Beginning the session / setting the scene
- Summarise where things have got to; check with the patient.
- Discover what has happened since last seen.
- Calibrate how the patient is thinking/feeling.
- Negotiate an agenda.

Sharing the information
- Assess the patient's understanding first: what the patient already knows, is thinking or has been told.
- Gauge how much the patient wishes to know.
- Give warning first that difficult information is coming, e.g. *'I'm afraid we have some work to do ...'* or *'I'm afraid it looks more serious than we had hoped ...'*
- Give basic information, simply and honestly; repeat important points.
- Relate your explanation to the patient's perspective.
- Do not give too much information too early; do not 'pussyfoot' but do not overwhelm.
- Give information in small 'chunks'; verbally categorise information.
- Watch the pace, check repeatedly for understanding and feelings as you proceed.
- Use language carefully with regard given to the patient's intelligence, reactions, emotions: avoid jargon.
- Be aware of your own non-verbal behaviour throughout.

Being sensitive to the patient
- Read and respond to the patient's non-verbal cues; face/body language, silences, tears.
- Allow for 'shutdown' (when the patient turns off and stops listening) and then give time and space: allow possible denial.
- Keep pausing to give patient opportunity to ask questions.
- Gauge patient's need for further information as you go and give more information as requested, i.e. listen to the patient's wishes as patients vary greatly and one individual's preferences may vary over time or from one situation to another.
- Encourage expression of feelings early, i.e. *'How does that news leave you feeling?' 'I'm sorry that was difficult for you'*, *'You seem upset by that'*.
- Respond to patient's feelings and predicament with acceptance, empathy and concern.
- Check patient's previous knowledge about information just given.
- Specifically elicit all the patient's concerns.
- Check understanding of information given (*'Would you like to run through what are you going to tell your wife?'*).
- Be aware of unshared meanings (i.e. what cancer means for the patient compared with what it means for the physician).
- Do not be afraid to show emotion or distress.

Planning and support
- Having identified all the patient's specific concerns, offer specific help by breaking down overwhelming feelings into manageable concerns, prioritising and distinguishing the fixable from the unfixable.
- Identify a plan for what is to happen next.
- Give a broad time frame for what may lie ahead.
- Give hope tempered with realism ('preparing for the worst and hoping for the best').
- Ally yourself with the patient (*'We can work on this together ... between us'*), i.e. emphasise partnership with the patient, confirm your role as advocate of the patient.
- Emphasise quality of life.
- Safety net.

Follow up and closing
- Summarise and check with patient for understanding, additional questions.
- Don't rush the patient to treatment.
- Set up early further appointment, offer telephone calls, etc.
- Identify support systems; involve relatives and friends.
- Offer to see/tell spouse or others.
- Make written materials available.

If the patient attends with a companion, read and respond to the companion's verbal and non-verbal cues, and allow pauses for questions, but remember that the patient is your first concern.

Throughout be aware of your own anxieties – with regard to giving information, previous experience, or failure to cure or help.

Building relationship with patients and significant others is not limited to any particular section in Box 8.1 but is clearly a most important part of the entire interaction. Notice how many of the suggestions above, and the skills from the Calgary–Cambridge Guides discussed in the next section, are related to establishing common ground, acknowledging and responding sensitively to the patient's perspective (thoughts and feelings), and demonstrating attentive verbal and non-verbal behaviour. In the context of disclosing bad news, these same skills are building blocks for creating and sustaining therapeutic relationships regardless of whether you and the patient are virtual strangers or know each other well.

Key skills of the Calgary–Cambridge Guides to apply with greater depth, intention and intensity

Breaking bad news is a context that changes both the content of the interview and the intensity, intention and awareness with which certain of the core communication process skills of the Calgary–Cambridge Guides need to be applied. Here is a description of these process skills tabulated under the appropriate headings of the Calgary–Cambridge Guides.

Skills from the Calgary–Cambridge Guides	Applying skills with greater depth, intention and intensity
Initiation	As in any other interview, success in setting the scene is crucial.
Preparation	How to set up the appointment: if the news is serious and complex information needs to be given, preparation requires special thought and planning. When and where should it be done, who should be there; are you as the doctor thoroughly prepared emotionally and factually? This is particularly important when disclosing the diagnosis of dementia to a patient and their family (Lecouturier *et al.* 2008). Pay attention to comfort and non-verbal skills; posture and tone of voice are vital (Bruera *et al.* 2007).
Greet patient Negotiate agenda	Interviewing more than one person at a time: many ill people, or people who know that they are going to be given difficult or complicated information, bring a relative or friend with them to see the doctor. You then have more than one person present with different ideas, concerns and expectations and different agendas. Focusing on the 'main' patient is essential. Yet it is also important to take the accompanying friend or relative into consideration. When there is time it is often helpful to agree to see the patient and relatives both separately and together. Note the results of Benson and Britten's (1996) study of patients with cancer, which showed that most rejected disclosure to others without their consent.
Explanation and planning	Breaking bad news is a special case of explanation and planning so it is not surprising that this difficult situation requires particularly masterful use of most of the skills associated with this phase of the interview.
Chunk and check	*Giving information in manageable chunks and checking for understanding* are key skills here, allowing the physician to calibrate where the patient is at any particular time as this part of the interview proceeds.
Assess the patient's starting point	*Discovering what the patient already knows,* is fearful of and is hoping for is difficult but vital, particularly when the patient is frightened. This may be even more complicated when a relative or friend is present. In their study of information giving during 'bad news' oncology interactions in the United States, Eggly *et al.* (2006) showed that companions asked significantly more questions than the patient and that positive ratings of the relationship between physicians and companions were correlated with fewer questions being asked by the latter. It may be that the patient is overwhelmed at the beginning of the interview and is happy to have a spokesperson to speak on their behalf. There are considerable rewards for obtaining an accurate picture of where the patient and their relatives are coming from before giving information such as prognosis or treatment options.

Continued

Skills from the Calgary–Cambridge Guides	Applying skills with greater depth, intention and intensity
Assess the patient's starting point (*cont.*)	The aim of the doctor is to understand and acknowledge both the patient and their relative's needs early on in order to set the scene for excellent relationships with patient and significant others in the future
Assess each person's individual information needs	*Discovering what the patient wants to know* is also critical. Most patients want to know that they have cancer (Meredith *et al.* 1996), including the elderly (Ajaj *et al.* 2001). Gauging how much the patient wishes to know requires high levels of skill. Understanding potential cultural influences is helpful here but it is most important to ascertain the needs and preferences of the individual patient or significant other. Various authors make different recommendations about how this task should be accomplished. Buckman (1994) suggests a direct preliminary question such as 'if this condition turns out to be something serious, are you the type of person who likes to know exactly what is going on?' Maguire and Faulkner (1988a) suggest a hierarchy of euphemisms for the bad news, pausing after each to gain the patient's reaction. Other authors suggest making a more direct start to giving the news after a warning shot and gauging how to proceed as you go: they argue that patients who wish to use denial mechanisms will still be able to blank out what they do not want to hear.
Use explicit categorisation or signposting	*Giving a warning shot* first is a special case of explicit categorisation or signposting of information that is about to be given, alerting the patient that all is not as they hoped. It may be useful to give a warning shot near the beginning of the interview, particularly when it is a follow-up interview. There are a number of ways to do this, and which one might be the best in the circumstance depends on the patient's situation and the doctor's style. For the patient with a terminal illness or the patient with a threatened miscarriage awaiting the result of a scan, it might be *'I'm afraid the news isn't as good as we hoped'* accompanied by appropriate non-verbal behaviour. The doctor can then pause and let the likelihood of the news being difficult for the patient sink in, before continuing the interview. To help patients focus their attention, the usual signposts are also important, e.g. *'There are two important things to remember. First ..., second ...'*
Relate explanations to patient's perspective	*Encouraging questions* from patients and their companions is important in building trust. The most frequently occurring topics were found by Eggly *et al.* (2006) to be diagnostic testing, diagnosis and prognosis. Older patients tended to ask fewer questions and educated patients to ask more.

Skills from the Calgary–Cambridge Guides	Applying skills with greater depth, intention and intensity
Encourage questions	*Give hope tempered with realism*
	This is easier for the doctor when the patient has a real hope of recovery or improvement, for example a patient recovering from a road traffic accident, or a patient who is found to have a renal calculus. It is much more difficult to give hope to a patient who has suffered a severe stroke, or in whom chemotherapy has failed. All patients and their families need hope. The key is to clarify the issues surrounding it. Inspiring and instilling hope is related to the patient working in partnership and affirming the patient's worth (Cutcliffe 1995). Accurate disclosure of prognosis by paediatricians to parents of a child with cancer can support hope even when the prognosis is poor (Mack *et al.* 2007). Clayton *et al.* (2008), in their review of communication with terminally ill patients and their families, have shown that encouraging patients to focus on hope for compassionate care and support, and specific goals such being to attend a daughter's wedding, or that expert pain control will be available, rather than long life is likely to be helpful.
Discuss options and opinions	*Discuss treatment options*
	Again this needs to be introduced when the patient is ready to hear the doctor's recommendations. Make it clear to the patient that they will be involved in decisions about treatment.
	Give a prognosis
	If the patient wants to discuss the future, avoid giving too definite a time scale; however, giving a broad framework may help the patient who wishes to plan ahead.
Building the relationship	Throughout the interview continuing to build relationship with the patient and any significant others in attendance is vital. If you do not know the patient or significant other well, laying down foundations for a trusting relationship needs to be done with intention at the very beginning of the interaction.
Pick up cues Demonstrate empathy	*Checking out non-verbal cues* allows the doctor to identify points at which the patient wants to ask a question or calibrate the patient's emotional state, and then to express empathy and compassion for the patient's position. It also gives the doctor space to enquire about further concerns and respond to the patient with feeling. *'I can see that you are very distressed to hear that the results of the tests confirm your worst fears … I am extremely sorry … (pause) … you mentioned your husband is disabled – have you any other concerns you wish to discuss now?'*

Continued

Skills from the Calgary–Cambridge Guides	Applying skills with greater depth, intention and intensity
Pick up cues Demonstrate empathy (*cont.*)	A special case of picking up cues is associated with the *shutdown* – a point at which the patient (or significant other) who is receiving bad news seems to block out or be unable to take in what you are saying. Acknowledging that the patient does not wish to hear any more requires chunking and checking of your information giving as you proceed and paying particular attention to the patient's verbal cues (e.g. changing the subject abruptly) or more commonly non-verbal cues (e.g. becoming tearful, silent or looking uncomfortable or angry).
Allow the patient to take in the seriousness of the bad news	Doctors find it very difficult to be silent while a patient and her family express strong feelings and emotion, often crying while taking in the news. Back *et al.* (2009) have studied the patterns of behaviours which doctors exhibit when 'told' to remain silent; how uncomfortable they often look and what negative non-verbal skills they can display. The authors advocate compassionate silence – where the doctor shows that she cares and will not leave the silence so long as to make the patient uncomfortable.
Provide support	*Partnership and advocacy*
	Support for the patient is essential. Overt statements such as, *'We need to work on this together'*, or *'I will speak to the specialist on your behalf'*, or *'You will not be left to cope with this on your own … how can we go forward now?'* may help patients and need to be emphasised.
Demonstrate appropriate non-verbal behaviour	*Doctors not hiding their own distress*
	Patients can be upset by doctors who remain unmoved by their distress at being given bad news (Woolley *et al.* 1989). Doctors should not fear displaying emotion (Fallowfield 1993). But how much of your own distress to share with a patient is a difficult judgement to make and must depend on individual personalities and specific situations. Clearly, it is not the patient's task to care for the doctor's distress. On the other hand, it is difficult for doctors not to show anxiety when performing this complex task and patients may pick up the doctor's non-verbal cues here. Retaining the patient's confidence and continuing to build the relationship with the patient is the overall objective here.
Closure	Time spent on this section of the interview pays dividends; often at this point in the consultation the doctor is able to summarise possible next steps with the patient and give the patient back some control.

Skills from the Calgary–Cambridge Guides	Applying skills with greater depth, intention and intensity
Contract with patient re next steps Safety net	*Clear follow-up plans*, setting an early date for the next appointment, offering to telephone the patient to check that all is well with the agreed plan and beginning to work out the next steps are seen as supportive and reassuring. Offering to contact significant others when the patient has expressed concern about informing others about a diagnosis or prognosis is often helpful, as is giving time for the patient to absorb bad news and to decide how long they need to consider treatment options. *Document what the patient and the relatives have been told*; this is extremely helpful, particularly when the family physician and the specialist communicate with each other, or in the event that the patient will be receiving care from a team of other healthcare providers.

This framework includes all the steps recommended by patients, doctors and nurses in a study designed to discover whether there is a consensus between patients and providers on guidelines for breaking bad news (Girgis *et al.* 1999). It also reflects the recommendations and skills presented in an evidence-based videotape produced in the United States, entitled *Cancer Disclosure: Communicating the Diagnosis to Patients*. This video, produced in 1986, remains an excellent teaching demonstration using numerous simulated examples and the personal narratives of both doctors and cancer patients.

Cultural and social diversity

The communication skills needed for exploring multicultural issues are a special case of the core skills used to understand the patient's perspective (both in gathering information and in explanation and planning) and building the relationship. The same could be said for issues of social diversity such as age, gender, socio-economic class, status and educational level.

Many of the concepts that form the basis for the disease–illness model (as discussed in Chapter 3) came originally from anthropological and cross-cultural studies. Multicultural interviews were viewed as an extreme example of all medical encounters and the lessons learned were later applied to doctors and patients working within a single culture. Here we are reversing the process and exploring how the core skills of discovering the patient's perspective apply to the specific difficulties of multicultural situations where doctors and patients often hold differing perspectives.

Increasingly we encounter ethnic complexities and mobility of peoples throughout the world. Johnson *et al.* (1995) have said that 'each culture is a textured pattern of beliefs and practices, some of which are coherent and consistent and others contested and contradictory'. They suggest that doctors must explore a patient's health beliefs and views of their symptoms and illness in every medical interview. If doctors ignore this advice, they risk making assumptions or value judgements and stereotyping patients. This can lead not only to conflict but also inaccuracy. In multicultural contexts – indeed, in all cases of diversity between physician and patient – discrimination is a potential problem. If most discrimination is unintentional, as Dovidio and Gaertner (1996) suggest, and if most doctors either are not aware that they discriminate or deny the possibility, as a Kaiser Family Foundation (1999) survey revealed, then we need to be particularly vigilant about diversity issues in healthcare and how we handle them.* For instance, in a study of colorectal cancer care, black minority patients were less likely to be satisfied with their overall care (Ayanian. 2010).

Johnson *et al.* (1995) make the following points that doctors may find useful when consulting with a patient who comes from a culture different from their own. A person's culture provides him or her with ideas about health and illness, notions about causality, notions about who controls healthcare decisions and how steps in seeking healthcare are made. They have also developed a useful explanatory model, which sets out common differences between Western-trained physicians and traditional ethnic patients. This approach is supported by a cross-cultural study by Chugh *et al.* (1993). Their main findings were that there were a number of barriers to patient satisfaction, to doctors giving diagnosis and treatment and to patients receiving it. The barriers were related to the patient's cultural experiences, ideas, beliefs and expectations as well as language difficulties.

Myerscough (1992) and Eleftheriadou (1996) have provided useful information about a number of problems related to culture commonly encountered by Western physicians. Examples given include the importance of the family structure and lifestyle, women's roles, attitudes towards women and their children, dress, religion, food and fasting, and life and death.

Ferguson and Candib (2002), in their review of culture, language and the doctor–patient relationship, found consistent evidence that minority patients with insufficient English were less likely to engender empathic responses from their physicians, were more likely to receive less information generally, and were unlikely to be encouraged to develop partnership in decision making.

The appropriate provision of a well-trained interpreter in the consultation is an important issue. Ngo-Metzger *et al.* (2003), in their study of Chinese and Vietnamese immigrants to the United States, found that patients preferred using professional interpreters to family members, and that the interpreter should be the same sex as themselves. In a study describing the content of talk about health problems and medications during clinical encounters involving professional interpreters or family members, Rosenberg *et al.* (2011) found that encounters involving interpreters were more likely than encounters with family to include discussions of emotions about the problem and indications for follow-up.

While best practices for interpreters are still being determined, the value of using a professional interpreter is becoming clearer. In a study of patients with limited English proficiency admitted to a tertiary care hospital (Lindholm *et al.* 2012), 39% received professional language interpretation on admission and discharge dates. Patients who did not receive interpretation had an increase in length of hospital stays. Interpretation at admission had the greatest impact on length of stay. Patients receiving interpretation at admission and/or discharge were less likely to be readmitted than those receiving no interpretation.

---

* With thanks to Charlene Pope for her insights on social psychology and for making us aware of this work.

On the other hand, however proficient the interpreter is, there is likely to be considerable conversational loss. Aranguri *et al.* (2006), in their study of primary care physicians and their Hispanic patients with dyslipidaemias, found that interpreters used virtually no small talk or rapport-building skills. We suggest that doctors need to pay special attention in particular to their non-verbal relationship-building skills while the interpreter is translating.

In her commentary introducing a series of articles on issues of diversity, Roter (2002) proposes relationship-centred care as an approach for meeting the needs of diverse patient populations, including diversity related to culture or ethnicity, gender, age, sexual orientation or religious beliefs as well as situations where physician and patient speak different languages.

Common issues and barriers in cross-cultural communication and social diversity

Box 8.2 offers a useful list of potential points of difference or barriers to effective interaction that require special attention when the cultural or social backgrounds of the physician and patient are different.

Box 8.2   Common issues and barriers in cross-cultural communication and social diversity

Use of language
- Use of foreign language (i.e. patient or physician must communicate in a language in which they are not fluent)
- Use of slang
- Accent/dialect
- Giving offence through over-familiarity, etc.

Use and interpretation of non-verbal communication
- Physical touch
- Body language
- Proximity – closeness/distance
- Eye contact
- Expression of affect/emotion

Cultural beliefs and healthcare
- Interpretation of symptoms – what is considered normal and abnormal
- Beliefs about causation
- Beliefs about efficacy of treatment alternatives
- Attitudes toward illness and disease
- Use of complementary or alternative sources of healthcare
- Gender and age expectations about roles and relationships
- Role of doctor and social interactions related to power and ways of showing respect
- Perceived responsibilities regarding adherence to medical recommendations
- Family life events (e.g. rituals and beliefs around arranged marriages,

pregnancy and childbirth, older adult care-giving, treatment of elders, death)
- Psychosocial issues (identifying common stressors, awareness of diversity in family/community supports)
- Role of the doctor in mental health and disability

Sensitive issues
- Sexuality – including sexual orientation, sexual practices and birth control
- Uneasiness regarding some physical examinations
- Use and abuse of alcohol and other substances
- Domestic violence and abuse
- Sharing bad news

Medical practice issues/barriers
- Extent of doctor/patient partnership, extent of family involvement; personal and family responsibility for healthcare and treatment
- Ethical issues in care
- Doctors' assumptions, stereotyping or prejudices
- Concurrent consulting with a practitioner of complementary or alternative medicine

Some knowledge of the different ethnic or cultural contexts in which a physician practises is useful, and in some cases it is vital. Such knowledge can give the doctor confidence and may allow some 'shortcuts' to be made. However, the core skills of understanding each individual patient and their particular health beliefs, whichever culture they come from, remain essential. For example, it is important not to assume that all patients wish their doctors to respect their autonomy and share decision making. For individuals in many cultures the norm is still to expect doctors to be paternalistic and more doctor-centred (Lamiani *et al.* 2008). Labelling the patient with the attitudes and outlook of a whole race or culture may be just as damaging as not being sensitive to cultural issues at all – the doctor's objective must be to find out each individual patient's unique perspective and experience of illness. This is equally important when both doctor and patient share the same culture. Kai *et al.* (2007) support this approach. Their study using focus groups from a cross-section of health workers in cancer care in the UK showed that many clinicians experience discomfort and uncertainty in responding to patients from a different cultural background. Despite being culturally aware, participants felt trapped by their inability to engage socially and emotionally with these patients.

There are therefore two slightly conflicting communication issues to be faced by the clinician: how to avoid making assumptions about a patient based on their ethnicity and how at the same time to value and be willing to explore and understand cultural differences that might make a considerable difference to how you care for the patient. It is not surprising that the development of mutual understanding and trust between a patient and doctor from different cultural backgrounds often takes time and effort from both parties.

Teal and Street (2009) have developed a useful model containing critical elements of cultural competence in the medical interview, which includes the importance of integrating core communication skills with situational awareness and adaptability together with knowledge about core cultural issues.

Key skills of the Calgary–Cambridge Guides that need applying with greater depth, intention and intensity

The examples of skills from the Calgary–Cambridge Guides that are singled out for particular attention here relate mainly to the physician eliciting and understanding the patient's perspective more accurately and responding to it more explicitly. Employing these skills carefully can also often help the patient to understand the physician's perspective.

Skills from the Calgary–Cambridge Guides	Applying these skills with greater depth, intention and intensity
Initiation	
Greet and make introductions	Check pronunciation of name and how patient would like to be addressed.
Demonstrate interest, concern and respect, and attend to the patient's physical comfort	Demonstrate sensitivity to patient's wish to be interviewed with a family member or by a male or female doctor.
	Offer the help of an interpreter and if agreed, include negotiations during the agenda setting process about the role the interpreter will play.
	Check preferred language to be used in the interview.
	Offer to postpone the interview if the language barrier is too great.
	Consider gender issues between doctor and patient in the interview and in the physical examination.
Gathering information	
Discover the patient's perspective: ideas, concerns, expectations, effects on life and feelings	Explore the patient's: • beliefs about causation • culturally determined expectations of treatment • family, marital, religious and social mores • understanding of social and community networks • use of complementary or alternative sources of healthcare.
	Patients from some cultural or social backgrounds may be less aware of links between psychosocial issues and their physical symptoms. Exploring underlying depression and somatisation in these circumstances is not easy and may depend on remaining open to the patient's point of view and building up trust over a long period of time. Physicians may have to judge when to accept the patient's healthcare choices or views of their illness, rather than risk challenging the patient unsuccessfully with consequent damage to trust or the doctor–patient relationship.
Involve the patient, encourage them to contribute and to ask questions	Patients need to be encouraged to ask questions. In a US study, black patients were less likely to ask questions of their oncologists and were less likely to have a companion with them (Eggly *et al.* 2011).

Continued

Skills from the Calgary–Cambridge Guides	Applying these skills with greater depth, intention and intensity
Building the relationship	
Demonstrate appropriate non-verbal behaviour	Be aware of possible cultural differences in non-verbal behaviour e.g. eye contact, touch, proximity.
Accept the patient's views and feelings non-judgementally	Value the patient's ideas and beliefs non-judgementally, without stereotyping or patronising the patient (e.g. accept the patient's and family's wishes for examination, investigation and referral). Avoid making assumptions, or check them out. Show sensitivity to cultural differences around issues such as sexual problems, use and abuse of alcohol or other substances, and domestic violence.
Provide support	Overtly express support.
Explanation and planning	
Assess the patient's starting point	Check out cultural context before giving information. This is particularly important when working with disabled patients where the research suggests that these patients feel less well listened to and respected, are given less information and are less commonly involved in planning treatment (Duggan *et al.* 2010).
	Work with an interpreter during the interview if necessary.
	Check that the interpreter has given information accurately and completely and that the patient understands.
Relate explanation to the patient's perspective	Check cultural context/linguistic ability before giving information. Check whether the patient's concerns have been addressed.
Check understanding	Checking understanding frequently is particularly important where there is a language problem, even if an interpreter is present.
	Give real choices based on the patient's background and situation.
Negotiate mutually acceptable plan	The patient who is unused to a collaborative and sharing partnership with the doctor may find this unfamiliar or difficult to cope with.

The following phrases are some examples of precise phrasing to help physicians explore and value cultural difference while at the same time avoid stereotyping and making assumptions. In general, if your initial questions or comments would work equally well for the majority culture, you are on the right track. Asking questions about the individual patient or the patient's family rather than about their culture helps personalise rather than label. Eloquent support for this straightforward approach comes from a gathering of some 60 immigrant women from numerous cultures and ethnic groups.* When we asked these women (whose experience living in Canada ranged from a few months to many years) what they most wanted

---

* With thanks to the participants of Multicultural Health for Immigrant Women: A Dialogue, sponsored by Alberta/Northwest Territories Network of Immigrant Women, Calgary, Alberta, March 1992.

us to teach doctors about cross-cultural communication, the first person to respond received enthusiastic and unanimous endorsement: 'Please teach them to treat us first as individuals rather than as representatives of a cultural group.' While the women certainly thought it helpful to understand cultural differences and the diversity of health beliefs, they stressed that without getting to know individual patients there simply was no way of knowing who fit generalisations about culture or ethnicity and who did not. The research of Chugh *et al.* (1994) offers further rationale for this basic principle of cross-cultural communication. It showed that health beliefs *within* ethnic groups in a diverse, multicultural Canadian city differed more than health beliefs *between* those same ethnic groups.

With each of the following examples, keep in mind that the non-verbal behaviour you use and your ability to pick up and respond to the patient's cues are at least as important as your choice of words.

'What effect is all this having on your life and on those around you?'

'Can you tell me a little about yourself and your family ...? Where do you live ...? Who is at home with you ...? Where was your family home ...? What are your parents' background ...? Do you practise a religion yourself?'

'I know that problems with fertility can cause tensions in families – has that been true at all for you?'

'Sometimes people's family or religious backgrounds are very important when discussing gynaecological problems – people who are Catholic, for instance, have strong religious views about contraception. Is there anything from your own background that affects how you think about your problem?'

Then follow up according to the patient's response:

'You mention that you are from Afghanistan. I don't know anything about Afghanistan's culture ... Is it OK, for instance, for a doctor to shake the hand of a patient? What is your preference for greeting?

'I can understand that it must be frustrating for you that I can't understand you as well as you would like. Would it help if we had an interpreter?'

'I'd like to know what sort of treatment you were expecting or hoping for. From what I know of Chinese culture, it might be quite different from what we offer here. If that is true for you, I'd like to help'.

'You tell me that your body hurts all over ... Do you have any ideas about why this may be?

Other useful phrases:

- When you don't know the patient or relative and are unsure whether to shake hands:
  - observe the person's response
  - apologise if they seem offended – you didn't mean to offend
  - make sure to do something else instead to build the relationship, such as asking if they would tell you the greeting with which they are most comfortable
- Ask permission if you wish to ask a sensitive question:
  - *'Would it be alright to ask you about this or not?'*
- Ask what would help:
  - *'I need to … Is there anything that will help you with this?'*
- Explain why:
  - *'This may be difficult for you – the reason I need to ask you/do this is …'*
  - *'Sometimes people have their own explanations for things and it helps to understand patient's views.'*
  - *'I know that sometimes women would prefer to be examined by a female doctor – is that important for you?'*

Eleftheriadou (1996) provides a concise and practical summary of what to consider when communicating with patients from different cultures and offers some particularly useful examples of how to improve that communication. Cole and Bird's (2000) book on the medical interview also contains a useful chapter on this topic. Kai's (2003) more recent book on ethnicity, health and primary care tackles a number of issues, including effective cross-cultural communication and interpreting and translating. He also underlines the importance of awareness of the iceberg model of cultural influences in health encounters – physicians may be aware of gender, age, ethnicity and nationality, but important cultural contexts such as socio-economic status, religion and sexual and political orientation may remain unrecognised. Through their insightful exploration of patient narratives and case studies, the work of Geist-Martin *et al.* (2003) moves us closer to patients' experiences and perceptions regarding cultural issues and other issues of diversity in healthcare. It also suggests useful approaches for enhancing communication in various contexts of diversity. Other useful descriptions can be found in Steele's account of overcoming cultural and language barriers (Steele 2002) and Fadiman's (1997) study of a Hmong child with epilepsy and how the medical culture in which she is treated collides with her family's belief systems.

Age-related issues

In this section we look at communication with older patients (and, where applicable, relatives or friends who are assisting them) and with young children and their parents. Here, and for the rest of the issues explored in this chapter, we include only representative examples of the skills from the guides that are relevant.

Communicating with older patients

Communication with older people demands special consideration. All over the world the numbers of seniors in the population have been rising steadily during the last 100 years. In the Western world, estimates indicate that 35% of the population will be over 60 by the year 2030. Here are some questions all doctors need to ask of themselves and the elderly patients who consult them, based on the work of Geisler (1991).

- What are the special psychological and physical problems related to aging in this person?
- Have hearing loss or neurological problems compromised this person's ability to communicate? If so, what do I need to do differently?
- What is the meaning of sickness or approaching death to this person?
- If the patient presents with symptoms of illness, is this a cue that the patient needs help in other ways? Are they depressed, lonely, or fearing disability and loss of independence, or death?
- What do I know about the world of this person and what has happened to this person in their life? Are there limitations of medical management and treatment in this person that I should consider?
- What does this person expect of me as their doctor?
- Are relatives or friends assisting this person? Do they need or want to be involved and, if so, how can I accommodate them?
- Are multiple healthcare providers involved with this patient? Is continuity of care an issue?

Wolff and Roter (2012) point to the need for special consideration with respect to older adults with poor mental health function accompanied by family companions. Their audiotaped, observational study found that when a family companion was present during routine office visits with these patients, the visits were shorter, the companion and the patient provided less psychosocial information, and physicians engaged in less question-asking, less partnership building and less patient-centred communication.

Key skills of the Calgary–Cambridge Guides to apply with greater depth, intention and intensity

The principle of treating people first as individuals rather than as 'elderly patients' pertains here just as it did in dealing with cultural issues. Unfortunately, ageism is common in healthcare. We would always encourage you to ask: 'Am I making and acting on inaccurate or inappropriate assumptions or generalisations based on the age of this patient rather than finding out about the individual? For example, based on age am I assuming that this person is more disabled or incapacitated or disinterested than they in fact are?' A small qualitative study of disclosing the diagnosis of dementia to patients and their families (Lecouturier *et al.* 2008) underlines the importance of the context of the dialogue. Patients want to know what is happening to them but how to disclose, to whom (the patient and/or their family) and over how long needs to be tailored to the individual and their concerns of the moment. Examples of some of the key skills that deserve particular attention when working with older people include the following.

Skills from the Calgary–Cambridge Guides	Applying these skills with greater depth, intention and intensity
Initiation	
Develop rapport	Special consideration needs to be given, for instance, to people who are frail, hearing impaired or partially sighted. Many older patients see the doctor with a relative or other caregiver – here rapport needs to be carefully developed with all parties.
Screen	The physician needs to remember that screening and prioritisation are particularly important with older people because of the potential presence of multiple problems or disabilities over time. Remember that: • the type and number of problems do not necessarily predict function • not all problems are current • not all problems need help • not all problems are on the patient's agenda.
Listen attentively	Gauging the patient's emotional state early and throughout the interview is very important when consulting with the elderly. Both anxiety and depression are common in the elderly and may not present overtly.
Gathering information	
Ask clarifying questions Time-frame Summarise	Often with older patients, the doctor listens to a complex narrative, with large amounts of seemingly elusive data – here the skills of clarification, time-framing, summarising and checking become very important. For example, explicitly requesting that the patient explain their problem from when it first began up to the present or over a particular time period can be helpful.
Pick up cues	The patient may be embarrassed but keen to discuss issues such as incontinence, a scrotal hernia or a breast lump – picking up, checking out, and responding to non-verbal or verbal cues is particularly important.
Use language appropriately	Clear language is required if the patient is confused, disoriented, upset or has speech or hearing difficulties. Begin by checking out assumptions about what is contributing to the communication difficulties. Are pain or other medications a factor? Are jargon or the language in which you are speaking a problem? When a patient is dysarthric or deaf, check their understanding and ascertain whether the patient would find it easier to communicate via the written word. In hospital check if the patient uses hearing aids and, if so, whether the aids are in place and in working order.
Discover the patient's perspective	The patient's perspective is all-important here. The effect that the condition has on the patient's life often predicts the patient's expectations or follow through regarding treatment and needs to be carefully taken into consideration.

Skills from the Calgary–Cambridge Guides	Applying these skills with greater depth, intention and intensity
Building the relationship	
Demonstrate appropriate non-verbal behaviour	Patience and time – going at the patient's pace is vital.
Demonstrate sensitivity, empathy, acceptance and support	Older patients and their significant others may need a great deal of emotional as well as practical support. Attempting to appreciate the predicament the patient is in may help you to understand what at first sight is awkward or unusual behaviour. The response to such embarrassing problems as incontinence should be empathic and respectful – offer practical help.
Structuring the interview	
Summarise Signpost	Using these two skills in tandem may be particularly useful with older patients, particularly those who have hearing difficulties and loss of memory. Elderly patients can become lost in their own complex narrative and need help in structuring their own account – summary and signposting therefore help both patient and doctor. Structuring the consultation allows the doctor to check out questions or plans with carers as well as the patient: *'I know that you find it hard to get out to do the shopping now … Can I just check with your daughter a moment … where do you live?'* A memory test can be a useful tool of assessment with elderly patients; this needs to be signposted carefully to avoid embarrassment or anger.
Explanation and planning	
Chunk and check Use diagrams	Chunk and check, using clear language free from jargon. Using diagrams and written instructions particularly in relation to medication is helpful for those with memory loss and their caregivers.

Stewart *et al.*'s (2000b) valuable review of 50 articles on older patient–physician communication underscores the benefits of increased collaboration and active participation on the part of older patients. The studies reviewed describe the influence of communication on older patients' expectations, decision making, recall, adherence, satisfaction, emotional health outcomes, physical health outcomes, and hospitalisation. Key communication dimensions which emerged from the studies reviewed were concordance between physician and older patient regarding expectations of the encounter, patient participation in question asking and information giving, information given in a timely and sensitive manner, inclusion of 'take home' information, mutual discussion of resources and responsibility, discussion of relevant aspects of the patients' life context, a caring attitude from the physician and continuity of care.

Encouragingly, Zaleta and Carpenter (2010), in their audio study of 54 patients where physicians disclosed the diagnosis of dementia in triadic interviews, showed that there were many instances of patient-centred consulting. However, another study (Wolff and Roter 2012) showed that with a subsection of older patients with poor mental health who had a companion with them, physicians demonstrated less patient-centred care and asked fewer questions of the patient. The lesson here is that doctors need to use the skills of triadic interviewing with all patients who are accompanied by a relative or friend, and that this is particularly true of the elderly and those who are mentally and physically frail. Both the patient and the companion need to be listened to and empathised with. They may both have quite different perspectives on the patient's illness. Both need to be questioned and given information and opportunity to ask questions. Both need to agree with a management plan. It is true that the companion may be able to provide a useful 'witness statement' but that doesn't negate the fact that the patient is the doctor's first concern.

Mader and Ford (1995) also provide useful insights into interviewing older patients. Geist-Martin *et al.* (2003) devote an entire section of their book to communicating in health across the life span, from infancy to old age, including insightful patient narratives and suggestions for more effective communication in a variety of health-related contexts.

Communicating with children and parents*

When communicating with children, it is vital to remember that the child is the patient but the parent is also a key person in many transactions. This triadic consultation, where the doctor has to communicate with both parents and children at the same time, is particularly challenging, as all parties will inevitably need individual attention. It is important to start the interview by addressing the child and not to direct all your attention to the parent(s) during a paediatric interview. Ask young children whether they would like to tell their story or prefer their parents to do so. Children often have their own needs, and addressing these can improve their satisfaction and adherence to treatment (Pantell 1982).

Many paediatric problems brought to medical attention are minor but can cause significant parental anxiety. Serious childhood illness is overwhelming for all parents. It is therefore not surprising that in both circumstances parental satisfaction is closely related to timely acknowledgement of parental concerns and expectations during a consultation (Korsch *et al.* 1968; Mangione-Smith *et al.* 2001).

Parents tend to interrupt their children during medical interviews (Tates and Meeuwesen 2000). They may disagree with their child's view of the problem and feel that they are wasting the doctor's time by letting their child talk, or they may be anxious about the doctor receiving an accurate view of the problem as they perceive it. It is very useful to pick up cues from both parents and children when there is disagreement, particularly when the problem is a behavioural one. You may need to negotiate separate time with both a teenager and her parent/s. It is important not to marginalise teenagers. Valuing children of all ages and respecting their views is more likely to encourage the development of successful relationships between you and your young patients (Dixon-Woods *et al.* 1999; Young *et al.* 2003).

Children of different ages bring different difficulties to the paediatric interview. Consultations concerning infants are in some sense the easiest, as most of the discourse is conducted with the parent(s). Toddlers and infants require special skills

---

* We are indebted to Dr Rachel Howells for her contributions and insights throughout this section.

to engage them, as they are naturally fearful of new environments and strangers. Older pre-adolescents can be very 'private' and self-conscious, and teenagers even more so. It is important not to patronise older children and adolescents, and to offer them opportunities to be involved fully in the information gathering and planning stages of the consultation (Lewis *et al.* 1988).

A basic appreciation of language and cognitive development flexibly applied is useful for developing paediatric communication skills – so, too, is a grasp of what children of different ages understand about illness (Ginsburg and Opper 1988; Bibace and Walsh 1981).

Most of the skills that underlie the successful paediatric consultation are based on the core skills of consultations with adult patients, although it is important to remember that insufficient research has been done on the interactional dynamics of the triadic consultation and the skills required for it to be a successful and effective encounter (Tates and Meeuwesen 2001). A review of the literature on communication in the paediatric interview in primary care (Cahill and Papageorgiou 2007a) has shown that children between the ages of 6 and 12 have little meaningful involvement in their consultations. Although the children in the reviewed studies sometimes took part during history taking and examination, they had much less involvement during explanation and planning discussions. Doctors were in a position to allocate turns. However, if a parent interrupted the interaction between the doctor and the child, the consultation tended to revert to adult–adult interaction; the adults dominated and controlled these consultations. In a study involving video analysis of communication in paediatric consultations again in primary care, Cahill and Papageorgiou (2007b) found that child involvement is improved if parents are encouraged to voice their concerns early on in the consultation and the child is then invited to speak.

A more recent video study done in the United States involving parents and children aged 2.5 and older, examined predictors of children answering questions in primary care paediatric visits. Stivers (2012) found that each year of a child's age increased the likelihood that he or she would answer, and that girls were much more likely to answer physicians' questions than boys. Parents' race and education were predictors of whether physicians selected children to answer questions, but were not associated with children's propensity for answering. Children who answered early in the encounter were more likely to continue to answer. Physicians improved the likelihood of children answering when they asked social questions early on, phrased questions that could be answered 'yes' or 'no', and directed their gaze directly at the child while asking a question.

Parents with babies admitted to neonatal units have special concerns. Alderson *et al.* (2006), in their study of parents with infants with either confirmed or potential neurological problems, reported missed opportunities for more dialogue with neonatal staff. Parents appreciated more information, two-way decision making and the feeling of drawing together with nurses and doctors, whereas doctors emphasised more distancing aspects of interviews.

The sections of the consultation that need special focus in this age group are initiating the interview and building the relationship. For instance, developing rapport in the early stages of the consultation with a toddler or pre-adolescent child is of prime importance, as it is this which will ensure the patient's comfort and assurance throughout the consultation and pave the way for what may be difficult or painful examinations or investigations later on.

Key skills of the Calgary–Cambridge Guides that need applying with greater depth, intention and intensity

Skills from the Calgary–Cambridge Guides	Applying these skills in greater depth, intention and intensity
Initiation	
Preparation	Create an appropriate environment for the child and the family including toys and books appropriate to age; pay attention to seating.
Establish initial rapport	Greet and establish the identities of adults and children present through the child if old enough.
	Engage the child through play, neutral chat or by establishing rapport with the parents. Gauge the child's initial comfort level with you and adjust your approach accordingly.
	Establish interest and concern and attend to the comfort of child and adult(s).
Identify the reason for the consultation	Establish from the child if possible who will 'lead' on the story and how others will contribute; will child or parent start?
Gathering information	
Listen, facilitate, use open and closed questions appropriately	Play and gather information at the same time for younger children.
	Actively encourage telling of story of problems in the child's and parents' own words.
	Use open and closed questioning techniques appropriate to the age of the child – closed questioning with choices works well with young children; narrative with older children. Determine and acknowledge ideas (beliefs regarding cause of illness may differ between parent and child). Establish both the parent's and the child's perspective where appropriate.
Understand the child's and parent's perspectives Establish background information – context	Encourage expression of feelings (parents may be able to describe a young child's feelings but provide space for children to describe their own).
	This includes the following: • pregnancy and birth history • immunisation and childhood illness history • growth and developmental history • drug and allergy history • family and social history.
Structuring	
Use internal summary and signposting	Use this skill frequently, especially when you are transferring your attention from the child to the parent(s) and back again. *'David, your mother has just told me all about your tummy pains and what she thinks they are ... now I want to hear from you; can you tell me exactly where this pain is ... can you point to it?'*

Skills from the Calgary–Cambridge Guides	Applying these skills in greater depth, intention and intensity
Physical examination	
Create an appropriate environment for examination	General physical examination in younger children: • choice of parent's lap/couch/at play • use of least invasive examination techniques first • use of play to facilitate examination • be opportunistic. General physical examination of older children: • anticipate that they may be embarrassed and require privacy • ask whom the patient wishes to stay with them.
Building the relationship	
Continue to build rapport	Continue to build rapport with children and their parents as appropriate. Children often appreciate fun, cheerfulness and jokes combined with gentleness.
Share your thinking	Share your thinking with parents – not always easy if you are keeping children happy at the same time. Adolescents sometimes find too much eye contact off-putting. Taking your full attention off the young person and for instance asking them to help you to draw a family tree will often help them to talk more freely.
Explanation and planning	
Provide correct amount and type of information Incorporate patient's perspective Involve the patient in decision making	Provide the correct amount and type of information suitable for both the child *and* the parent to understand. It may be appropriate for the parent to explain to a younger child on your behalf. Incorporate both the parent's *and* the child's perspective when giving information. Involve both the parents *and* the child in decision making where appropriate.
Closing the session	
Safety-netting	Safety-netting is very important for parental satisfaction and to ensure accurate understanding.

In two publications on this topic, Perrin and Geritty (1981) and Santrock (1998) contribute insights into interviewing children and their families. A useful video-tape by Korsch (2002) demonstrates effective communication between paediatric patient and doctor, with a particular focus on reducing the power gap. Levetown (2008) has written an excellent review of the literature about communicating with children and families. Howells *et al.* (2010) have recently developed a useful tool for assessing paediatric consultation skills based on the Calgary–Cambridge Guide.

The telephone interview

The telephone interview is now becoming a common mode of doctor–patient communication. Triaging, managing minor or administrative problems or follow up for both acute and chronic conditions can all be effectively achieved on the telephone (Pinnock *et al.* 2003). Car and Sheik's (2003) review of telephone consultations has shown that patient satisfaction with this medium of consulting is high. Patients value speed and improvement of access, reduced travel time and costs, as well as the possibility of increased frequency of contact. However, until recently there has been little study of the skills needed to consult effectively on the telephone, nor of the training doctors need to use this medium with skill and confidence, which is vital if quality and safety are to be ensured (Toon 2002). Browne and Eberle (1974) and Ott *et al.* (1974) found that medical histories taken over the telephone are seriously incomplete. A recent study in the UK comparing consulting modes between face-to-face and telephone consultations in general practice has shown that telephone consultations were shorter, with less questioning by both doctors and patients and less disclosure of and discussion of problems by patients (McKinstry *et al.* 2010). A qualitative study undertaken by Hewitt *et al.* (2010) to clarify some of these differences used conversational analysis to look at the data. Also involving general practice in the UK, this study showed that telephone consultations tend to be mono-topical. Doctors used similar skills when eliciting information and patients' concerns; patients tended to spontaneously volunteer their problems more easily than in face-to-face consultations and they were also less likely to raise new problems towards the end of the consultation. In other words, patients were more focused on the telephone. The authors point out the importance of careful verbal examination in a telephone consultation and equally careful 'safety-netting' and follow-up planning. They also encourage doctors to explain the significance of the possible development of symptoms and the rationale for the patient or parent to seek help appropriately.

In a randomised controlled study of patients' and interpreters' views on interpreting for the patient during telephone versus video connection, Locatis *et al.* (2010) showed that patients found an interpreter to be helpful but that there were no differences from the patients' point of view between being interpreted via video connection with both picture and sound and using the telephone only. On the other hand, the interpreters much preferred using the video connection for interpreted consultations. A study by Agha *et al.* (2009) supported these findings.

Although the core skills for communication with patients pertain to consulting on the telephone, there are some important differences between this and face-to-face communication. Here again some skills need to be used with greater depth and accuracy, particularly if the patient lacks confidence on the telephone.

Understanding can be compromised because visual non-verbal cues that normally are important for sending and interpreting messages are unavailable to both physician and patient. In emergency work, it is common for someone else to telephone on behalf of an ill or elderly patient so that communication may have to be conducted through a third party. Careful active listening, frequent checking for understanding and an interested response are paramount if the telephone interview is to be effective. Encouraging the patient to speak requires the use of verbal rather than non-verbal facilitation, '*mm … mm …, aha … yep …*', or the clearer, '*I see … go on … tell me a bit more … yes … yes …*'. Discovering the patient's concerns, ideas, and hopes for the consultation is vital. If patients are ill at ease with telephone consultations, this is often due to difficulties with previous telephone experiences, which have not always been in a medical context (Hopton *et al.* 1996). Overtly picking up the patient's cues enables the doctor to enter this arena in an efficient and empathic manner. *'It sounds as if you are very concerned ... I can hear from your voice that you are anxious about ...'* Sometimes a careful challenge needs to be made: *'You don't sound satisfied with what I've just said'.* Hearing-impaired individuals may find telephoning difficult.

Paradoxically, consultations on the telephone should be no shorter than face-to-face ones because of the necessity of clarifying, without doubt, both the disease and illness content of the interview. It is easy to cut corners and fail to clarify specific parts of the patient's story and miss an important diagnosis. Asking what the patient can see or feel (*'What does the rash look like?'* or *'How alert is your baby?'*) may allow the clinician to manage the problem safely without seeing the patient. Giving information needs to be clear and simple, with chunking and checking throughout. Repetition and summarising the management plan more than once is useful. Asking the patient to reiterate important details back to the doctor is a particularly useful form of repetition here. Offering options often enables the patient and the doctor to move towards mutual common ground (*see* Chapter 6) and allows negotiation to proceed more smoothly. Closing the consultation will be difficult if the patient feels that their needs have not been met, and in particular if follow-up plans are unclear or the patient has not agreed to the doctor's suggestions. Accurate recording of the interview is crucial.

Out-of-hours consultations in primary care practice where the doctor does not know the patient may present special problems. Males' (1998) qualitative study of UK family doctors' experiences of giving telephone advice suggests that guideline development, rehearsal using role-play and greater initial supervision of residents is likely to be effective.

Key skills of the Calgary–Cambridge Guides that need applying with greater depth, intention and intensity

Skills from the Calgary–Cambridge Guides	Applying these skills with greater depth, intention and intensity
Initiation	
Preparation	Answer the telephone or return calls promptly.
	When you are initiating the call, check that you have all the relevant information in front of you before picking up the telephone.
Make introductions	Check that you are talking to the correct patient – you may not recognise the patient's voice, even if you know the patient well.
Develop rapport	If you are using an interpreter and video calling, make sure that you have planned the consultation in terms of timing and personnel, and that the IT equipment is in working order. Use tone of voice and supporting statements early in order to develop rapport – appropriate smiling while talking will be 'heard' by the patient.

Continued

Skills from the Calgary–Cambridge Guides	Applying these skills with greater depth, intention and intensity
Gathering information	
Listen actively	Give verbal encouragement to continue rather than listening in silence.
Gauge the patient's emotional state	Pick up cues and respond clearly and verbally to them. This is obviously easier when video calling is used.
Clarify	Carefully clarify the clinical story, using appropriate direct questions in order not to miss important data.
Discover the patient's framework	Clarify that the patient's ideas, concerns and expectations have been obtained before proceeding to explanation and planning; check this carefully if you are using an interpreter.
Building the relationship	
Demonstrate empathy, acceptance, sensitivity Provide support	These need to be demonstrated verbally and repeatedly, using the appropriate non-verbal skills, particularly when you are being interpreted or when video calling is used.
Structuring the interview	
Use internal summary Signpost	Use these two skills in tandem more frequently when you cannot see the patient, in order to clarify transitions between open and closed questions, the disease and illness frameworks and explanation and planning.
Explanation and planning	
Chunk and check	Check understanding and agreement verbally rather than using a nod of the head, for example.
Use clear language free from jargon and moderate pace	This is particularly important if the telephone connection is of poor quality. Giving some ideas about the prognosis is particularly helpful early in an illness, especially when the doctor and the patient have decided that a face-to-face consultation is not necessary.
Offer options	Offer options before trying to agree on a management plan. This might work particularly successfully where an interpreter is used; don't forget that however professional the interpreter is, the more they understand the structure of the consultation and that the doctor is aligning herself with the patient, the more accurately the interpreter is likely to help the patient feel that they and the doctor have reached mutual common ground.
Negotiate a management plan	Check that the management plan is acceptable. This is more likely to reassure the patient who has agreed that they do not need to see a doctor on this occasion. Encourage the patient to repeat the advice given. Ask if there are any outstanding questions or concerns.

Skills from the Calgary–Cambridge Guides	Applying these skills with greater depth, intention and intensity
Closing	
Summarise and check Safety-net	These three skills need particular attention on the telephone, and where there is an interpreter working with the patient on the phone too, in order to be clinically safe and to maintain rapport and the patient's confidence.

Patients with mental illness

Interviewing patients with mental illness demonstrates the importance of the core skills of gathering information (in particular of taking an accurate clinical history) and building the relationship. Encouragingly, there have been more studies of communication with patients with mental illness in the last few years. In a recent study of interviewing 104 patients with mental illness, Del Piccolo *et al.* (2012) showed that female patients are more likely to drop cues and that female psychiatrists are more likely to 'pick them up', but that they tend to give the patient space rather than explore the cue in detail. The patient here may need silence to start to make sense of what is happening to them. On the other hand, silence could be felt as pressurising, especially when the patient is ill, and in this study empathic responses from the psychiatrists were infrequent. Another study (Castillo *et al.* 2012) exploring the difference between residents' consultations and those of more experienced psychiatrists discovered that the residents' visits were twice as long as psychiatrists' visits, and that residents devoted a significantly greater proportion of their talk to relationship-building and activating/partnering aspects of communication, whereas the psychiatrists devoted a greater proportion to biomedically related data-gathering/counselling/patient education. Analysis of voice tones in this study revealed that residents were perceived as sounding significantly friendlier and more sympathetic, while the psychiatrists disappointingly were rated as sounding more dominant and rushed.

A British study (de Las Cuevas *et al.* 2012) of senior psychiatrists showed that the psychiatrists were favourable in their attitude to involving patients in a process of reciprocal communication where patients' preferences, values, and expectations were considered, but they were more cautious in their attitude to sharing decisions with patients. This result is disappointing when you consider that shared partnership is the key to helping patients with serious mental illness comply with management and medication.

However, communicating effectively when addressing psychiatric and psychological problems in everyday practice can be difficult. A recent book, *Communication Skills in Mental Health Care: An Introduction* (Coll *et al.* 2012), provides a clear and concise guide on how to run consultations, using the Calgary–Cambridge model. The model is applied to an extensive variety of mental health conditions, ranging from taking a good psychiatric history to specialist scenarios such as working with families and young people or breaking bad news in mental health. There are also practical and comprehensive chapters on anxiety, depression, psychosis, risk to self, and the all-important subject of mental capacity. The book also discusses dealing with emotions and mental health consultations in primary care. There is a useful accompanying DVD.

Uncovering hidden depression and assessing suicidal risk

Depression is a frequently occurring psychiatric disorder that is easily missed in medical practice. Accurate diagnosis depends on the skill of the doctor. Here the process skills need to be highlighted, not only to help the patient tell their story more easily and discover their perspective, but also in order to elicit the all-important content of this specific psychiatric interview – namely, how depressed the patient is and whether they are suicidal or not.

The psychiatric interview differs from all other medical interviews in that the mental health examination is an integral part of the interviewing process – the interview is the 'history' and the 'examination' at one and the same time. Using the process skills of the guides accurately and compassionately in order to cover the content of the psychiatric interview, is one of the most demanding and difficult tasks in medicine. The interviewer not only has to establish initial rapport and discover the patient's story as far as possible but also has to make a formal assessment of the patient's mental state and assess the patient's risk of harm to himself.

Many depressed patients feel that they do not deserve to take up the doctor's time. It is often part of their illness that they feel that it is not possible for physicians to listen to and fully understand them. As a consequence, they may receive less effective care than they need and deserve (Gask *et al.* 2003). Focusing on building the relationship right from the beginning of the interview will encourage patients to 'open up' and tell their story in their own words, as well as sharing their feelings about the situation that they find themselves in, an important part of the therapeutic approach. Building rapport, expressing empathy and support and asking difficult questions sensitively should help the physician to elicit key facts such as whether the depressed patient has a severe and sustained disturbance of mood accompanied by feelings of worthlessness, loss of interest and morbid guilt together with alterations in appetite, weight and sleep pattern. It is essential to discover whether patients who are thought to be at suicidal risk have thoughts of hopelessness, self-harm or suicide. Both open questions and precision in closed questioning technique (reversing the 'open-to-closed' cone) are therefore important and must of course be combined with a compassionate approach and the willingness to witness what the patient is experiencing.

Again, flexibility with open and closed questions is very important. Patients who are very depressed may respond well to open questions and empathic statements that help them to express their feelings and may reveal all the information the doctor needs. But they may also need the physician to use a series of directed questions to help them tell a story, parts of which may be difficult for them to disclose (e.g. details of suicidal intent). The physician may have to make a judgement on how long to persevere with trying to 'open up' a severely depressed patient in an attempt to build rapport and obtain all the information required or when to move to more closed questions to elucidate how depressed the patient is, how likely the patient is to attempt suicide again and whether it is safe to allow the patient to return home.

Key skills of the Calgary–Cambridge Guides that need applying with greater depth, intention and intensity

Skills from the Calgary–Cambridge Guides	Applying these skills with greater depth, intention and intensity
Initiation	
Develop initial rapport	How you greet a patient who is overtly depressed is crucial. Matching the patient's pace and mood and picking up and responding to verbal and non-verbal cues is a very important part of developing initial rapport. Look especially for facial expression and tone and pace of talk and match it.
Gathering information	
Listen, facilitate Gauge the patient's emotional state	Listen to the patient's opening statement without interruption, showing concern and compassion. Express empathy and continue to pick up and respond to verbal and non-verbal cues.
Use open and closed questions appropriately	Direct the patient into an open question about feelings: this will often get you to the root of the problem quickly. Allowing the patient to express feelings is often cathartic, although it is a question of careful timing when to signpost the interview into directive questions to enable the patient to tell more of the story and feel more in control. Directive questions about why the patient feels he is depressed, what the main concerns are, the effect on personal life and work, and any hopes or expectations from the doctor, are highly important.
Clarify	Repetition, paraphrasing and the use of silence all help to 'open up' a patient who is feeling hopeless, worthless and guilty.
Discover the patient's perspective	Directive questions about why the patient feels he is depressed, what the main concerns are, the effect on personal life and work, and any hopes or expectations from the doctor, are important and again may also help to clarify the story and help with risk assessment.
Building the relationship	*The skills from this key section of the interview need to be used flexibly at every stage* (see also *above*)
Demonstrate empathy	It is important to be skilful in how you express empathy. Patients will quickly detect if your tone of voice does not match what you say: *'How can you know what I'm feeling …?'* Tears demand the special response of a combination of supportive body language including touch, silence, empathy and knowing when to 'move on'.
Accept	Accept non-judgementally what the patient says and how they feel. Avoid premature reassurance: *'I'm sure you will be better soon …'*
Provide support	Discover the patient's support systems and offer support and continuity of care yourself where possible.

Examples of specific phrasing for uncovering depression/suicidal risk include:

'I'm wondering how low you really are … can you bear to tell me?'

'You look depressed today … would you like to tell me about how you are feeling?'

'You've told me that you feel hopeless and guilty about your situation … do you feel we can help at all?'

'You are wondering if you are depressed. I'd like to ask you some specific questions about your mood, concentration, appetite and sleeping patterns, which will help us …'

'Do you ever feel that there's a light at the end of the tunnel?'

'You've told me how difficult it is to sleep. What is going through your mind when you are lying tossing and turning?'

'Some people feel that they can't go on when they are depressed. Have you had thoughts like that … that you'd like to end it all? Have you made any plans?'

'You took a serious overdose of paracetamol last night. How are you feeling about that now? Are you glad or disappointed that it failed?'

The psychotic patient

Patients with delusions and hallucinations present considerable communication challenges. Here the patient is in some way out of touch with reality – this may be quite a subtle state or the patient may be acutely ill, not making sense, suspicious and possibly violent, with little insight. Not only may such patients be unable to function normally but also their communication skills are often impaired and they are commonly frightened and untrusting. In fact, it may be impossible to form a relationship with the patient – any attempts to get close to the patient may be misinterpreted and feel threatening. On the other hand, patients with mental illness greatly value being understood.

The beginning of an interview with a psychotic patient is crucial – lack of mutual trust and rapport in the first minute or two can quickly lead to conflict and difficulties. Anxious and sometimes angry relatives and friends may complicate the interviewing process. Davies (1997) has suggested that the use of open questions initially is vital in elucidating the nature of the presenting problem and establishing rapport. Asking direct or closed questions is not easy, yet, as Cox (1989) demonstrated, more information may be elicited if the interviewer makes specific probes in her direct questioning and uses the open-to-closed cone (*see* Chapter 3) flexibly.

Engaging the patient in a therapeutic alliance may be very difficult when there is lack of insight or when the patient has only agreed to see the physician because of family pressure or under duress from the law. Negotiating treatment with a psychotic patient is particularly challenging and may be impossible – for instance, when there is a need for compulsory admission to hospital.

The challenge for the doctor is to overcome these barriers to communication while simultaneously gathering information, often from diverse cues, of the presence and extent of a psychotic disorder. Gathering information in a sensitive and empathic manner when possibly the physician is ill at ease requires communication skills of a high order. Do not underestimate the effect of anxiety, fear and discomfort on both doctor and patient. The first interview a patient and their family have with a doctor where there is a possibility of severe mental illness is akin to receiving bad news and is likely to be remembered for the whole of the patient's life. It is vital that the interview is effective, that fears are aired and stigma avoided. This will help to set the scene constructively for any future interviews and assessments.

Key skills of the Calgary–Cambridge Guides that need applying with greater depth, intention and intensity

Skills from the Calgary–Cambridge Guides	Applying these skills with greater depth, intention and intensity
Initiation	
Preparation	It is particularly important to gather information from patient records and from those with prior knowledge of the patient before starting the interview – not only do you need to know as much as possible about the patient's past history but also you need to establish risk to yourself and others. For example, is the patient potentially dangerous?
Make introductions	Introducing yourself as a doctor or psychiatrist and explaining why you are there may be difficult – the patient may not have sought this interview. On the one hand there is a need for a clear explanation of who the doctor is and why they have been asked to see the patient. On the other, if the patient is thought disordered, full explanation of your psychiatric role can immediately increase suspicion and impair rapport.
	Establish early whether there is a risk of violence and position yourself accordingly.
Gathering information	
Listen, facilitate Gauge the patient's emotional state	Listen to the patient's perspective of their problems rather than asking about thought disorders directly, picking up the patient's non-verbal cues and asking sensitively how the patient is feeling may give you information about not only the patient's concerns (e.g. that the neighbours are being a nuisance) but also how suspicious and paranoid the patient is. It may also allow you to assess the extent of the patient's delusions or hallucinations.
	You can help build rapport by exploring the patient's 'external' problems (the effect on their life) rather than 'internal' problems first. Eliciting the patient's concerns – staying initially with the patient's world view and problems rather than attempting to explore thought disorders too early in the interview – will help build rapport.

Continued

Skills from the Calgary–Cambridge Guides	Applying these skills with greater depth, intention and intensity
Listen, facilitate Gauge the patient's emotional state (*cont.*)	The patient may not think they are 'ill' and the doctor needs to reflect back the patient's experiences and develop a shared understanding of the patient's perspective of how these experiences are affecting the patient's life.
Discover the patient's perspective	Discover the patient's beliefs. Acknowledging them but not colluding with the patient is a difficult skill that we explore shortly.
Move between open and closed questioning: reverse the open-closed cone if necessary	Flexibility in applying the open-closed cone is vital. Either too early open-ended questioning or very directed questions about psychosis can increase anxiety – sometimes the open-to-closed cone needs reversing here (*see* following section, 'The open-to-closed cone').
Clarify	You may need to try a variety of approaches if the patient does not follow your lead and 'open up' – for example, try an educated guess to clarify the situation. Once you have the patient's trust, and they are willing to talk, you can follow the patient's lead and ask further clarifying questions that link and make sense to him or her.
Pick up cues	Picking up verbal and non-verbal cues but not necessarily overtly responding to them is sometimes necessary; reflecting back verbal and non-verbal cues immediately may increase suspicion.
Building the relationship	
Demonstrate appropriate non-verbal behaviour	Keep calm, and be careful with pace. Flexibility with regard to eye contact is important – too much eye contact may agitate the patient and increase paranoia. Sit down and sit still. Be careful about the use of touch, which can be misinterpreted.
Demonstrate acceptance	Try not to show surprise; offer non-judgemental acceptance.
Demonstrate empathy	Take care not to express empathy insincerely – most physicians find it difficult to put themselves in a psychotic patient's shoes, and patients know this.
Provide support	Offer realistic help without collusion.
Structuring the interview	
Use internal summary Signpost	Carefully summarising the story back to the patient and signposting what the physician needs to discover next may calm the patient, particularly when used in conjunction with offers of help. Structuring the interview with signposting and sequencing can help a patient with thought disorder. Signposting is vital as the patient may not be concentrating and misunderstand reasons for focused questions.

Skills from the Calgary–Cambridge Guides	Applying these skills with greater depth, intention and intensity
Explanation and planning	
Shared decision making	Being truthful to a patient about unpleasant side effects of an antipsychotic drug, when the patient is reluctant to take medication is not easy. However, building rapport and achieving concordance in the patient who is at risk of psychosis is essential (Seale *et al.* 2006). A full discussion where the doctor shares his thinking about why the patient needs to take the medication may depend on how much insight the patient has. The goal here is for the patient to take the medication and to trust the doctor, but the balance of achieving mutual common ground may not be easy.

Examples of specific phrasing

The open-to-closed cone

Attempts to assess the extent of the patient's thoughts, beliefs and thinking processes can be difficult and requires judicial use of open and closed questions. Often the technique of 'following' with closed questions rather than open ones will clarify how thought-disordered the patient is without confrontation and will allow you to perform a mental health assessment of the patient while you obtain the clinical history:

> Patient: *'I can see people at the window.'*
> Doctor: *'Mmm … can you tell me who are they? … What are they saying?'* (rather than *'Tell me all about them'*, which may upset and agitate the patient and produce the response *'Can't you see them?'*).

The patient may then follow your line of questioning and clarify that he has visual and auditory hallucinations. However, patients who are less suspicious often want to talk about their psychotic symptoms in some detail. Addressing their concerns about their illness will be perceived as more supportive and may help the patient to engage with the psychiatric services more easily (McCabe *et al.* 2002).

Empathy without collusion

It is important not to confront delusions as false beliefs – empathise with the patient's situation and legitimise their experience without necessarily agreeing or colluding with their interpretation of reality. Do not rebuff the patient but remain interested in their view and offer empathy and help with their problems:

> *'I can certainly understand that you would feel so upset because you think you are being poisoned.'*

In response to *'Don't you believe me?'*, you could respond as follows:

> *'You ask if I believe you about whether you are being poisoned. I can tell you for sure that I am not poisoning you. I can't tell for sure right now whether anyone else my be poisoning you, but I'd like to listen to you and help in any way that I can.'*

Combining advocacy and support with challenge

This is a difficult balancing act with a psychotic patient. Offering explanations that accept the patient's experiences as valid, and showing empathy but providing an alternative view is a difficult balancing act with a psychotic patient, particularly if they challenge you and ask you if you think that they are mad. It is helpful for the doctor to find phrases that work well in different circumstances and to practise them.

> *'I know that you feel that you are not ill at the moment, but I am concerned about you today ... I think that you need some treatment, and I would like to help.'*

Gathering information from others

It is often very important to get accurate information from others who know the patient well – including other professionals, for instance – to determine whether the patient is improving or deteriorating. Obtaining such witness statements can be perceived as threatening and unsupportive to a paranoid person with disordered thinking. If the doctor is aiming to achieve a collaborative relationship, it is important to have the patient's permission if possible. In these circumstances relatives and friends are often anxious and sometimes angry, which may also complicate the interviewing process. It may be important to allow extra time to talk with the patient's significant others who may naturally be overwhelmed by what is happening to their relative.

For more insights on how to interview the mentally ill, see Gask (1998) and Johnstone *et al.* (1998).

Interviewing the older patient with mental illness

Interviewing older patients with mental illness or those who are frail and may have some cognitive impairment is particularly challenging. In contrast to what might be expected, Wolff and Roter (2012) have noted in a study of elderly infirm patients with psychiatric symptoms that accompanied patients' visits were shorter and less patient-centred than unaccompanied visits. Perhaps consultations with the mentally infirm should start after introductions, with the psychiatrist and the patient alone, and then the accompanying adult should be interviewed either with the patient or separate from the patient when a good witness statement can be taken as to how the patient is coping alone, and so forth. A particularly helpful handbook by McKillop and Petrini (2011) notes that

> it can be very difficult to communicate with people with dementia. Each case requires its own unique handling. Not every scenario can be covered, as many

times your own judgment is what will work best according to the circumstances.
These can even change from dawn to evening as well from day to day. Never
assume things will be the way they were the last time you communicated. Be on
your guard. Be adaptable.

Medically unexplained symptoms

This issue is one in which doctors express considerable difficulty and frustration.
They often describe patients with medically unexplained symptoms as 'heart-sink'
patients and may respond to these patients whose symptoms appear baffling, with
little interest, empathy or support. In a study of family practice in the UK, Salmon
et al. (2009) demonstrated that, contrary to the common view of general practitioners that patients wish to have their symptoms investigated, patients actively wish
to explore psychological issues and obtain a clear explanation of their symptoma-
tology. Patients provided many cues concerning psychosocial difficulties and their
need for emotional support and were guarded in expressing a desire for physical
intervention. In another study of general practitioners in the UK, the explanation
of the high level of physical interventions for medically unexplained symptoms lay
in the doctors' responses rather than the patients' demands (Ring *et al.* 2004). It is
vital to pick up and explore patients' cues during the first consultation and provide
explanations tailored to the patient's need concerning their physical symptoms.
The objective is to prevent symptoms from becoming 'fixed' and to make a trusting and supportive relationship with the patient. Launer (2009) has suggested that
'medically unexplored stories' would be a more helpful wording for the acronym
MUS (medically unexplained symptoms) for both patients and doctors. Taking a
more narrative-based approach is likely to provide more opportunity for effective
psychological interventions.

In a focus group study dealing with how general practitioners manage patients
with unexplained symptoms, doctors adopted ritualistic ways of conducting the
consultation – that of regularly seeing and examining the patients. They found it
difficult to explain the symptoms their patients were experiencing (Olde Hartman
et al. 2009). In another study analysing conversational behaviours (Monzoni
et al. 2011) between neurologists and patients with symptoms thought to be of
emotional origin, it was evident that doctors faced huge interactional challenges,
particularly where there was resistance to the physicians' explanations.

However, in a study of patients with fibromyalgia and the cues and concerns
they expressed, Eide *et al.* (2011) underline the importance of a patient-centred
style. Doctors picking up patients' cues and concerns and expressing empathy
resulted in fewer cues from patients, not more. In an interesting study of why
general practitioners decline training for help with their patients with medically
unexplained symptoms (Salmon *et al.* 2007), those general practitioners who
declined training devalued their psychological interventions, whereas those who
accepted training did not. The authors suggest that, 'whereas negative attitudes
to patients have previously been regarded as the main barrier to involvement in
measures to improve patient management, GPs devaluing of their own psychological skills with these patients may be more important'.

In one of a number of recent books on treating medically unexplained symptoms, Wolfolk and Allen (2006) describe various affective cognitive behavioural

approaches to help patients explain and manage their symptoms. General practitioners have found positive interventions valuable in helping to make consultations more comfortable, and understand their patients' sufferings better, but they also found it very difficult to initiate change in their patients' behaviour (Aiarzaguena *et al.* 2009). Again a recent book, *Communication Skills in Mental Health Care: An Introduction* (Coll *et al.* 2012), provides some help to physicians here and the skills suggested are based on the Calgary–Cambridge model.

A review of experts' opinions of the management of unexplained symptoms in primary care (Heijmans *et al.* 2011) has shown little evidence of the effectiveness of any interventions for these patients and underline the need for research into this difficult issue for doctors when communicating in a consultation. However, the UK Royal College of Psychiatrists (2013) has advocated the use of cognitive behavioural therapy for anxiety symptoms as well as its use in depression. The UK government has recently invested heavily in cognitive behavioural therapy counsellors in primary care (see Whitfield and Williams' (2003) review article for the use of cognitive behavioural therapy in depression in busy clinical settings and Nezu *et al.* (2001) who have published a useful review of the efficacy of cognitive behavioural therapy in medically unexplained symptoms, anxiety, fibromyalgia and other difficult to treat illnesses).

The key, however, to the success and acceptance by patients of all these specialised treatments in psychological conditions and mental illness is that the practitioner uses all the basic skills of building the relationship: listening, clarifying, expressing empathy, sharing her thinking with the patient, and giving clear explanations before moving on to planning the treatment and what to do next.

And, of course, each practitioner needs to have the capacity to care for this group of patients who are often extremely ill and frightened, and who may have had less than satisfactory management in the past.

Other communication issues

Many other communication issues in medicine can be usefully explored in a similar way. The following list contains key communication issues and challenges for learners and teachers:

- ethical issues
- gender issues
- informed consent
- interviewing patients with a sexual or genito-urinary problem
- prevention and health promotion issues/changing behaviour
- explaining risk
- talking with patients who have sensory impairment
- low literacy patients
- communication during ward rounds
- death, dying and bereavement
- anger and aggression
- communicating via mobile phone, SMS (texting), Skype, FaceTime, or video link
- handling complaints
- malpractice

- interviewing and intervention for alcohol and substance abuse
- talking with patients in intensive care – acute life-threatening disease or injury
- ending the doctor–patient relationship.

Further reading

Additional sources that cover many of the issues mentioned here and which the reader may find useful include the following:

- Brewin T (1996) *Relating to the Relatives: breaking bad news, communication and support.* Radcliffe Medical Press, Oxford.
- Corney R (ed) (1991) *Developing Communication and Counselling Skills in Medicine.* Tavistock/Routledge, London.
- Fielding R (1995) *Clinical Communication Skills.* Hong Kong University Press, Hong Kong.
- Hope T, Fulford KM and Yates A (1996) *The Oxford Practice Skills Course: ethics, law and communication skills in health care education.* Oxford University Press, Oxford.
- Keithley J and Marsh G (eds) (1995) *Counselling in Primary Health Care.* Oxford General Practice Series. Oxford University Press, Oxford.
- Kleinman A, Eisenberg L and Good B (1998). Culture, illness, and care: clinical lessons from anthropologic and cross-cultural research. *Ann Intern Med.* **88**: 251–8.
- Kubler-Ross E (1967) *On Death and Dying.* Tavistock Publications, London.
- Lipkin M, Putman SM and Lazare A (eds) (1995) *The Medical Interview: clinical care, education and research.* Springer-Verlag, New York.
- Lloyd M and Bor R (1996) *Communication Skills for Medicine.* Churchill Livingstone, London.
- Myerscough PR (1992) *Talking with Patients: a basic clinical skill.* Oxford University Press, Oxford.
- Parkes CM (1972) *Bereavement: studies of grief in adult life.* International Universities Press, New York, NY.
- Platt FW and Gordon GH (2004) *The Field Guide to the Difficult Patient Interview* (2e) Lippincott, Williams and Wilkins, Philadelphia, PA.
- Professional Education and Training Committee (PETC) of New South Wales Cancer Council and the Post Graduate Medical Council (PGMC) of New South Wales, The (1992) *Communicating With Your Patients: an interactional skills training manual for junior medical officers.* PETC and PGMC, Sydney.
- Spitzer J (2003) *Caring for Jewish Patients.* Radcliffe Medical Press, Oxford.
- Tate P (2010) *The Doctor's Communication Handbook* (6th ed). Radcliffe Publishing, Oxford.

References

Abdel-Tawab N and Roter D (2002) The relevance of client-centered communication to family planning settings in developing countries: lessons from the Egyptian experience. *Soc Sci Med.* **54**(9): 1357–68.

Adams CL and Kurtz SM (2006) Building on existing models from human medical education to develop a communication curriculum in veterinary medicine. *J Vet Med Educ.* **33**(1): 28–37.

Adams CL and Ladner LD (2004) Implementing a simulated client program: bridging the gap between theory and practice. *J Vet Med Educ.* **31**(2): 138–45.

Adamson TE, Bunch WH, Baldwin DC Jr and Oppenberg A (2000) The virtuous orthopaedist has fewer malpractice suits. *Clin Orthop Relat Res.* (378): 104–9.

Agha Z, Schapira RM, Laud PW, McNutt G and Roter DL (2009) Patient satisfaction with physician–patient communication during telemedicine. *Telemed J E Health.* **15**(9): 830–9.

Agledahl KM, Gulbrandsen P, Forde R and Wifstad A (2011) Courteous but not curious: how doctors' politeness masks their existential neglect; a qualitative study of video-recorded patient consultations. *J Med Ethics.* **37**(11): 650–4.

Ahalt C, Walter LC, Yourman L, Eng C, Perez-Stable EJ and Smith AK (2012) 'Knowing is better': preferences of diverse older adults for discussing prognosis. *J Gen Intern Med.* **27**(5): 568–75.

Aiarzaguena JM, Gaminde I, Grandes G, Salazar A, Alonso I and Sanchez A (2009) Somatisation in primary care: experiences of primary care physicians involved in a training program and in a randomised controlled trial. *BMC Fam Pract.* **10**: 73.

Aita V, McIlvain H, Backer E, McVea K and Crabtree B (2005) Patient-centered care and communication in primary care practice: what is involved? *Patient Educ Couns.* **58**(3): 296–304.

Ajaj A, Singh MP and Abdulla AJ (2001) Should elderly patients be told they have cancer? Questionnaire survey of older people. *BMJ.* **323**(7322): 1160.

Akabayashi A, Kai I, Takemura H and Okazaki H (1999) Truth telling in the case of a pessimistic diagnosis in Japan. *Lancet.* **354**(9186): 1263.

Alamo MM, Moral RR and Perula de Torres LA (2002) Evaluation of a patient-centred approach in generalized musculoskeletal chronic pain/fibromyalgia patients in primary care. *Patient Educ Couns.* **48**(1): 23–31.

Alderson P, Hawthorne J and Killen M (2006) Parents' experiences of sharing neonatal information and decisions: consent, cost and risk. *Soc Sci Med.* **62**(6): 1319–29.

Aljubran AH (2010) The attitude towards disclosure of bad news to cancer patients in Saudi Arabia. *Ann Saudi Med.* **30**(2): 141–4.

Als AB (1997) The desk-top computer as a magic box: patterns of behaviour connected with the desk-top computer; GPs' and patients' perceptions. *Fam Pract.* **14**(1): 17–23.

Ambady N, Koo J, Rosenthal R and Winograd CH (2002a) Physical therapists' nonverbal communication predicts geriatric patients' health outcomes. *Psychol Aging.* **17**(3): 443–52.

Ambady N, Laplante D, Nguyen T, Rosenthal R, Chaumeton N and Levinson W (2002b) Surgeons' tone of voice: a clue to malpractice history. *Surgery.* **132**(1): 5–9.

Anderson S and Marlett N (2004) The language of recovery: how effective communication of information is crucial to restructuring post-stroke life. *Top Stroke Rehabil.* **11**(4): 55–67.

Apter AJ, Paasche-Orlow MK, Remillard JT, Bennett IM, Ben-Joseph EP, Batista RM, Hyde J and Rudd RE (2008) Numeracy and communication with patients: they are counting on us. *J Gen Intern Med.* **23**(12): 2117–24.

Aranguri C, Davidson B and Ramirez R (2006) Patterns of communication through interpreters: a detailed sociolinguistic analysis. *J Gen Intern Med.* **21**(6): 623–9.

Arborelius E and Bremberg S (1992) What can doctors do to achieve a successful consultation? Videotaped interviews analysed by the 'consultation map' method. *Fam Pract.* **9**(1): 61–6.

Argyle M (1975) *Bodily Communication*. International Universities Press, New York, NY.

Audrey S, Abel J, Blazeby JM, Falk S and Campbell R (2008) What oncologists tell patients about survival benefits of palliative chemotherapy and implications for informed consent: qualitative study. *BMJ.* **337**: a752.

Ayanian JZ (2010) Racial disparities in outcomes of colorectal cancer screening: biology or barriers to optimal care? *J Natl Cancer Inst.* **102**(8): 511–13.

Bachmann C, Abramovitch H, Barbu CG, Cavaco AM, Elorza RD, Haak R, Loureiro E, Ratajska A, Silverman J, Winterburn S and Rosenbaum M (2012) A European consensus on learning objectives for a core communication curriculum in health care professions. *Patient Educ Couns.* Epub Nov 28.

Back AL, Bauer-Wu SM, Rushton CH and Halifax J (2009) Compassionate silence in the patient–clinician encounter: a contemplative approach. *J Palliat Med.* **12**(12): 1113–17.

Back AL, Trinidad SB, Hopley EK, Arnold RM, Baile WF and Edwards KA (2011) What patients value when oncologists give news of cancer recurrence: commentary on specific moments in audio-recorded conversations. *Oncologist.* **16**(3): 342–50.

Bagley CH, Hunter AR and Bacarese-Hamilton IA (2011) Patients' misunderstanding of common orthopaedic terminology: the need for clarity. *Ann R Coll Surg Engl.* **93**(5): 401–4.

Baile WF, Buckman R, Lenzi R, Glober G, Beale EA and Kudelka AP (2000) SPIKES: a six-step protocol for delivering bad news; application to the patient with cancer. *Oncologist.* **5**(4): 302–11.

Baile WF, Kudelka AP, Beale EA, Glober GA, Myers EG, Greisinger AJ, Bast RC Jr, Goldstein MG, Novack D and Lenzi R (1999) Communication skills training in oncology. Description and preliminary outcomes of workshops on breaking bad news and managing patient reactions to illness. *Cancer.* **86**(5): 887–97.

Baker SJ (1955) The theory of silences. *J Gen Psychol.* **53**(1): 145–67.

Baker LH, O'Connell D and Platt FW (2005) 'What else?' Setting the agenda for the clinical interview. *Ann Intern Med.* **143**(10): 766–70.

Barbour A (2000) *Making Contact or Making Sense: functional and dysfunctional ways of relating.* Humanities Institute Lecture 1999–2000 Series, University of Denver, Denver, CO.

Barnett PB (2001) Rapport and the hospitalist. *Am J Med.* **111**(9B): S31–5.

Barrows HS and Tamblyn RM (1980) *Problem-Based Learning: an approach to medical education.* Springer, New York, NY.

Barry CA, Bradley CP, Britten N, Stevenson FA and Barber N (2000) Patients' unvoiced agendas in general practice consultations: qualitative study. *BMJ.* **320**(7244): 1246–50.

Barry CA, Stevenson FA, Britten N, Barber N and Bradley CP (2001) Giving voice to the life-world. More humane, more effective medical care? A qualitative study of doctor–patient communication in general practice. *Soc Sci Med.* **53**(4): 487–505.

Barsevich AM and Johnson JE (1990) Preference for information and involvement, information seeking and emotional responses of women undergoing colposcopy. *Res Nurs Health.* **13**: 1–7.

Barsky AJ 3rd (1981) Hidden reasons some patients visit doctors. *Ann Intern Med.* **94**(4 Pt. 1): 492–8.

Bass LW and Cohen RL (1982) Ostensible versus actual reasons for seeking pediatric attention: Another look at the parental ticket of admission. *Pediatrics.* **70**(6): 870–4.

Bastiaens H, Van Royen P, Pavlic DR, Raposo V and Baker R (2007) Older people's preferences for involvement in their own care: a qualitative study in primary health care in 11 European countries. *Patient Educ Couns.* **68**(1): 33–42.

Bayer Institute for Health Care Communication (1999) *P.R.E.P.A.R.E. to be Partners (Program for Patients).* Bayer Institute for Health Care Communication, New Haven, CT.

Beach MC, Duggan PS and Moore RD (2007) Is patients' preferred involvement in health decisions related to outcomes for patients with HIV? *J Gen Intern Med.* **22**(8): 1119–24.

Beach MC and Inui T (2006) Relationship-centered care: a constructive reframing. *J Gen Intern Med.* **21**(Suppl. 1): S3–8.

Beach MC, Roter DL, Wang NY, Duggan PS and Cooper LA (2006) Are physicians' attitudes of respect accurately perceived by patients and associated with more positive communication behaviors? *Patient Educ Couns.* **62**(3): 347–54.

Beaver K, Luker KA, Owens RG, Leinster SJ, Degner LF and Sloan JA (1996) Treatment decision making in women newly diagnosed with breast cancer. *Cancer Nurs.* **19**(1): 8–19.

Becker MH (1974) The health belief model and sick role behaviour. *Health Educ Monogr.* **2**: 409–19.

Beckman HB and Frankel RM (1984) The effect of physician behaviour on the collection of data. *Ann Intern Med.* **101**(5): 692–6.

Beckman HB and Frankel RM (1994) The use of videotape in internal medicine training. *J Gen Intern Med.* **9**(9): 517–21.

Beckman HB, Frankel RM and Darnley J (1985) Soliciting the patients complete agenda: a relationship to the distribution of concerns. *Clin Res.* **33**: 714A.

Beisecker A and Beisecker T (1990) Patient information-seeking behaviours when communicating with doctors. *Med Care.* **28**(1): 19–28.

Belcher VN, Fried TR, Agostini JV and Tinetti ME (2006) Views of older adults on patient participation in medication-related decision making. *J Gen Intern Med.* **21**(4): 298–303.

Bell RA, Kravitz RL, Thom D, Krupat E and Azari R (2002) Unmet expectations for care and the patient-physician relationship. *J Gen Intern Med.* **17**(11): 817–24.

Bellet PS and Maloney MJ (1991) The importance of empathy as an interviewing skill in medicine. *JAMA.* **266**(13): 1831–2.

Bensing J (1991) Doctor–patient communication and the quality of care. *Soc Sci Med.* **32**(11): 1301–10.

Bensing JM, Deveugele M, Moretti F, Fletcher I, van Vliet L, Van Bogaert M and Rimondini M (2011) How to make the medical consultation more successful from a patient's perspective? Tips for doctors and patients from lay people in the United Kingdom, Italy, Belgium and the Netherlands. *Patient Educ Couns.* **84**(3): 287–93.

Bensing JM, Tromp F, van Dulmen S, van den Brink-Muinen A, Verheul W and Schellevis FG (2006) Shifts in doctor–patient communication between 1986 and 2002: a study of videotaped general practice consultations with hypertension patients. *BMC Fam Pract.* **7**: 62.

Bensing JM, Verheul W, Jansen J and Langewitz WA (2010) Looking for trouble: the added value of sequence analysis in finding evidence for the role of physicians in patients' disclosure of cues and concerns. *Med Care.* **48**(7): 583–8.

Benson J and Britten N (1996) Respecting the autonomy of cancer patients when talking with their families: qualitative analysis of semi-structured interviews with patients. *BMJ.* **313**: 729–31.

Berg JS, Dischler J, Wagner DJ, Raia JJ and Palmer-Shevlin N (1993) Medication compliance: a healthcare problem. *Ann Pharmacother.* **27**(9 Suppl): S1–24.

Bertakis KD (1977) The communication of information from physician to patient: a method for increasing patient retention and satisfaction. *J Fam Pract.* **5**(2): 217– 22.

Bertakis KD, Roter D and Putnam SM (1991) The relationship of physician medical interview style to patient satisfaction. *J Fam Pract.* **32**(2): 175–81.

Bibace R and Walsh M (1981) *Children's Conceptions of Health, Illness and Bodily Functions.* Jossey-Bass, San Francisco, CA.

Blacklock SM (1977) The symptom of chest pain in family medicine. *J Fam Pract.* **4**(3): 429–33.

Blanchard CG, Labrecque MS, Ruckdeschel JC and Blanchard EB (1988) Information and decision making preferences of hospitalised adult cancer patients. *Soc Sci Med.* **27**: 1139.

Blatt B, LeLacheur SF, Galinsky AD, Simmens SJ and Greenberg L (2010) Does perspective-taking increase patient satisfaction in medical encounters? *Acad Med.* **85**(9): 1445–52.

Bonvicini KA, Perlin MJ, Bylund CL, Carroll G, Rouse RA and Goldstein MG (2009) Impact of communication training on physician expression of empathy in patient encounters. *Patient Educ Couns.* **75**(1): 3–10.

Booth N, Kohannejad J and Robinson R (2002) *Information in the Consulting Room (iiCR) Final Project Report.* Sowerby Centre for Health, Newcastle upon Tyne.

Boreham P and Gibson D (1978) The informative process in private medical consultations: a preliminary investigation. *Soc Sci Med.* **12**(5A): 409–16.

Bourhis RY, Roth S and MacQueen G (1989) Communication in the hospital setting: a survey of medical and everyday language use amongst patients, nurses and doctors. *Soc Sci Med.* **28**(4): 339–46.

Bowes P, Stevenson F, Ahluwalia S and Murray E (2012) I need her to be a doctor: patients experiences of presenting health information from the internet in GP consultations. *Br J Gen Pract.* **62**(604): e732–8.

Bracci R, Zanon E, Cellerino R, Gesuita R, Puglisi F, Aprile G, Barbieri V, Misuraca D, Venuta S, Carle F and Piga A (2008) Information to cancer patients: a questionnaire survey in three different geographical areas in Italy. *Support Care Cancer.* **16**(8): 869–77.

Braddock CH, Fihn SD, Levinson W, Jonsen AR and Pearlman RA (1997) How doctors and patients discuss routine clinical decisions: informed decision making in the outpatient setting. *J Gen Intern Med.* **12**(6): 339–45.

Bradshaw PW, Ley P, Kincey JA and Bradshaw J (1975) Recall of medical advice: comprehensibility and specificity. *Br J Soc Clin Psychol.* **14**: 55–62.

Branch WT and Malik TK (1993) Using 'windows of opportunities' in brief interviews to understand patients' concerns. *JAMA.* **269**(13): 1667–8.

Bravo BN, Postigo JML, Segura LR, Selva JPS, Trives JJR, Córcoles MJ, López MN and Hidalgo JLT (2010) Effect of the evaluation of recall on the rate of information recalled by patients in primary care. *Patient Educ Couns.* **81**(2): 272–4.

Brewin T (1996) *Relating to the Relatives: breaking bad news; communication and support.* Radcliffe Medical Press, London.

Briggs GW and Banahan BF (1979) A training workshop in psychological medicine for teachers of family medicine. Handouts 1–3: therapeutic communication. Society of Teachers of Family Medicine, Denver, CO.

Britten N (1994) Patients' ideas about medicines: a qualitative study in a general practice population. *Br J Gen Pract.* **44**(387): 465–8.

Britten N (2003) Concordance and compliance. In: R Jones, N Britten, L Culpepper, D Gass, R Grol, D Mant and C Silagy (eds) *Oxford Textbook of Primary Medical Care.* Oxford University Press, Oxford.

Britten N, Stevenson FA, Barry CA, Barber N and Bradley CP (2000) Misunderstandings in prescribing decisions in general practice: qualitative study. *BMJ.* **320**(7233): 484–8.

Brock DM, Mauksch LB, Witteborn S, Hummel J, Nagasawa P and Robins LS (2011) Effectiveness of intensive physician training in upfront agenda setting. *J Gen Intern Med.* **26**(11): 1317–23.

Brod TM, Cohen MM and Weinstock E (1986) *Cancer Disclosure: communicating the diagnosis to patients* [video recording]. Medcom Inc, Garden Grove, CA.

Brody DS (1980) The patient's role in clinical decision-making. *Ann Intern Med.* **93**: 718–22.

Brody DS and Miller SM (1986) Illness concerns and recovery from a URI. *Med Care.* **24**(8): 742–8.

Brody DS, Miller SM, Lerman CE, Smith DG and Caputo GC (1989) Patient perception of involvement in medical care: relationship to illness attitudes and outcomes. *J Gen Intern Med.* **4**: 506–11.

Bronshtein O, Katz V, Freud T and Peleg R (2006) Techniques for terminating patient–physician encounters in primary care settings. *Isr Med Assoc J.* **8**(4): 266–9.

Brown CE, Roberts NJ and Partridge MR (2007) Does the use of a glossary aid patient understanding of the letters sent to their general practitioner? *Clin Med.* **7**(5): 457–60.

Brown RF, Butow PN, Dunn SM and Tattersall MH (2001) Promoting patient participation and shortening cancer consultations: a randomised trial. *Br J Cancer.* **85**(9): 1273–9.

Brown RF, Butow PN, Ellis P, Boyle F and Tattersall MHN (2004) Seeking informed consent to cancer clinical trials: describing current practice. *Soc Sci Med.* **58**(12): 2445–57.

Brown SB and Eberle BJ (1974) Use of the telephone by pediatric house staff: a technique for pediatric care not taught. *J Pediatr.* **84**(1): 117–19.

Brown VA, Parker PA, Furber L and Thomas AL (2011) Patient preferences for the delivery of bad news: the experience of a UK Cancer Centre. *Eur J Cancer Care (Engl).* **20**(1): 56–61.

Broyles S, Sharp C, Tyson J and Sadler J (1992) How should parents be informed about major procedures? An exploratory trial in the neonatal period. *Early Hum Dev.* **31**(1): 67–75.

Bruera E, Palmer JL, Pace E, Zhang K, Willey J, Strasser F and Bennett MI (2007) A randomized, controlled trial of physician postures when breaking bad news to cancer patients. *Palliat Med.* **21**(6): 501–5.

Buckman R (1994) *How to Break Bad News: a guide for health care professionals.* Papermac, London.

Buckman R (2002) Communications and emotions. *BMJ.* **325**(7366): 672.

Buller MK and Buller DB (1987) Physicians' communication style and patient satisfaction. *J Health Soc Behav.* **28**(4): 375–88.

Bunge M, Muhlhauser I and Steckelberg A (2010) What constitutes evidence-based patient information? Overview of discussed criteria. *Patient Educ Couns.* **78**(3): 316–28.

Burack RC and Carpenter RR (1983) The predictive value of the presenting complaint. *J Fam Pract.* **16**(4): 749–54.

Burton D, Blundell N, Jones M, Fraser A and Elwyn G (2010) Shared decision-making in cardiology: do patients want it and do doctors provide it? *Patient Educ Couns.* **80**(2): 173–9.

Butler C, Rollnick S and Stott N (1996) The practitioner, the patient and resistance to change: recent ideas on compliance. *CMAJ.* **154**(9): 1357–62.

Butow PN, Brown RF, Cogar S, Tattersall MH and Dunn SM (2002) Oncologists' reactions to cancer patients' verbal cues. *Psychooncology.* **11**(1): 47–58.

Butow PN, Dunn SM, Tattersall MHN and Jones QJ (1994) Patient participation in the cancer consultation: evaluation of a question prompt sheet. *Ann Oncol.* **5**: 199–204.

Bylund CL, Gueguen JA, Sabee CM, Imes RS, Li Y and Sanford AA (2007) Provider–patient dialogue about Internet health information: an exploration of strategies to improve the provider–patient relationship. *Patient Educ Couns.* **66**(3): 346–52.

Bylund CL and Makoul G (2002) Empathic communication and gender in the physician-patient encounter. *Patient Educ Couns.* **48**(3): 207–16.

Bylund CL and Makoul G (2005) Examining empathy in medical encounters: an observational study using the empathic communication coding system. *Health Commun.* **18**(2): 123–40.

Byrne PS and Long BEL (1976) *Doctors Talking to Patients.* Her Majesty's Stationery Office, London.

Cahill P and Papageorgiou A (2007a) Triadic communication in the primary care paediatric consultation: a review of the literature. *Br J Gen Pract.* **57**(544): 904–11.

Cahill P and Papageorgiou A (2007b) Video analysis of communication in paediatric consultations in primary care. *Br J Gen Pract.* **57**(544): 866–71.

Campion P, Foulkes J, Neighbour R and Tate P (2002) Patient centredness in the MRCGP video examination: analysis of large cohort. Membership of the Royal College of General Practitioners. *BMJ.* **325**(7366): 691–2.

Campion PD, Butler NM and Cox AD (1992) Principle agendas of doctors and patients in general practice consultations. *Fam Pract.* **9**(2): 181–90.

Canale, S. D., D. Z. Louis, et al. (2012). "The Relationship Between Physician Empathy and Disease Complications: An Empirical Study of Primary Care Physicians and Their Diabetic Patients in Parma, Italy." *Acad Med.* **87**(9): 1243–9 1210.1097/ACM.1240b1013e3182628fbf.

Car J and Sheikh A (2003) Telephone consultations. *BMJ.* **326**(7396): 966–9.

Carroll JG and Monroe J (1979) Teaching medical interviewing: a critique of educational research and practice. *J Med Educ.* **54**(6): 498–500.

Cassata DM (1978) Health communication theory and research: an overview of the communication specialist interface. In: BD Ruben (ed) *Communication Yearbook.* Transaction Books, New Brunswick, NJ.

Cassell EJ (1985) *Talking with Patients: Volume 2. Clinical Technique.* MIT Press, Cambridge, MA.

Cassileth B, Zupkis R and Sutton-Smith K (1980) Information and participation preferences among cancer patients. *Ann Intern Med.* **92**(6): 832–6.

Castillo EG, Pincus HA, Wieland M, Roter D, Larson S, Houck P, Reynolds CF and Cruz M (2012) Communication profiles of psychiatric residents and attending physicians in medication-management appointments: a quantitative pilot study. *Acad Psychiatry*. **36**(2): 96–103.

Castro CM, Wilson C, Wang F and Schillinger D (2007) Babel babble: physicians' use of unclarified medical jargon with patients. *Am J Health Behav*. **31** (Suppl 1): S85–95.

Cegala DJ (1997) A study of doctors' and patients' communication during a primary care consultation: implications for communication training. *J Health Commun*. **2**(3): 169–94.

Cegala DJ (2003) Patient communication skills training: a review with implications for cancer patients. *Patient Educ Couns*. **50**(1): 91–4.

Cegala DJ, Chisolm DJ and Nwomeh BC (2012) Further examination of the impact of patient participation on physicians' communication style. *Patient Educ Couns*. **89**(1): 25–30.

Cegala DJ and Post DM (2009) The impact of patients' participation on physicians' patient-centered communication. *Patient Educ Couns*. **77**(2): 202–8.

Chan WS, Stevenson M and McGlade K (2008) Do general practitioners change how they use the computer during consultations with a significant psychological component? *Int J Med Inform*. **77**(8): 534–8.

Charles C, Gafni A and Whelan T (1997) Shared decision-making in the medical encounter: what does it mean? (or it takes at least two to tango) *Soc Sci Med*. **44**(5): 681–92.

Charles C, Gafni A and Whelan T (1999a) Decision-making in the physician–patient encounter: revisiting the shared treatment decision-making model. *Soc Sci Med*. **49**(5): 651–61.

Charles C, Whelan T and Gafni A (1999b) What do we mean by partnership in making decisions about treatment? *BMJ*. **319**(7212): 780–2.

Chewning B, Bylund CL, Shah B, Arora NK, Gueguen JA and Makoul G (2012) Patient preferences for shared decisions: a systematic review. *Patient Educ Couns*. **86**(1): 9–18.

Chugh U, Agger-Gupta N, Dillmann E, Fisher D, Gronnerud P, Kulig JC, Kurtz S and Stenhouse A (1994) *The Case for Culturally Sensitive Health Care: a comparative study of health beliefs related to culture in six north-east Calgary communities*. Citizenship and Heritage Secretariat, Alberta Community Development & Calgary Catholic Immigration Society, Calgary, AB.

Chugh U, Dillman E, Kurtz SM, Lockyer J and Parboosingh J (1993) Multicultural issues in medical curriculum: implications for Canadian physicians. *Med Teach*. **15**: 83–91.

Claramita M, Utarini A, Soebono H, Van Dalen J and Van der Vleuten C (2011) Doctor–patient communication in a Southeast Asian setting: the conflict between ideal and reality. *Adv Health Sci Educ*. **16**(1): 69–80.

Clayton JM, Butow PN, Tattersall MHN, Devine RJ, Simpson JM, Aggarwal G, Clark KJ, Currow DC, Elliott LM, Lacey J, Lee PG and Noel MA (2007) Randomized controlled trial of a prompt list to help advanced cancer patients and their caregivers to ask questions about prognosis and end-of-life care. *J Clin Oncol*. **25**(6): 715–23.

Clayton JM, Hancock K, Parker S, Butow PN, Walder S, Carrick S, Currow D, Ghersi D, Glare P, Hagerty R, Olver IN and Tattersall MH (2008) Sustaining hope when communicating with terminally ill patients and their families: a systematic review. *Psychooncology*. **17**(7): 641–59.

Coambs RB, Jensen P, Hoa Her M, Ferguson BS, Jarry JL, Wong JS and Abrahamsohn RV (1995) *Review of the Scientific Literature on the Prevalence, Consequences, and Health Costs of Noncompliance and Inappropriate Use of Prescription Medication in Canada*. Pharmaceutical Manufacturers Association of Canada (University of Toronto Press), Ottawa, ON.

Cocksedge S, George B, Renwick S and Chew-Graham CA (2013) Touch in primary care consultations: qualitative investigation of doctors' and patients' perceptions. *Br J Gen Pract*. **63**(609): 283–90.

Cocksedge S, Greenfield R, Nugent GK and Chew-Graham C (2011) Holding relationships in primary care: a qualitative exploration of doctors' and patients' perceptions. *Br J Gen Pract*. **61**(589): e484–91.

Cocksedge S and May C (2005) The listening loop: a model of choice about cues within primary care consultations. *Med Educ*. **39**(10): 999–1005.

Cohen H and Britten N (2003) Who decides about prostate cancer treatment? A qualitative study. *Fam. Pract*. **20**(6): 724–9.

Cohen-Cole (1991) *The Medical Interview: a three function approach*. Mosby-Year Book, St. Louis, MO.

Cole S and Bird J (2000) *The Medical Interview: the three function approach* (2nd ed). Mosby, St. Louis, MO.

Coleman C (2011) Teaching health care professionals about health literacy: a review of the literature. *Nurs Outlook*. **59**(2): 70–8.

Coll X, Papageorgiou A, Stanley A and Tarbuck A (2012) *Communication Skills in Mental Health Care: an introduction*. Radcliffe Publishing, Oxford.

Colletti L, Gruppen L, Barclay M and Stern D (2001) Teaching students to break bad news. *Am J Surg*. **182**(1): 20–3.

Collins DL and Street RL Jr (2009) A dialogic model of conversations about risk: coordinating perceptions and achieving quality decisions in cancer care. *Soc Sci Med*. **68**(8): 1506–12.

Corney R (ed) (1991) *Developing Communication and Counselling Skills in Medicine*. Tavistock/Routledge, London.

Coulehan JL, Platt FW, Egener B, Frankel R, Lin CT, Lown B and Salazar WH (2001) 'Let me see if I have this right …': words that help build empathy. *Ann Intern Med*. **135**(3): 221–7.

Coulter A (1999) Paternalism or partnership? Patients have grown up: and there's no going back. *BMJ*. **319**(7212): 719–20.

Coulter A (2002) After Bristol: putting patients at the centre. *BMJ*. **324**(7338): 648–51.

Coulter A (2009) *Implementing Shared Decision Making in the UK*. Health Foundation, London.

Coulter A (2012) Patient engagement: what works? *J Ambul Care Manage*. **35**(2): 80–9.

Coulter A, Entwistle V and Gilbert D (1999) Sharing decisions with patients: is the information good enough? *BMJ*. **318**(7179): 318–22.

Coulter A, Peto V and Doll H (1994) Patients' preferences and general practitioners' decisions in the treatment of menstrual disorders. *Fam Pract*. **11**(1): 67–74.

Cousin G, Schmid Mast M, Roter DL and Hall JA (2012) Concordance between physician communication style and patient attitudes predicts patient satisfaction. *Patient Educ Couns*. **87**(2): 193–7.

Cox A (1989) Eliciting patients' feelings. In: Stewart M and Roter D (eds) *Communicating with Medical Patients*. Sage Publications, Newbury Park, CA.

Cox A, Hopkinson K and Rutter M (1981a) Psychiatric interviewing techniques II: naturalistic study. *Br J Psychiatry*. **138**: 283–91.

Cox A, Rutter M and Holbrook D (1981b) Psychiatric interviewing techniques V: experimental study. *Br J Psychiatry*. **139**: 29–37.

Cox, M. E., W. S. Yancy, *et al.* (2011) Effects of counseling techniques on patients' weight-related attitudes and behaviors in a primary care clinic. *Patient Educ Couns*. **85**(3): 363–8.

Croom A, Wiebe DJ, Berg CA, Lindsay R, Donaldson D, Foster C, Murry M and Swinyard MT (2011) Adolescent and parent perceptions of patient-centered communication while managing type 1 diabetes. *J Pediatr Psychol*. **36**(2): 206–15.

Cushing AM and Jones A (1995) Evaluation of a breaking bad news course for medical students. *Med Educ*. **29**: 430–5.

Cutcliffe, J. R. (1995). "How do nurses inspire and instil hope in terminally ill HIV patients?" *J Adv Nurs*. **22**(5): 888–95.

Dance FEX (1967) Toward a theory of human communication. In: FEX Dance (ed) *Human Communication Theory: original essays*. Holt, Rhinehart & Winston; New York, NY.

Dance FEX and Larson CE (1972) *Speech Communication: concepts and behaviour*. Holt, Rinehart & Winston; New York, NY.

Davies T (1997) ABC of mental health: mental health assessment. *BMJ*. **314**: 1536–9.

Davis MA, Hoffman JR and Hsu J (1999) Impact of patient acuity on preference for information and autonomy in decision making. *Acad Emerg Med*. **6**(8): 781–5.

Deber R (1994) The patient–physician partnership: changing roles and the desire for information. *CMAJ*. **151**(2): 171–6.

Deber R, Kraetschmer N and Irvine J (1996) What role do patients wish to play in treatment decision making. *Arch Int Med*. **156**: 1414–20.

Degner LF, Kristjanson LJ, Bowman D, Sloan JA, Carriere KC, O'Neil J, Bilodeau B, Watson

P and Mueller B (1997) Information needs and decisional preferences in women with breast cancer. *JAMA.* **277**(18): 1485–92.

Degner LF and Sloan JA (1992) Decision making during serious illness: what role do patients really want to play? *J Clin Epidemiol.* **45**(9): 941–50.

De Haes H and Bensing J (2009) Endpoints in medical communication research, proposing a framework of functions and outcomes. *Patient Educ Couns.* **74**(3): 287–94.

De Las Cuevas C, Rivero-Santana A, Perestelo-Perez L, Perez-Ramos J, Gonzalez-Lorenzo M, Serrano-Aguilar P and Sanz EJ (2012) Mental health professionals' attitudes to partnership in medicine taking: a validation study of the Leeds Attitude to Concordance Scale II. *Pharmacoepidemiol Drug Saf.* **21**(2): 123–9.

Del Piccolo L, Mazzi MA, Dunn G, Sandri M and Zimmermann C (2007) Sequence analysis in multilevel models: a study on different sources of patient cues in medical consultations. *Soc Sci Med.* **65**(11): 2357–70.

Del Piccolo L, Mazzi MA, Goss C, Rimondini M and Zimmermann C (2012) How emotions emerge and are dealt with in first diagnostic consultations in psychiatry. *Patient Educ Couns.* **88**(1): 29–35.

Del Piccolo L, Saltini A, Zimmermann C and Dunn G (2000) Differences in verbal behaviours of patients with and without emotional distress during primary care consultations. *Psychol Med.* **30**(3): 629–43.

De Morgan SE, Butow PN, Lobb EA, Price MA and Nehill C (2011) Development and pilot testing of a communication aid to assist clinicians to communicate with women diagnosed with ductal carcinoma in situ (DCIS). *Support Care Cancer.* **19**(5): 717–23.

DeVito JA (1988) *Human Communication: the basic course* (4th ed). Harper & Row, New York, NY.

Deyo RA and Diehl AK (1986) Patient satisfaction with medical care for low back pain. *Spine.* **11**(1): 28–30.

DiMatteo MR (2004) Variations in patients' adherence to medical recommendations. *Med Care.* **42**(3): 200–9.

DiMatteo MR, Hays RD and Prince LM (1986) Relationship of physicians' nonverbal communication skill to patient satisfaction, appointment noncompliance and physician workload. *Health Psychol.* **5**(6): 581–94.

DiMatteo MR, Taranta A, Friedman HS and Prince LM (1980) Predicting patient satisfaction from physicians' nonverbal communication skill. *Med Care.* **18**(4): 376–87.

Dimoska A, Butow PN, Dent E, Arnold B, Brown RF and Tattersall MHN (2008a) An examination of the initial cancer consultation of medical and radiation oncologists using the Cancode interaction analysis system. *Br J Cancer.* **98**(9): 1508–14.

Dimoska A, Butow PN, Lynch J, Hovey E, Agar M, Beale P and Tattersall MHN (2012) Implementing patient question-prompt lists into routine cancer care. *Patient Educ Couns.* **86**(2): 252–8.

Dimoska A, Tattersall MHN, Butow PN, Shepherd H and Kinnersley P (2008b) Can a 'prompt list' empower cancer patients to ask relevant questions? *Cancer.* **113**(2): 225–37.

Dixon-Woods M, Young B and Heney D (1999) Partnerships with children. *BMJ.* **319**(7212): 778–80.

Donovan JL (1995) Patient decision making: the missing ingredient in compliance research. *Int J Technol Assess Health Care.* **11**(3): 443–55.

Donovan JL and Blake DR (2000) Qualitative study of interpretation of reassurance among patients attending rheumatology clinics: 'just a touch of arthritis, doctor?' *BMJ.* **320**(7234): 541–4.

Dornan T and Carroll C (2003) Medical communication and diabetes. *Diabet Med.* **20**(2): 85–7.

Dosanjh S, Barnes J and Bhandari M (2001) Barriers to breaking bad news among medical and surgical residents. *Med Educ.* **35**(3): 197–205.

Dovidio J and Gaertner S (1996) Affirmative action, unintentional biases and intergroup relations. *J Soc Issues.* **52**(4): 51–75.

Dowell J, Jones A and Snadden D (2002) Exploring medication use to seek concordance with 'non-adherent' patients: a qualitative study. *Br J Gen Pract.* **52**(474): 24–32.

Duggan A, Bradshaw YS and Altman W (2010) How do I ask about your disability? An examination of interpersonal communication processes between medical students and patients with disabilities. *J Health Commun.* **15**(3): 334–50.

Duke P, Reis S and Frankel RMA (Submitted for publication) A skills-based approach for integrating the electronic health record and patient-centered communication into the medical visit. *Teach Learn Med.*

Dunn SM, Butow PN, Tattersall MH, Jones QJ, Sheldon JS, Taylor JJ and Sumich MD (1993) General information tapes inhibit recall of the cancer consultation. *J Clin Oncol.* **11**(11): 2279–85.

Dyche L and Swiderski D (2005) The effect of physician solicitation approaches on ability to identify patient concerns. *J Gen Intern Med.* **20**(3): 267–70.

Dye NE and DiMatteo MR (1995) Enhancing cooperation with the medical regimen. In: M Lipkin Jr, SM Putnam and A Lazare (eds) *The Medical Interview: clinical care, education and research.* Springer-Verlag, New York, NY.

Eddy DM (1990) Clinical decision making: from theory to practice: anatomy of a decision. *JAMA.* **263**: 441–3.

Edwards A (2004) Flexible rather than standardised approaches to communicating risks in health care. *Qual Saf Health Care.* **13**(3): 169–70.

Edwards A and Elwyn G (2001a) *Evidence-Based Patient Choice: inevitable or impossible?* Oxford University Press, Oxford.

Edwards A and Elwyn GJ (2001b) Risks: listen and don't mislead. *Br J Gen Pract.* **51**(465): 259–60.

Edwards A, Elwyn G and Mulley A (2002) Explaining risks: turning numerical data into meaningful pictures. *BMJ.* **324**(7341): 827–30.

Edwards A, Elwyn G, Wood F, Atwell C, Prior L and Houston H (2005) Shared decision making and risk communication in practice: a qualitative study of GPs' experiences. *Br J Gen Pract.* **55**(510): 6–13.

Edwards A, Hood K, Matthews E, Russell D, Russell I, Barker J, Bloor M, Burnard P, Covey J, Pill R, Wilkinson C and Stott N (2000) The effectiveness of one-to-one risk communication interventions in health care: a systematic review. *Med Decis Making.* **20**(3): 290–7.

Egan G (1990) *The Skilled Helper: a systematic approach to effective helping.* Brooks/Cole, Pacific Grove, CA.

Egbert LD, Batitt GE, Welch CE and Bartlett MK (1964) Reduction of postoperative pain by encouragement and instruction of patients. *N Engl J Med.* **270**: 825–7.

Eggly S, Penner LA, Greene M, Harper FW, Ruckdeschel JC and Albrecht TL (2006) Information seeking during 'bad news' oncology interactions: question asking by patients and their companions. *Soc Sci Med.* **63**(11): 2974–85.

Eggly, S., F. W. K. Harper, et al. (2011). Variation in question asking during cancer clinical interactions: A potential source of disparities in access to information. *Patient Educ Couns.* **82**(1): 63–8.

Eide H, Graugaard P, Holgersen K and Finset A (2003) Physician communication in different phases of a consultation at an oncology outpatient clinic related to patient satisfaction. *Patient Educ Couns.* **51**(3): 259–66.

Eide H, Sibbern T, Egeland T, Finset A, Johannessen T, Miaskowski C and Rustoen T (2011) Fibromyalgia patients' communication of cues and concerns: interaction analysis of pain clinic consultations. *Clin J Pain.* **27**(7): 602–10.

Eisenthal S, Emery R, Lazare A and Udin H (1979) 'Adherence' and the negotiated approach to parenthood. *Arch Gen Psych.* **36**(4): 393.

Eisenthal S, Koopman C and Stoeckle JD (1990) The nature of patients' requests for physicians'. *Help Acad Med.* **65**(6): 401–5.

Eisenthal S and Lazare A (1976) Evaluation of the initial interview in a walk-in clinic: the patient's perspective on a 'customer approach'. *J Nerv Mental Dis.* **162**(3): 169–76.

Ekdahl AW, Andersson L and Friedrichsen M (2010) 'They do what they think is the best for me.' Frail elderly patients' preferences for participation in their care during hospitalization. *Patient Educ Couns.* **80**(2): 233–40.

Ekman P, Friesen WV and Ellsworth P (1972) *Emotion in the Human Face: guidelines for research.* Pergamon, New York, NY.

Eleftheriadou Z (1996) Communicating with patients of different backgrounds. In: M Lloyd and R Bor (eds) *Communication Skills for Medicine.* Churchill Livingstone, London.

Elstein AS and Schwarz A (2002) Clinical problem solving and diagnostic decision making: selective review of the cognitive literature. *BMJ.* **324**(7339): 729–32.

Elwyn G, Edwards A and Britten N (2003a) 'Doing prescribing': how doctors can be more effective. *BMJ.* **327**(7419): 864–7.

Elwyn G, Edwards A, Gwyn R and Grol R (1999a) Towards a feasible model for shared decision making: focus group study with general practice registrars. *BMJ.* **319**(7212): 753–6.

Elwyn G, Edwards A and Kinnersley P (1999b) Shared decision-making in primary care: the neglected second half of the consultation. *Br J Gen Pract.* **49**(443): 477–82.

Elwyn G, Edwards A, Kinnersley P and Grol R (2000) Shared decision making and the concept of equipoise: the competences of involving patients in healthcare choices. *Br J Gen Pract.* **50**(460): 892–9.

Elwyn G, Edwards A, Mowle S, Wensing M, Wilkinson C, Kinnersley P and Grol R (2001a) Measuring the involvement of patients in shared decision-making: a systematic review of instruments. *Patient Educ Couns.* **43**(1): 5–22.

Elwyn G, Edwards A, Wensing M, Hood K, Atwell C and Grol R (2003b) Shared decision making: developing the OPTION scale for measuring patient involvement. *Qual Saf Health Care.* **12**(2): 93–9.

Elwyn G, Joshi H, Dare D, Deighan M and Kameen F (2001b) Unprepared and anxious about 'breaking bad news': a report of two communication skills workshops for GP registrars. *Educ Gen Pract.* **12**: 34–40.

Elwyn G, Kreuwel I, Durand MA, Sivell S, Joseph-Williams N, Evans R and Edwards A (2011) How to develop web-based decision support interventions for patients: a process map. *Patient Educ Couns.* **82**(2): 260–5.

Elwyn TS, Fetters MD, Sasaki H and Tsuda T (2002) Responsibility and cancer disclosure in Japan. *Soc Sci Med.* **54**(2): 281–93.

Ely JW, Levinson W, Elder NC, Mainous AG 3rd and Vinson DC (1995) Perceived causes of family physicians' errors see comments. *J Fam Pract.* **40**(4): 337–44.

Ende J, Kazis L, Ash AB and Moskovitz MA (1989) Measuring patients' desire for autonomy. *J Gen Intern Med.* **4**: 23–30.

Epstein RM (2000) The science of patient-centered care. *J Fam Pract.* **49**(9): 805–7.

Epstein RM, Alper BS and Quill TE (2004) Communicating evidence for participatory decision making. *JAMA.* **291**(19): 2359–66.

Epstein RM, Franks P, Shields CG, Meldrum SC, Miller KN, Campbell TL and Fiscella K (2005) Patient-centered communication and diagnostic testing. *Ann Fam Med.* **3**(5): 415–21.

Epstein RM, Morse DS, Frankel RM, Frarey L, Anderson K and Beckman HB (1998) Awkward moments in patient–physician communication about HIV risk. *Ann Intern Med.* **128**(6): 435–42.

Epstein RM and Peters E (2009) Beyond information: exploring patients' preferences. *JAMA.* **302**(2): 195–7.

Epstein RM, Quill TE and McWhinney IR (1999) Somatization reconsidered: incorporating the patient's experience of illness. *Arch Intern Med.* **159**(3): 215–22.

Evans BJ, Stanley RO, Mestrovic R and Rose L (1991) Effects of communication skills training on students' diagnostic efficiency. *Med Educ.* **25**(6): 517–26.

Faden R, Becker C, Lewis C, Freeman A and Faden A (1981) Disclosure of information to patients in medical care. *Med Care.* **19**(7): 718–33.

Fadiman A (1997) *The Spirit Catches You and You Fall Down.* Farrer, Strauss & Giroux, New York, NY.

Fallowfield L (1993) Giving sad and bad news. *Lancet.* **341**: 476–8.

Fallowfield LJ (2008) Treatment decision-making in breast cancer: the patient–doctor relationship. *Breast Cancer Res Treat.* **112**(Suppl. 1): 5–13.

Fallowfield LJ, Hall A, Maguire GP and Baum M (1990) Psychological outcomes of different treatment policies in women with early breast cancer outside a clinical trial. *BMJ*. **301**: 575–80.

Fallowfield LJ and Lipkin M (1995) Delivering sad or bad news. In: M Lipkin (ed) *The Medical Interview: clinical care; education and research*. Springer-Verlag, New York, NY.

Ferguson WJ and Candib LM (2002) Culture, language and the doctor–patient relationship. *Fam Med*. **34**(5): 353–61.

Field D (1995) Education for palliative care: formal education about death and dying and bereavement in UK medical schools in 1983 and 1994. *Med Educ*. **29**: 414–19.

Fielding R (1995) *Clinical Communication Skills*. Hong Kong University Press, Hong Kong.

Fink AS, Prochazka AV, Henderson WG, Bartenfeld D, Nyirenda C, Webb A, Berger DH, Itani K, Whitehill T, Edwards J, Wilson M, Karsonovich C and Parmelee P (2010) Enhancement of surgical informed consent by addition of repeat back: a multicenter, randomized controlled clinical trial. *Ann Surg*. **252**(1): 27–36.

Finlay I and Dallimore D (1991) Your child is dead. *BMJ*. **302**: 1524–5.

Fleissig A, Glasser B and Lloyd M (2000) Patients need more than written prompts for communication to be successful. *BMJ*. **320**(7230): 314–15.

Floyd M, Lang F, Beine KLB and McCord E (1999) Evaluating interviewing techniques for the sexual practices history: use of trigger tapes to assess patient comfort. *Arch Fam Med*. **8**(3): 218–23).

Floyd MR, Lang F, McCord RS and Keener M (2005) Patients with worry: presentation of concerns and expectations for response. *Patient Educ Couns*. **57**(2): 211–16.

Ford S, Schofield T and Hope T (2003) What are the ingredients for a successful evidence-based patient choice consultation? A qualitative study. *Soc Sci Med*. **56**(3): 589–602.

Ford S, Schofield T and Hope T (2006) Observing decision-making in the general practice consultation: who makes which decisions? *Health Expect*. **9**(2): 130–7.

Fowler FJ Jr, Gallagher PM, Bynum JP, Barry MJ, Lucas FL and Skinner JS (2012) Decision-making process reported by Medicare patients who had coronary artery stenting or surgery for prostate cancer. *J Gen Intern Med*. **27**(8): 911–16.

Francis V, Korsch B and Morris M (1969) Gaps in doctor–patient communication. *N Engl J Med*. **280**(10): 535–40.

Frankel R (1995) Some answers about questions in clinical interviews. In: G Morris and R Chenail (eds) *The Talk of the Clinic: explorations in the analysis of medical and therapeutic discourse*. Lawrence Erlbaum Associates, Hillsdale, NJ.

Frankel R, Altschuler A, George S, Kinsman J, Jimison H, Robertson NR and Hsu J (2005) Effects of exam-room computing on clinician–patient communication: a longitudinal qualitative study. *J Gen Intern Med*. **20**(8): 677–82.

Frankel R and Stein T (1999) Getting the most out of the clinical encounter: the four habits model. *Permanente Journal*. **3**(3): 79–88.

Frankel RM (2009) Empathy research: a complex challenge. *Patient Educ Couns*. **75**(1): 1–2.

Freidson E (1970) *Professional Dominance*. Atherton Press, Chicago, IL.

Friedman HS (1979) Non-verbal communication between patient and medical practitioners. *J Soc Issues*. **35**(1): 82–99.

Gafaranga J and Britten N (2003) 'Fire away': the opening sequence in general practice consultations. *Fam Pract*. **20**(3): 242–7.

Gafni A, Charles C and Whelan T (1998) The physician–patient encounter: the physician as a perfect agent for the patient versus the informed treatment decision-making model. *Soc Sci Med*. **47**(3): 347–354.

Gaissmaier W and Gigerenzer G (2008) Statistical illiteracy undermines informed shared decision making. *Z Evid Fortbild Qual Gesundhwes*. **102**(7): 411–13.

Garden R (2009) Expanding clinical empathy: an activist perspective. *J Gen Intern Med*. **24**(1): 122–5.

Garg A, Buckman R and Kason Y (1997) Teaching medical students how to break bad news. *CMAJ*. **156**(8): 1159–64.

Gask L (1998) Psychiatric interviewing. In: E Johnstone, C Freeman and A Zealley (eds) *Companion to Psychiatric Studies* (6th ed). Churchill Livingstone, Edinburgh.

Gask L, Rogers A, Oliver D, May C and Roland M (2003) Qualitative study of patients' perceptions of the quality of care for depression in general practice. *Br J Gen Pract*. **53**(489): 278–83.

Gattellari M, Butow PN and Tattersall MH (2001) Sharing decisions in cancer care. *Soc Sci Med*. **52**(12): 1865–78.

Gazda GM, Asbury FR, Balzer FJ, Childers WC, Phelps RE and Walters RP (1995) *Human Relations Development: a manual for educators* (5th ed). Allyn & Bacon, Boston, MA.

Geisler L (1991) *Doctor and Patient: a partnership through dialogue*. Pharma Verlag, Frankfurt.

Geist-Martin P, Ray EB and Sharf BF (2003) *Communicating Health: personal, cultural, and political complexities*. Wadsworth, Belmont, CA.

Gibb JR (1961) Defensive communication. *J Commun*. **11**(3): 141–8.

Gick ML (1986) Problem-solving strategies. *Educ Psychol*. **21**(1–2): 99–120.

Gigerenzer G (2002) *Reckoning with Risk*. Penguin Books, London.

Gigerenzer G and Edwards A (2003) Simple tools for understanding risks: from innumeracy to insight. *BMJ*. **327**(7417): 741–4.

Gill VT, Pomerantz A and Denvir P (2010) Pre-emptive resistance: patients' participation in diagnostic sense-making activities. *Sociol Health Illn*. **32**(1): 1–20.

Ginsberg H and Opper S (1988) *Piaget's Theory of Intellectual development* (3rd ed). Prentice Hall: Englewood Cliffs, NJ.

Girgis A, Sanson-Fisher RW and Schofield MJ (1999) Is there consensus between breast cancer patients and providers on guidelines for breaking bad news? *Behav Med*. **25**(2): 69–77.

Godolphin W (2009) Shared decision-making. *Healthc Q*. 12 Spec No Patient; e186–90.

Godolphin W, Towle A and McKendry R (2001) Evaluation of the quality of patient information to support informed shared decision making. *Health Expect*. **4**: 235–242.

Goldberg D, Steele JJ, Smith C and Spivey L (1983) *Training Family Practice Residents to Recognise Psychiatric Disturbances*. National Institute of Mental Health, Rockville, MD.

Goleman D (2011) *The Brain and Emotional Intelligence: new insights*. More Than Sound, Northampton, MA.

Good MJD and Good BJ (1982) *Patient Requests in Primary Care Clinics*. D Reidel, Boston, MA.

Goodwin C (1981) *Conversation Organisation: interaction between speakers and hearers*. Academic Press, New York, NY.

Gorawara-Bhat R and Cook MA (2011) Eye contact in patient-centered communication. *Patient Educ Couns*. **82**(3): 442–7.

Gordon GH, Joos SK and Byrne J (2000) Physician expressions of uncertainty during patient encounters. *Patient Educ Couns*. **40**(1): 59–65.

Greatbatch D, Heath C, Campion P and Luff P (1995) How do desk-top computers affect the doctor–patient interaction? *Fam Pract*. **12**(1): 32–6.

Greatbach D, Luff P, Heath C and Campion P (1993) Interpersonal communication and Human-computer interaction: an examination of the use of computers in medical consultations. *Interact Comput*. **5**(2): 193–216.

Greene J and Hibbard JH (2012) Why does patient activation matter? An examination of the relationships between patient activation and health-related outcomes. *J Gen Intern Med*. **27**(5): 520–6.

Greenfield S, Kaplan SH and Ware JE (1985) Expanding patient involvement in care. *Ann Intern Med*. **102**(4): 520–8.

Greenhill N, Anderson C, Avery A and Pilnick A (2011) Analysis of pharmacist–patient communication using the Calgary–Cambridge guide. *Patient Educ Couns*. **83**(3): 423–31.

Griffin SJ, Kinmonth AL, Veltman MW, Gillard S, Grant J and Stewart M (2004) Effect on health-related outcomes of interventions to alter the interaction between patients and practitioners: a systematic review of trials. *Ann Fam Med*. **2**(6): 595–608.

Griffith CH 3rd, Wilson JF, Langer S and Haist SA (2003) House staff nonverbal communication skills and standardized patient satisfaction. *J Gen Intern Med*. **18**(3): 170–4.

Grol R, van Beurden W, Binkhorst T and Toemen T (1991) Patient education in family practice: the consensus reached by patients, doctors and experts. *Fam Pract*. **8**: 133–9.

Groopman J (2007) *How Doctors Think*. Houghton Mifflin, Boston, MA.

Guadagnoli E and Ward P (1998) Patient participation in decision-making. *Soc Sci Med*. **47**(3): 329–39.

Haas LJ, Glazer K, Houchins J and Terry S (2006) Improving the effectiveness of the medical visit: a brief visit-structuring workshop changes patients' perceptions of primary care visits. *Patient Educ Couns.* **62**(3): 374–8.

Hack TF, Degner LF and Dyck DG (1994) Relationship between preferences for decision control and illness information among women with breast cancer. *Soc Sci Med.* **39**: 279–89.

Hack TF, Pickles T, Bultz BD, Ruether JD and Degner LF (2007) Impact of providing audiotapes of primary treatment consultations to men with prostate cancer: a multi-site, randomized, controlled trial. *Psychooncology.* **16**(6): 543–52.

Hadlow J and Pitts M (1991) The undersanding of common terms by doctors, nurses and patients. *Soc Sci Med.* **32**(2): 193–6.

Hagerty RG, Butow PN, Ellis PA, Lobb EA, Pendlebury S, Leighl N, Goldstein D, Lo SK and Tattersall MH (2004) Cancer patient preferences for communication of prognosis in the metastatic setting. *J Clin Oncol.* **22**(9): 1721–30.

Haidet P and Paterniti DA (2003) 'Building' a history rather than 'taking' one: a perspective on information sharing during the medical interview. *Arch Intern Med.* **163**(10): 1134–40.

Hall JA, Harrigan JA and Rosenthal R (1995) Non-verbal behaviour in clinician–patient interaction. *Appl Prev Psychol.* **4**(1): 21–35.

Hall JA, Roter DL and Katz NR (1987) Task versus socioemotional behaviour in physicians. *Med Care.* **25**(5): 399–412.

Hall JA, Roter DL and Katz NR (1988) Meta-analysis of correlates of provider behaviour in medical encounters. *Med Care.* **26**(7): 657–75.

Hall JA, Roter DL and Rand CS (1981) Communication of affect between patient and physician. *J Health Soc Behav.* **22**(1): 18–30.

Halvorsen PA, Selmer R and Kristiansen IS (2007) Different ways to describe the benefits of risk-reducing treatments: a randomized trial. *Ann Intern Med.* **146**(12): 848–56.

Hampton JR, Harrison MJ, Mitchell JR, Prichard JS and Seymour C (1975) Relative contributions of history-taking, physical examination and laboratory investigation to diagnosis and management of medical outpatients. *Br Med J.* **2**(5969): 486–9.

Hannawa AF (2012) 'Explicitly implicit': examining the importance of physician nonverbal involvement during error disclosures. *Swiss Med Wkly.* **142**: w13576.

Hanson JL (2008) Shared decision making: have we missed the obvious? *Arch Intern Med.* **168**(13): 1368–70.

Harrigan JA, Oxman TE and Rosenthal R (1985) Rapport expressed through nonverbal behaviour. *J Nonverbal Behav.* **9**(2): 95–110.

Harrington J, Noble LM and Newman SP (2004) Improving patients' communication with doctors: a systematic review of intervention studies. *Patient Educ Couns.* **52**(1): 7–16.

Harrison ME and Walling A (2010) What do we know about giving bad news? A review. *Clin Pediatr (Phila).* **49**(7): 619–26.

Haskard K, Williams S, DiMatteo M, Heritage J and Rosenthal R (2008) The provider's voice: patient satisfaction and the content-filtered speech of nurses and physicians in primary medical care. *J Nonverbal Behav.* **32**(1): 1–20.

Haug M and Lavin B (1983) *Consumerism in Medicine: challenging physician authority.* Sage Publications, Thousand Oaks, CA.

Hay MC, Cadigan RJ, Khanna D, Strathmann C, Lieber E, Altman R, McMahon M, Kokhab M and Furst DE (2008) Prepared patients: internet information seeking by new rheumatology patients. *Arthritis Rheum.* **59**(4): 575–82.

Haynes RB, McKibbon KA and Kanani R (1996) Systematic review of randomised trials of interventions to assist patients to follow prescriptions for medications. *Lancet.* **348**(9024): 383–6.

Haynes RB, Taylor DW and Sackett DL (1979) *Compliance in Health Care.* Johns Hopkins University Press, Baltimore, MD.

Headache Study Group of the University of Western Ontario, The (1986) Predictors of outcome in headache patients presenting a family physicians: a one year prospective study. *Headache.* **26**(6): 285–94.

Health Canada (1996) *It Helps to Talk.* Health Canada, Ottawa, ON.

Health Informatics Unit, Royal College of Physicians (2008) *A Clinician's Guide to Record*

Standards. Part 2: Standards for the structure and contentof medical records and communications when patients are admitted to hospital. Academy of Royal Medical Colleges, London.

Heath C (1984) Participation in the medical consultation: the co-ordination of verbal and non-verbal behaviour between the doctor and the patient. *Sociol Health Illn.* **6**(3): 311–38.

Hecker KG, Adams CL and Coe JB (2012) Assessment of first-year veterinary students' communication skills using an objective structured clinical examination: the importance of context. *J Vet Med Educ.* **39**(3): 304–10.

Heijmans, M., T. C. olde Hartman, et al. (2011). Experts' opinions on the management of medically unexplained symptoms in primary care. A qualitative analysis of narrative reviews and scientific editorials. *Family Practice.* **28**(4): 444–55.

Heisler M, Cole I, Weir D, Kerr EA and Hayward RA (2007) Does physician communication influence older patients' diabetes self-management and glycemic control? Results from the Health and Retirement Study (HRS). *J Gerontol A Biol Sci Med Sci.* **62**(12): 1435–42.

Helman CG (1978) Free a cold, starve a fever: folk models of infection in an English suburban community and their relation to medical treatment. *Cult Med Psychiatry.* **2**(2): 107–37.

Helman CG (1981) Disease versus illness in general practice. *J R Coll Gen Pract* **31**: 548–52.

Henbest RJ and Stewart M (1990a) Patient-centredness in the consultation. 1: A method of measurement. *Fam Pract.* **6**(4): 249–53.

Henbest RJ and Stewart M (1990b) Patient-centredness in the consultation. 2: Does it really make a difference? *Fam Pract.* **7**(1): 28–33.

Heritage J (2011) The interaction order and clinical practice: some observations on dysfunctions and action steps. *Patient Educ Couns.* **84**(3): 338–43.

Heritage J and Robinson JD (2006) The structure of patients' presenting concerns: physicians' opening questions. *Health Commun.* **19**(2): 89–102.

Heritage J, Robinson JD, Elliott MN, Beckett M and Wilkes M (2007) Reducing patients' unmet concerns in primary care: the difference one word can make. *J Gen Intern Med.* **22**(10): 1429–33.

Heritage J and Stivers T (1999) Online commentary in acute medical visits: a method of shaping patient expectations. *Soc Sci Med.* **49**(11): 1501–17.

Herman JM (1985) The use of patients' preferences in family practice. *J Fam Pract.* **20**: 153–6.

Hewitt H, Gafaranga J and McKinstry B (2010) Comparison of face-to-face and telephone consultations in primary care: qualitative analysis. *Br J Gen Pract.* **60**(574): e201–12.

Hoffer Gittel J (2003) How relational coordination works in other industries: the case of health care. In: *The Southwest Airlines Way: using the power of relationships to achieve high performance.* McGraw-Hill, New York, NY.

Hoffer Gittel J, Fairfield K, Beirbaum B, Head W, Jackson R, Kelly M, Laskin R, Lipson S, Siliski J, Thornhill T and Zuckerman J (2000) Impact of relationalship coordination on quality of care, post-operative pain and functioning and the length of stay: a nine-hospital study of surgical patients. *Med Care.* **38**(8): 807–19.

Hojat M, Louis DZ, Markham FW, Wender R, Rabinowitz C and Gonnella JS (2011) Physicians' empathy and clinical outcomes for diabetic patients. *Acad Med.* **86**(3): 359–64.

Hojat M, Vergare MJ, Maxwell K, Brainard G, Herrine SK, Isenberg GA, Veloski J and Gonnella JS (2009) The devil is in the third year: a longitudinal study of erosion of empathy in medical school. *Acad Med.* **84**(9): 1182–91.

Holmes-Rovner M, Valade D, Orlowski C, Draus C, Nabozny-Valerio B and Keiser S (2000) Implementing shared decision-making in routine practice: barriers and opportunities. *Health Expect.* **3**(3): 182–91.

Hope RA, Fulford KWM and Yates A (1996) *The Oxford Practice Skills Course: ethics, law, and communication skills in health care education.* Oxford University Press, Oxford.

Hope T (1996) *Evidence Based Patient Choice.* King's Fund Publishing, London.

Hopton J, Hogg R and McKee I (1996) Patients' accounts of calling the doctor out of hours: qualitative study in one general practice. *BMJ.* **313**(7063): 991–4.

Horder J, Byrne P, Freeling P, Harris C, Irvine D and Marinker M (1972) *The Future General Practitioner. Learning and Teaching.* Royal College Of General Practitioners, London.

Howells RJ, Davies HA, Silverman JD, Archer JC and Mellon AF (2010) Assessment of doctors' consultation skills in the paediatric setting: the Paediatric Consultation Assessment Tool. *Arch Dis Child*. **95**(5): 323–9.

Hsu I, Saha S, Korthuis PT, Sharp V, Cohn J, Moore RD and Beach MC (2012) Providing support to patients in emotional encounters: a new perspective on missed empathic opportunities. *Patient Educ Couns*. **88**(3): 436–42.

Hudak PL, Armstrong K, Braddock C 3rd, Frankel RM and Levinson W (2008) Older patients' unexpressed concerns about orthopaedic surgery. *J Bone Joint Surg Am*. **90**(7): 1427–35.

Hudak PL, Clark SJ and Raymond G (2011) How surgeons design treatment recommendations in orthopaedic surgery. *Soc Sci Med*. **73**(7): 1028–36.

Hulka BS (1979) Patient–clinician interaction. In: RB Haynes, DW Taylor and DL Sackett (eds) *Compliance in Health Care*. Johns Hopkins University Press, Baltimore, MD.

Inui TS, Yourtee EL and Williamson JW (1976) Improved outcomes in hypertension after physician tutorials. *Ann Intern Med*. **84**: 646–51.

Jansen J, Butow PN, van Weert JC, van Dulmen S, Devine RJ, Heeren TJ, Bensing JM and Tattersall MH (2008) Does age really matter? Recall of information presented to newly referred patients with cancer. *J Clin Oncol*. **26**(33): 5450–7.

Janssen NB, Oort FJ, Fockens P, Willems DL, de Haes HC and Smets EM (2009) Under what conditions do patients want to be informed about their risk of a complication? A vignette study. *J Med Ethics*. **35**(5): 276–82.

Jenkins V, Solis-Trapala I, Langridge C, Catt S, Talbot DC and Fallowfield LJ (2011) What oncologists believe they said and what patients believe they heard: an analysis of phase I trial discussions. *J Clin Oncol*. **29**(1): 61–8.

Jenkins V, Fallowfield L and Saul J (2001) Information needs of patients with cancer: results from a large study in UK cancer centres. *Br J Cancer*. **84**(1): 48–51.

Johnson TM, Hardt EJ and Kleinman A (1995) Cultural factors. In: M Lipkin Jr, SM Putnam, A Lazare A (eds) *The Medical Interview: clinical care, education and research*. Springer-Verlag, New York, NY.

Johnstone EC, Freeman CPL and Zealley AK (1998) *Companion to Psychiatric Studies* (6th ed). Churchill Livingstone, Edinburgh.

Joos SK, Hickam DH and Borders LM (1993) Patients' desires and satisfaction in general medical clinics. *Public Health Rep*. **108**(6): 751–9.

Joos SK, Hickam DH, Gordon GH and Baker LH (1996) Effects of a physician communication intervention on patient care outcomes. *J Gen Int Med*. **11**(3): 147–55.

Kai J (2003) *Ethnicity, Health and Primary Care*. Oxford Medical Publications, Oxford University Press, Oxford.

Kai J, Beavan J, Faull C, Dodson L, Gill P and Beighton A (2007) Professional uncertainty and disempowerment responding to ethnic diversity in health care: a qualitative study. *PLoS Med*. **4**(11): e323.

Kaiser Family Foundation (1999) National Survey of Physicians: Part 1. Doctors on disparities in medical care. Henry J Kaiser Family Foundation, Menlo Park, CA.

Kale E, Finset A, Eikeland HL and Gulbrandsen P (2011) Emotional cues and concerns in hospital encounters with non-Western immigrants as compared with Norwegians: an exploratory study. *Patient Educ Couns*. **84**(3): 325–31.

Kalet A, Pugnaire MP, Cole-Kelly K, Janicik R, Ferrara E, Schwartz MD, Lipkin M Jr and Lazare A (2004) Teaching communication in clinical clerkships: models from the Macy Initiative in Health Communication. *Acad Med*. **79**(6): 511–20.

Kaner E, Heaven B, Rapley T, Murtagh M, Graham R, Thomson R and May C (2007) Medical communication and technology: a video-based process study of the use of decision aids in primary care consultations. *BMC Med Inform Decis Mak*. **7**: 2.

Kaplan CB, Siegel B, Madill JM and Epstein RM (1997) Communication and the medical interview: strategies for learning and teaching. *J Gen Intern Med*. **12**(Suppl. 2): S49–55.

Kaplan SH, Greenfield S, Gandek B, Rogers WH and Ware JE (1996) Characteristics of physicians with participatory decision-making styles. *Ann Intern Med*. **124**: 497–504.

Kaplan SH, Greenfield S and Ware JE (1989) Assessing the effects of physician–patient interactions on the outcomes of chronic disease. *Med Care*. **27**(3 Suppl): S110–27.

Karnieli-Miller O and Eisikovits Z (2009) Physician as partner or salesman? Shared decision-making in real-time encounters. *Soc Sci Med.* **69**(1): 1–8.

Kassirer JP (1983) Teaching clinical medicine by iterative hypothesis testing. *N Engl J Med.* **309**(15): 921–3.

Kassirer JP and Gorry GA (1978) ClinicKeithley J and Marsh G (1995) *Counselling in Primary Health Care.* Oxford Medical Publications, Oxford University Press, Oxford.

Keithley J and Marsh G (eds) (1995) *Counselling in Primary Health Care.* Oxford General Practice Series. Oxford University Press, Oxford.

Keller VF and Carroll JG (1994) A new model for physician–patient communication. *Patient Educ Couns.* **23**(2): 131–40.

Keller VF and Kemp-White M (2001) Choices and changes: a new model for influencing patient health behavior. *J Clin Outcomes Manag.* **4**(6, Special publication): 33–6.

Kemp EC, Floyd MR, McCord-Duncan E and Lang F (2008) Patients prefer the method of 'tell back-collaborative inquiry' to assess understanding of medical information. *J Am Board Fam Med.* **21**(1): 24–30.

Kessel N (1979) Reassurance. *Lancet.* **1**(8126): 1128–33.

Kiesler DJ and Auerbach SM (2006) Optimal matches of patient preferences for information, decision-making and interpersonal behavior: evidence, models and interventions. *Patient Educ Couns.* **61**(3): 319–41.

Kim SS, Kaplowitz S and Johnston MV (2004) The effects of physician empathy on patient satisfaction and compliance. *Eval Health Prof.* **27**(3): 237–51.

Kindelan K and Kent G (1987) Concordance between patients' information preferences and general practitionars' perceptions. *Psychol Health.* **1**(4): 399–409.

Kinmonth AL, Woodcock A, Griffin S, Spiegal N and Campbell MJ (1998) Randomised controlled trial of patient centred care of diabetes in general practice: impact on current wellbeing and future disease risk. Diabetes Care from Diagnosis Research Team. *BMJ.* **317**(7167): 1202–8.

Kinnersley P and Edwards A (2008) Complaints against doctors. *BMJ.* **336**(7649): 841–2.

Kinnersley P, Edwards A, Hood K, Ryan R, Prout H, Cadbury N, MacBeth F, Butow P and Butler C (2008) Interventions before consultations to help patients address their information needs by encouraging question asking: systematic review. *BMJ.* **337**: a485.

Kinnersley P, Stott N, Peters TJ and Harvey I (1999) The patient-centredness of consultations and outcome in primary care. *Br J Gen Pract.* **49**(446): 711–16.

Kleinman A (1980) *Patients and Healers in the Context of Culture.* University of California Press, Berkeley, CA.

Kleinman A, Eisenberg L and Good B. (1978) Culture, illness, and care: clinical lessons from anthropologic and cross-cultural research. *Ann Intern Med.* **88**(2): 251–8.

Kleinman A, Eisenberg L and Good B (1998). Culture, illness, and care: clinical lessons from anthropologic and cross-cultural research. *Ann Intern Med.* **88**: 251–8.

Koch R (1971) The teacher and nonverbal communication. *Theory Pract.* **10**(4): 231–42.

Koch-Weser S, Dejong W and Rudd RE (2009) Medical word use in clinical encounters. *Health Expect.* **12**(4): 371–82.

Korsch B and Harding C (1997) *The Intelligent Patient's Guide to the Doctor–Patient Relationship.* Oxford University Press, New York, NY.

Korsch BM (2002) Patient-centered communication in pediatric practice: reducing the power gap [video recording]. Medical Audio Visual Communications, Niagra Falls, NY.

Korsch BM, Gozzi EK and Francis V (1968) Gaps in doctor–patient communication. *Pediatrics.* **42**(5): 855–71.

Kravitz RL, Cope DW, Bhrany V and Leake B (1994) Internal medicine patients' expectations for care during office visits. *J Gen Intern Med.* **9**(2): 75–81.

Kripalani S and Weiss BD (2006) Teaching about health literacy and clear communication. *J Gen Intern Med.* **21**(8): 888–90.

Krupat E, Frankel R, Stein T and Irish J (2006) The Four Habits Coding Scheme: validation of an instrument to assess clinicians' communication behavior. *Patient Educ Couns.* **62**(1): 38–45.

Kubler-Ross E (1967) *On Death and Dying.* Tavistock, London.

Kuhl D (2002) *What Dying People Want: practical wisdom for the end of life*. Doubleday, Toronto, ON.

Kupst M, Dresser K, Schulman JL and Paul MH (1975) Evaluation of methods to improve communication in the physician-patient relationship. *Am J Orthopsychiatry*. **45**(3): 420.

Kurtz S, Silverman J, Benson J and Draper J (2003) Marrying content and process in clinical method teaching: enhancing the Calgary–Cambridge Guides. *Acad Med*. **78**(8): 802–9.

Kurtz SM (1989) Curriculum structuring to enhance communication skills development. In: M Stewart and D Roter (eds) *Communicating with Medical Patients*. Sage Publications, Newbury Park, CA.

Kurtz SM and Silverman JD (1996) The Calgary–Cambridge Observation Guides: an aid to defining the curriculum and organising the teaching in communication training programmes. *Med Educ*. **30**(2): 83–9.

Kurtz S, Silverman J and Draper J (1998) *Teaching and Learning Communication Skills in Medicine* (1e). Radcliffe Medical Press, Oxford.

Laidlaw TS, MacLeod H, Kaufman DM, Langille DB and Sargeant J (2002) Implementing a communication skills programme in medical school: needs assessment and programme change. *Med Educ*. **36**(2): 115–24.

Lamiani G, Meyer EC, Rider EA, Browning DM, Vegni E, Mauri E, Moja EA and Truog RD (2008) Assumptions and blind spots in patient-centredness: action research between American and Italian health care professionals. *Med Educ*. **42**(7): 712–20.

Lang F, Floyd MR and Beine KL (2000) Clues to patients' explanations and concerns about their illnesses: a call for active listening. *Arch Fam Med*. **9**(3): 222–7.

Lang F, Floyd MR, Beine KL and Buck P (2002) Sequenced questioning to elicit the patient's perspective on illness: effects on information disclosure, patient satisfaction and time expenditure. *Fam Med*. **34**(5): 325–30.

Langewitz W, Denz M, Keller A, Kiss A, Ruttimann S and Wossmer B (2002) Spontaneous talking time at start of consultation in outpatient clinic: cohort study. *BMJ*. **325**(7366): 682–3.

Langseth MS, Shepherd E, Thomson R and Lord S (2012) Quality of decision making is related to decision outcome for patients with cardiac arrhythmia. *Patient Educ Couns*. **87**(1): 49–53.

Larsen KM and Smith CK (1981) Assessment of nonverbal communication in the patient–physician interview. *J Fam Pract*. **12**(3): 481–8.

Launer J (2002) *Narrative-Based Primary Care: a practical guide*. Radcliffe Medical Press, Oxford.

Launer J (2009) Medically unexplored stories. *Postgrad Med J*. **85**: 503–4.

Lazare A, Eisenthal S and Wasserman L (1975) The customer approach to patienthood: attending to patient requests in a walk-in clinic. *Arch Gen Psychiatry*. **32**(5): 553–8.

Lecouturier J, Bamford C, Hughes JC, Francis JJ, Foy R, Johnston M and Eccles MP (2008) Appropriate disclosure of a diagnosis of dementia: identifying the key behaviours of 'best practice'. *BMC Health Serv Res*. **8**: 95.

Leopold N, Cooper J and Clancy C (1996) Sustained partnership in primary care. *J Fam Pract*. **42**(2): 129–37.

Levenstein JH, Belle Brown J, Weston WW, Stewart M, McCracken EC and McWhinney I (1989) Patient centred clinical interviewing. In: M Stewart and D Roter (eds) *Communicating with Medical Patients*. Sage Publications, Newbury Park, CA.

Levetown M (2008) Communicating with children and families: from everyday interactions to skill in conveying distressing information. *Pediatrics*. **121**(5): e1441–60.

Levinson W, Gorawara-Bhat R and Lamb J (2000) A study of patient clues and physician responses in primary care and surgical settings. *JAMA*. **284**(8): 1021–7.

Levinson W, Hudak PL, Feldman JJ, Frankel RM, Kuby A, Bereknyei S and Braddock C 3rd (2008) 'It's not what you say …': racial disparities in communication between orthopedic surgeons and patients. *Med Care*. **46**(4): 410–16.

Levinson W, Kao A, Kuby A and Thisted RA (2005) Not all patients want to participate in decision making. A national study of public preferences. *J Gen Intern Med*. **20**(6): 531–5.

Levinson W and Pizzo PA (2011) Patient–physician communication: it's about time. *JAMA*. **305**(17): 1802–3.

Levinson W and Roter D (1995) Physicians psychosocial beliefs correlate with their patient communication skills. *J Gen Inter Med*. **10**(7): 375–9.

Levinson W, Roter DL, Mullooly JP, Dull VT and Frankel RM (1997) Physician–patient communication: the relationship with malpractice claims among primary care physicians and surgeons. *JAMA*. **277**(7): 553–9.

Levinson W, Stiles WB, Inui TS and Engle R (1993) Physician frustration in communicating with patients. *Med Care*. **31**(4): 285–95.

Lewin S, Skea Z, Entwistle VA, Zwarenstein M and Dick J (2012) Interventions for providers to promote a patient-centred approach in clinical consultations. *Cochrane Database Syst Rev*. (4): CD003267.

Lewis C, Knopf D, Chastain-Lorber K, Ablin A, Zoger S, Matthay K, Glasser M and Pantell R (1988) Patient, parent and physician perspectives on pediatric oncology rounds. *J Pediatr*. **112**(3): 378–84.

Ley P (1988) *Communication with Patients: improving satisfaction and compliance*. Croom Helm, London.

Li HZ, Krysko M, Desroches NG and Deagle G (2004) Reconceptualizing interruptions in physician–patient interviews: cooperative and intrusive. *Commun Med*. **1**(2): 145–57.

Lindholm M, Hargraves JL, Ferguson WJ and Reed G (2012) Professional language interpretation and inpatient length of stay and readmission rates. *J Gen Intern Med*. **27**(10): 1294–9.

Lipkin M Jr (1987) The medical interview and related skills. In: WT Branch (ed) *The Office Practice of Medicine*. WB Saunders, Philadelphia, PA.

Lipkin M Jr, Putnam SM and Lazare A (1995) *The Medical Interview: clinical care, education and research*. Springer-Verlag, New York, NY.

Little P, Dorward M, Warner G, Moore M, Stephens K, Senior J and Kendrick T (2004) Randomised controlled trial of effect of leaflets to empower patients in consultations in primary care. *BMJ*. **328**(7437): 441.

Little P, Everitt H, Williamson I, Warner G, Moore M, Gould C, Ferrier K and Payne S (2001b) Preferences of patients for patient centred approach to consultation in primary care: observational study. *BMJ*. **322**(7284): 468–72.

Little P, Williamson I, Warner G, Gould C, Gantley M and Kinmonth AL (1997) Open randomised trial of prescribing strategies in managing sore throat. *BMJ*. **314**(7082): 722–7.

Lloyd M and Bor R (1996) *Communication Skills for Medicine*. Churchill Livingstone, London.

Locatis C, Williamson D, Gould-Kabler C, Zone-Smith L, Detzler I, Roberson J, Maisiak R and Ackerman M (2010) Comparing in-person, video, and telephonic medical interpretation. *J Gen Intern Med*. **25**(4): 345–50.

Longman T, Turner RM, King M and McCaffery KJ (2012) The effects of communicating uncertainty in quantitative health risk estimates. *Patient Educ Couns*. **89**(2): 252–9.

Low LL, Sondi S, Azman AB, Goh PP, Maimunah AH, Ibrahim MY, Hassan MR and Letchuman R (2011) Extent and determinants of patients' unvoiced needs. *Asia Pac J Public Health*. **23**(5): 690–702.

Lussier MT and Richard C (2008) Because one shoe doesn't fit all: a repertoire of doctor–patient relationships. *Can Fam Physician*. **54**(8): 1089–92, 1096–9.

MacDonald K (2009) Patient–clinician eye contact: social neuroscience and art of clinical engagement. *Postgrad Med*. **121**(4): 136–44.

Mack JW, Wolfe J, Cook EF, Grier HE, Cleary PD and Weeks JC (2007) Hope and prognostic disclosure. *J Clin Oncol*. **25**(35): 5636–42.

Mader SL and Ford AB (1995) The geriatric interview. In: M Lipkin Jr, SM Putman and A Lazare (eds) *The Medical Interview: clinical care, education and research*. Springer-Verlag, New York, NY.

Maguire P, Booth K, Elliott C and Jones B (1996a) Helping health professionals involved in cancer care acquire key interviewing skills: the impact of workshops. *Eur J Cancer*. **32A**(9): 1486–9.

Maguire P, Fairbairn S and Fletcher C (1986a) Consultation skills of young doctors: 1. Benefits of feedback training in interviewing as students persists. *BMJ*. **292**(6535): 1573–6.

Maguire P, Fairbairn S and Fletcher C (1986b) Consultation skills of young doctors: II. Most young doctors are bad at giving information. *BMJ*. **292**(6535): 1576–8.

Maguire P and Faulkner A (1988a) Communicate with cancer patients: 1. Handling bad news and difficult questions. *BMJ*. **297**: 907–9.

Maguire P, Faulkner A, Booth K, Elliott C and Hillier V (1996b) Helping cancer patients disclose their concern. *Eur J Cancer*. **32A**(1): 78–81.

Maguire P and Rutter D (1976) History-taking for medical students: 1. Deficiencies in performance. *Lancet*. **2**(7985): 556–8.

Maiman LA, Becker MH, Liptak GS, Nazarian LF and Rounds KA (1988) Improving pediatricians' compliance enhancing practices: a randomized trial. *Am J Dis Child*. **142**: 773–9.

Makoul G (1998) Medical student and resident perspectives on delivering bad news. *Acad Med*. **73**(10 Suppl.): S35–7.

Makoul G (2001) The SEGUE Framework for teaching and assessing communication skills. *Patient Educ Couns*. **45**(1): 23–34.

Makoul G (2003) The interplay between education and research about patient–provider communication. *Patient Educ Couns*. **50**(1): 79–84.

Makoul G, Arnston P and Scofield T (1995) Health promotion in primary care: physician–patient communication and decision about prescription medications. *Soc Sci Med*. **41**(9): 1241–54.

Makoul G and Clayman ML (2006) An integrative model of shared decision making in medical encounters. *Patient Educ Couns*. **60**(3): 301–12.

Makoul G, Curry RH and Tang PC (2001) The use of electronic medical records: communication patterns in outpatient encounters. *J Am Med Inform Assoc*. **8**(6): 610–15.

Makoul G and Schofield T (1999) Communication teaching and assessment in medical education: an international consensus statement. Netherlands Institute of Primary Health Care. *Patient Educ Couns*. **37**(2): 191–5.

Males T (1998) Experiences and perceived learning in out-of-hours telephone advice: interview study of ten GPs in a co-operative. *Educ Gen Pract*. **9**: 470–7.

Mandin H, Jones A, Woloshuk W and Harasym P (1997) Helping students learn to think like experts when solving clinical problems. *Acad Med*. **72**(3): 173–9.

Mangione-Smith R, Elliott MN, Stivers T, McDonald LL and Heritage J (2006) Ruling out the need for antibiotics: are we sending the right message? *Arch Pediatr Adolesc Med*. **160**(9): 945–52.

Mangione-Smith R, McGlynn EA, Elliott MN, Krogstad P and Brook RH (1999) The relationship between perceived parental expectations and pediatrician antimicrobial prescribing behavior. *Pediatrics*. **103**(4): 711–18.

Mangione-Smith R, McGlynn EA, Elliott MN, McDonald L, Franz CE and Kravitz RL (2001) Parent expectations for antibiotics, physician–parent communication and satisfaction. *Arch Pediatr Adolesc Med*. **155**(7): 800–6.

Manning P and Ray GB (2002) Setting the agenda: an analysis of negotiation strategies in clinical talk. *Health Commun*. **14**(4): 451–73.

Margalit AP, Glick SM, Benbassat J and Cohen A (2004) Effect of a biopsychosocial approach on patient satisfaction and patterns of care. *J Gen Intern Med*. **19**(5 Pt. 2): 485–91.

Margalit RS, Roter D, Dunevant MA, Larson S and Reis S (2006) Electronic medical record use and physician-patient communication: an observational study of Israeli primary care encounters. *Patient Educ Couns*. **61**(1): 134–41.

Marinker M, Blenkinsopp A, Bond C, Britten N, Feely M and George C (1997) *From Compliance to Concordance: achieving shared goals in medicine taking*. Royal Pharmaceutical Society of Great Britain, London.

Marinker M and Shaw J (2003) Not to be taken as directed. *BMJ*. **326**(7385): 348–9.

Marvel MK, Epstein RM, Flowers K and Beckman HB (1999) Soliciting the patient's agenda: have we improved? *JAMA*. **281**(3): 283–7.

Matthys J, Elwyn G, Van Nuland M, Van Maele G, De Sutter A, De Meyere M and Deveugele M (2009) Patients' ideas, concerns and expectations (ICE) in general practice: impact on prescribing. *Br J Gen Pract*. **59**(558): 29–36.

Mauksch LB, Dugdale DC, Dodson S and Epstein R (2008) Relationship, communication and efficiency in the medical encounter: creating a clinical model from a literature review. *Arch Intern Med*. **168**(13): 1387–95.

Mauri E, Vegni E, Lozza E, Parker PA and Moja EA (2009) An exploratory study on the Italian patients' preferences regarding how they would like to be told about their cancer. *Support Care Cancer.* **17**(12): 1523–30.

Maynard DW (1990) Bearing bad news. *Med Encounter.* **7**: 2–3.

Mazur DJ (2000) Information disclosure and beyond: how do patients understand and use the information they report they want? *Med Decis Making.* **20**(1): 132–4.

Mazzullo JM, Lasagna L and Griner PF (1974) Variations in interpretation of prescription instructions. *JAMA.* **227**(8): 929–31.

McCabe R, Heath C, Burns T and Priebe S (2002) Engagement of patients with psychosis in the consultation: conversation analytic study. *BMJ.* **325**(7373): 1148–51.

McConnell D, Butow PN and Tattersall MH (1999) Audiotapes and letters to patients: the practice and views of oncologists, surgeons and general practitioners. *Br J Cancer.* **79**(11–12): 1782–8.

McCroskey JC, Larson CE and Knapp ML (1971) *An Introduction to Interpersonal Communication.* Prentice Hall, Englewood Cliffs, NJ.

McGrath JM, Arar NH and Pugh JA (2007) The influence of electronic medical record usage on nonverbal communication in the medical interview. *Health Inform J.* **13**(2): 105–18.

McKillop J and Petrini C (2011) Communicating with people with dementia. *Ann Ist Super Sanita.* **47**(4): 333–6.

McKinlay JB (1975) Who is really ignorant: physician or patient? *J Health Soc Behav.* **16**(1): 3–11.

McKinley RK and Middleton JF (1999) What do patients want from doctors? Content analysis of written patient agendas for the consultation. *Br J Gen Pract.* **49**(447): 796–800.

McKinstry B, Hammersley V, Burton C, Pinnock H, Elton R, Dowell J, Sawdon N, Heaney D, Elwyn G, Sheikh A (2010) The quality, safety and content of telephone and face-to-face consultations: a comparative study. *Qual Saf Health Care.* **19**(4): 298–303.

McWhinney I (1989) The need for a transformed clinical method. In: M Stewart and D Roter (eds) *Communicating with Medical Patients.* Sage Publications, Newbury Park, CA.

Mehrabian A (1972) *Nonverbal Communication.* Aldine Atherton, Chicago, IL.

Mehrabian A and Ksionsky S (1974) *A Theory of Affiliation.* Lexington Books, DC Health, Lexington, MA.

Meichenbaum D and Turk DC (1987) *Facilitating Treatment Adherence: a practitioner's guidebook.* Plenum Press, New York, NY.

Meitar D, Karnieli-Miller O and Eidelman, S (2009) The impact of senior medical students' personal difficulties on their communication patterns in breaking bad news. *Acad Med.* **84**(11): 1582–94.

Meredith C, Symonds P, Webster L, Lamont D, Pyper E, Gillis CR and Fallowfield L (1996) Information needs of cancer patients in west Scotland: cross sectional survey of patients' views. *BMJ.* **313**(7059): 724–6.

Middleton JF (1995) Asking patients to write lists: feasibility study. *BMJ.* **311**(6996): 34.

Miller SM and Mangan CE (1983) Interacting effects of information and coping style in adapting to gynecologic stress: should the doctor tell all? *J Pers Soc Psychol.* **45**(1): 223–36.

Miller W (1983) Motivational interviewing with problem drinkers. *Behav Psychother.* **11**: 147–52.

Miller W and Rollnick S (1991) *Motivational Interviewing: preparing people to change addictive behaviour.* Guildford Press, New York, NY.

Miller WR and Rollnick S (2002) *Motivational Interviewing: preparing people for change* (2nd ed). Guilford Press, New York, NY.

Minhas R (2007) Does copying clinical or sharing correspondence to patients result in better care? *Int J Clin Pract.* **61**(8): 1390–5.

Mishler EG (1984) *The Discourse of Medicine: dialectics of medical interviews.* Ablex, Norwood, NJ.

Mitchell E and Sullivan F (2001) A descriptive feast but an evaluative famine: systematic review of published articles in primary care computing during 1980–97. *BMJ.* **322**(7281): 279–82.

Mitchison D, Butow P, Sze M, Aldridge L, Hui R, Vardy J, Eisenbruch M, Iedema R and

Goldstein D (2012) Prognostic communication preferences of migrant patients and their relatives. *Psychooncology*. **21**(5): 496–504.

Mjaaland TA, Finset A, Jensen BF and Gulbrandsen P (2011a) Patients' negative emotional cues and concerns in hospital consultations: a video-based observational study. *Patient Educ Couns*. **85**(3): 356–62.

Mjaaland TA, Finset A, Jensen BF and Gulbrandsen P (2011b) Physicians' responses to patients' expressions of negative emotions in hospital consultations: a video-based observational study. *Patient Educ Couns*. **84**(3): 332–7.

Monzoni CM, Duncan R, Grunewald R and Reuber M (2011) How do neurologists discuss functional symptoms with their patients: a conversation analytic study. *J Psychosom Res*. **71**(6): 377–83.

Moore M (2009) What do Nepalese medical students and doctoMorse DS, Edwardsen EA and Gordon HS (2008) Missed opportunities for interval empathy in lung cancer communication. *Arch Intern Med*. **168**(17): 1853–8.

Morse DS, Edwardsen EA and Gordon HS (2008) Missed opportunities for interval empathy in lung cancer communication. *Arch Intern Med*. **168**(17): 1853–8.

Muller-Engelmann M, Keller H, Donner-Banzhoff N and Krones T (2011) Shared decision making in medicine: the influence of situational treatment factors. *Patient Educ Couns*. **82**(2): 240–6.

Mulley AG, Trimble C and Elwyn G (2012) Stop the silent misdiagnosis: patients' preferences matter. *BMJ*. **345**: e6572.

Mumford E, Schlesinger HJ and Glass GV (1982) The effect of psychological intervention on recovery from surgery and heart attacks: an analysis of the literature. *Am J Public Health*. **72**(2): 141–51.

Munro JF and Campbell Ian W (2000) *Macleod's Clinical Examination* (10th ed). JF Munro, IW Campbell (eds). Churchill Livingstone, Edinburgh.

Murphy SM, Donnelly M, Fitzgerald T, Tanner WA, Keane FBV and Tierney S (2004) Patients' recall of clinical information following laparoscopy for acute abdominal pain. *Br J Surg*. **91**(4): 485–8.

Myers RE, Daskalakis C, Kunkel EJ, Cocroft JR, Riggio JM, Capkin M and Braddock CH 3rd (2011) Mediated decision support in prostate cancer screening: a randomized controlled trial of decision counseling. *Patient Educ Couns*. **83**(2): 240–6.

Myerscough PR (1992) *Talking with Patients: a basic clinical skill*. Oxford University Press, Oxford.

National Council for Hospice and Specialist Palliative Care Services HS UK. (2003) *Breaking Bad News … Regional Guidelines Developed from Partnerships in Caring (2000) DHSSPS February 2003*. Department of Health, Social Services & Public Safety, Belfast. February 2003 Ref: 261/02

Neighbour R (1987) *The Inner Consultation: how to develop an effective and intutive consulting style*. MTP Press, Lancaster, England.

Nelson WL, Han PK, Fagerlin A, Stefanek M and Ubel PA (2007) Rethinking the objectives of decision aids: a call for conceptual clarity. *Med Decis Making*. **27**(5): 609–18.

Neumann M, Bensing J, Mercer S, Ernstmann N, Ommen O and Pfaff H (2009) Analyzing the 'nature' and 'specific effectiveness' of clinical empathy: a theoretical overview and contribution towards a theory-based research agenda. *Patient Educ Couns*. **74**(3): 339–46.

Newton BW, Barber L, Clardy J, Cleveland E and O'Sullivan P (2008) Is there hardening of the heart during medical school? *Acad Med*. **83**(3): 244–9.

Nezu AM, Nezu CM and Lombardo ER (2001) Cognitive-behavior therapy for medically unexplained symptoms: a critical review of the treatment literature. *Behav Ther*. **32**(3): 537–83.

Ngo-Metzger Q, Massagli MP, Clarridge BR, Manocchia M, Davis RB, Iezzoni LI and Phillips RS (2003) Linguistic and cultural barriers to care. *J Gen Intern Med*. **18**(1): 44–52.

Noordman J, Verhaak P, van Beljouw I and van Dulmen S (2010) Consulting room computers and their effect on general practitioner–patient communication. *Fam Pract*. **27**(6): 644–51.

Norfolk T, Birdi K and Walsh D (2007) The role of empathy in establishing rapport in the consultation: a new model. *Med Educ.* **41**(7): 690–7.

Novack DH, Dube C and Goldstein MG (1992) Teaching medical interviewing: a basic course on interviewing and the physician–patient relationship. *Arch Intern Med.* **152**(9): 1814–20.

Novelli WD, Halvorson GC and Santa J (2012) Recognizing an opinion: Findings from the IOM Evidence Communication Innovation Collaborative. *JAMA.* **308**(15): 1531–2.

O'Brien MA, Whelan TJ, Villasis-Keever M, Gafni A, Charles C, Roberts R, Schiff S and Cai W (2009) Are cancer-related decision aids effective? A systematic review and meta-analysis. *J Clin Oncol.* **27**(6): 974–85.

O'Connor AM and Edwards A (2001) The role of decsion aids in promoting evidence based patient choice. In: A Edwards and G Elwyn (eds) *Evidence-Based Patient Choice.* Oxford University Press, Oxford.

O'Connor AM, Legare F and Stacey D (2003) Risk communication in practice: the contribution of decision aids. *BMJ.* **327**(7417): 736–40.

O'Connor AM, Rostom A, Fiset V, Tetroe J, Entwistle V, Llewellyn-Thomas H, Holmes-Rovner M, Barry M and Jones J (1999) Decision aids for patients facing health treatment or screening decisions: systematic review. *BMJ.* **319**(7212): 731–4.

O'Connor AM, Stacey D, Rovner D, Holmes-Rovner M, Tetroe J, Llewellyn-Thomas H, Entwistle V, Rostom A, Fiset V, Barry M and Jones J (2001) Decision aids for people facing health treatment or screening decisions. *Cochrane Database Syst Rev.* (3): CD001431.

O'Keefe M, Roberton D, Sawyer M and Baghurst P (2003) Medical student interviewing: a randomized trial of patient-centredness and clinical competence. *Fam Pract.* **20**(2): 213–19.

Olde Hartman TC, Hassink-Franke LJ, Lucassen PL, van Spaendonck KP and van Weel C (2009) Explanation and relations: how do general practitioners deal with patients with persistent medically unexplained symptoms; a focus group study. *BMC Fam Pract.* **10**: 68.

Orlander JD, Fincke BG, Hermanns D and Johnson GA (2002) Medical residents' first clearly remembered experiences of giving bad news. *J Gen Intern Med.* **17**(11): 825–31.

Orth JE, Stiles WB, Scherwitz L, Hennrikus D and Vallbona C (1987) Patient exposition and provider explanation in routine interviews and hypertensive patients' blood pressure control. *Health Psychol.* **6**(1): 29–42.

Ott JE, Bellaire J, Machotka P and Moon JB (1974) Patient management by telephone by child health associates and pediatric house officers. *J Med Educ.* **49**(6): 596–600.

Pantell RH, Stewart TJ, Dias JK, Wells P and Ross AW (1982) Physician communication with children and parents. *Pediatrics.* **70**(3): 396–402.

Parkes CM (1972) *Bereavement: studies of grief in adult life.* International Universities Press, New York, NY.

Parsons T (1951) *The Social System.* The Free Press, New York, NY.

Participants in the Bayer-Fetzer Conference on Physician–Patient Communication in Medical Education (2001) Essential elements of communication in medical encounters: the Kalamazoo consensus statement. *Acad Med.* **76**(4): 390–3.

Pearce C, Trumble S, Arnold M, Dwan K and Phillips C (2008) Computers in the new consultation: within the first minute. *Fam Pract.* **25**(3): 202–8.

Peltenburg M, Fischer JE, Bahrs O, van Dulmen S and van den Brink-Muinen A (2004) The unexpected in primary care: a multicenter study on the emergence of unvoiced patient agenda. *Ann Fam Med.* **2**(6): 534–40.

Pendleton D, Schofield T, Tate P and Havelock P (1984) *The Consultation: an approach to learning and teaching.* Oxford University Press, Oxford.

Pendleton D, Schofield T, Tate P and Havelock P (2003) *The New Consultation.* Oxford University Press, Oxford.

Peppiatt R (1992) Eliciting patients' views of the cause of their problem: a practical strategy for GPs. *Fam Pract.* **9**(3): 295–8.

Peräkylä A (2002) Agency and authority: extended responses to diagnostic statements in primary care encounters. *Res Lang Soc Interact.* **35**(2): 219–47.

Perrin EC and Gerrity PS (1981) There's a demon in your belly: children's understanding of illness. *Pediatrics.* **67**: 841–9.

Peterson MC, Holbrook J, VonHales D, Smith NL and Staker LV (1992) Contributions of the history, physical examination and laboratory investigation in making medical diagnoses. *West J Med*. **156**(2): 163–5.

Pilnick A and Dingwall R (2011) On the remarkable persistence of asymmetry in doctor/patient interaction: a critical review. *Soc Sci Med*. **72**(8): 1374–82.

Pinder R (1990) *The Management of Chronic Disease: patient and doctor perspectives on Parkinson's disease*. MacMillan Press, London.

Pinnock H, Bawden R, Proctor S, Wolfe S, Scullion J, Price D and Sheikh A (2003) Accessibility, acceptability and effectiveness in primary care of routine telephone review of asthma: pragmatic, randomised controlled trial. *BMJ*. **326**(7387): 477–9.

Platt FW, Gaspar DL, Coulchan JL, Fox L, Adler AJ, Weston WW, Smith RC and Stewart M (2001) 'Tell me about yourself': The patient-centered interview. *Ann Intern Med*. **134**(11): 1079–85.

Platt FW and Gordon GH (2004) *The Field Guide to the Difficult Patient Interview* (2e) Lippincott, Williams and Wilkins, Philadelphia, PA.

Platt FW and Keller VF (1994) Empathic communication: a teachable and learnable skill. *J Gen Intern Med*. **9**(4): 222–6.

Platt FW and McMath JC (1979) Clinical hypocompetence: the interview. *Ann Intern Med*. **91**(6): 898–902.

Platt FW and Platt CM (2003) Two collaborating artists produce a work of art. *Arch Intern Med*. **163**(10): 1131–2.

Politi MC, Clark MA, Ombao H and Legare F (2011b) The impact of physicians' reactions to uncertainty on patients' decision satisfaction. *J Eval Clin Pract*. **17**(4): 575–8.

Politi MC, Han PK and Col NF (2007) Communicating the uncertainty of harms and benefits of medical interventions. *Med Decis Making*. **27**(5): 681–95.

Poole AD and Sanson-Fisher RW (1979) Understanding the patient: a neglected aspect of medical eduction. *Soc Sci Med Med Psychol Med Sociol*. **13A**(1): 37–43.

Price EL, Bereknyei S, Kuby A, Levinson W and Braddock CH 3rd (2012) New elements for informed decision making: a qualitative study of older adults' views. *Patient Educ Couns*. **86**(3): 335–41.

Priest V and Speller V (1991) *The Risk Factor Management Manual*. Radcliffe Medical Press, Oxford.

Prochaska JO and DiClemente CC (1986) Towards a comprehensive model of change. In: R Miller and N Heather (eds) *Treating Addictive Behaviours*. Plenum Press, New York, NY.

Professional Education and Training Committee (PETC) of New South Wales Cancer Council and the Post Graduate Medical Council (PGMC) of New South Wales, The (1992) *Communicating With Your Patients: an interactional skills training manual for junior medical officers*. PETC and PGMC, Sydney.

Ptacek JT and Eberhardt TL (1996) Breaking bad news: a review of the literature. *JAMA*. **276**: 496–502.

Putnam SM, Stiles WB, Jacob MC and James SA (1988) Teaching the medical interview: an intervention study. *J Gen Intern Med*. **3**(1): 38–47.

Quilligan S and Silverman J (2012) The skill of summary in clinician–patient communication: a case study. *Patient Educ Couns*. **86**(3): 354–9.

Quill TE (1983) Partnerships in patient care: a contractual approach. *Ann Intern Med*. **98**: 228–34.

Quill TE and Brody H (1996) Physician recommendations and patient autonomy: finding a balance between physician power and patient choice. *Ann Intern Med*. **125**(9): 763–9.

Rabinowitz I, Luzzati R, Tamir A and Reis S (2004) Length of patient's monologue, rate of completion and relation to other components of the clinical encounter: observational intervention study in primary care. *BMJ*. **328**(7438): 501–2. [Erratum appears in *BMJ*. 2004 May 22; **328**(7450): 1236. Lazzatti, Rachel [corrrected to Lazzati, Rachel]].

Radford A, Stockley P, Silverman J, Taylor I, Turner R and Gray C (2006) Development, teaching and evaluation of a consultation structure model for use in veterinary education. *J Vet Med Educ*. **33**(1): 38–44.

Rakel D, Barrett B, Zhang Z, Hoeft T, Chewning B, Marchand L and Scheder J (2011)

Perception of empathy in the therapeutic encounter: effects on the common cold. *Patient Educ Couns*. **85**(3): 390–7.

Reilly S and Muzarkara B (1978) *Mixed message resolution by disturbed adults and children. Behavioral Sciences Clinical Research Center. Philadelphia State Hospital.* Paper presented at the International Communication Association Annual Conference, Chicago, Illinois, April 1978.

Rhoades DR, McFarland KF, Finch WH and Johnson AO (2001) Speaking and interruptions during primary care office visits. *Fam Med*. **33**(7): 528–32.

Rhodes KV, Vieth T, He T, Miller A, Howes DS, Bailey O, Walter J, Frankel R and Levinson W (2004) Resuscitating the physician–patient relationship: emergency department communication in an academic medical center. *Ann Emerg Med*. **44**(3): 262–7.

Riccardi VM and Kurtz SM (1983) *Communication and Counselling in Health Care*. Charles C Thomas Publisher, Springfield, IL.

Richard C and Lussier MT (2006a) MEDICODE: an instrument to describe and evaluate exchanges on medications that occur during medical encounters. *Patient Educ Couns*. **64**(1–3): 197–206.

Richard C and Lussier MT (2007) Measuring patient and physician participation in exchanges on medications: dialogue ratio, preponderance of initiative and dialogical roles. *Patient Educ Couns*. **65**(3): 329–41.

Richard R and Lussier MT (2003) *Dialogic Index: a description of physician and patient participation in discussions of medications*. Paper presented at the National Association of Primary Care Research Group Annual Conference, Banff, Alberta, 21–25 October 2003.

Ring A, Dowrick C, Humphris G and Salmon P (2004) Do patients with unexplained physical symptoms pressurise general practitioners for somatic treatment? A qualitative study. *BMJ*. **328**(7447): 1057.

Robins L, Witteborn S, Miner L, Mauksch L, Edwards K and Brock D (2011) Identifying transparency in physician communication. *Patient Educ Couns*. **83**(1): 73–9.

Robinson A and Thomson R (2001) Variability in patient preferences for participating in medical decision making: implication for the use of decision support tools. *Qual Health Care*. **10**(Suppl, 1): i34–8.

Robinson J (2001) Soliciting patients' presenting concerns. In: J Heritage and D Maynard (eds) *Practicing Medicine: structure and process in primary care encounters*. Cambridge University Press, Cambridge.

Robinson JD (1998) Getting down to business: talk, gaze and body organisation during openings of doctor patient consultations. *Health Commun*. **25**(1): 97–123.

Robinson JD (2001) Closing medical encounters: two physician practices and their implications for the expression of patients' unstated concerns. *Soc Sci Med*. **53**(5): 639–56.

Robinson JD and Heritage J (2006) Physicians' opening questions and patients' satisfaction. *Patient Educ Couns*. **60**(3): 279–85.

Rodriguez HP, Anastario MP, Frankel RM, Odigie EG, Rogers WH, von Glahn T and Safran DG (2008) Can teaching agenda-setting skills to physicians improve clinical interaction quality? A controlled intervention. *BMC Med Educ*. **8**: 3.

Rogers CR (1980) *A Way of Being*. Houghton-Mifflin, Boston, MA.

Rogers MS and Todd CJ (2000) The 'right kind' of pain: talking about symptoms in outpatient oncology consultations. *Palliat Med*. **14**(4): 299–307.

Rollnick S, Butler CC, Kinnersley P, Gregory J and Mash B (2010) Motivational interviewing. *BMJ*. **340**: c1900.

Rollnick S, Butler CC and Stott N (1997) Helping smokers make decisions: the enhancement of brief intervention for general medical practice. *Patient Educ Couns*. **31**(3): 191–203.

Rollnick S, Mason P and Butler C (1999) *Health Behavior Change: a guide for practitioners*. Churchill Livingstone, Edinburgh.

Rosenberg E, Richard C, Lussier MT and Shuldiner T (2011) The content of talk about health conditions and medications during appointments involving interpreters. *Fam Pract*. **28**(3): 317–22.

Rost KM, Flavin KS, Cole K and McGill JB (1991) Change in metabolic control and functional status after hospitalisation. *Diabetes Care*. **14**: 881–9.

Roter D (2000) The enduring and evolving nature of the patient–physician relationship. *Patient Educ Couns.* **39**(1): 5–15.

Roter D (2002) Three blind men and an elephant: reflections on meeting the challenges of patient diversity in primary care practice. *Fam Med.* **34**(5): 390–3.

Roter DL (1977) Patient participation in the patient–provider interaction: the effects of patient question asking on the quality of interaction, satisfaction and compliance. *Health Educ Monogr.* **5**: 281–315.

Roter DL, Frankel RM, Hall JA and Sluyter D (2006) The expression of emotion through nonverbal behavior in medical visits: mechanisms and outcomes. *J Gen Intern Med.* **21**(Suppl. 1): S28–34.

Roter DL and Hall JA (1987) Physicians' interviewing styles and medical information obtained from patients. *J Gen Intern Med.* **2**(5): 325–9.

Roter DL and Hall JA (1992) *Doctors Talking with Patients/Patients Talking with Doctors.* Auburn House, Westport, CT.

Roter DL, Hall JA, Kern DE, Barker R, Cole KA and Roca RP (1995) Improving physicians' interviewing skills and reducing patients' emotional distress. *Arch Intern Med.* **155**(17): 1877–84.

Roter DL, Stewart M, Putnam SM, Lipkin M Jr, Stiles W and Inui TS (1997) Communication patterns of primary care physicians. *JAMA.* **277**(4): 350–6.

Rowe MB (1986) Wait time: slowing down may be a way of of speeding up. *J Teach Educ.* **37**(1): 43–50.

Ruiz Moral R, Parras Rejano JM and Perula De Torres LA (2006) Is the expression 'Oh, by the way …' a problem that arises in the early moments of a consultation? *Eur J Gen Pract.* **12**(1): 40–1.

Rutter M and Cox A (1981) Psychiatric interviewing techniques I: methods and measures. *Br J Psychiatry.* **138**: 273–82.

Ruusuvuori J (2001) Looking means listening: coordinating displays of engagement in doctor–patient interaction. *Soc Sci Med.* **52**(7): 1093–108.

Salmon P, Dowrick CF, Ring A and Humphris GM (2004) Voiced but unheard agendas: qualitative analysis of the psychosocial cues that patients with unexplained symptoms present to general practitioners. *Br J Gen Pract.* **54**(500): 171–6.

Salmon P, Mendick N and Young B (2011) Integrative qualitative communication analysis of consultation and patient and practitioner perspectives: towards a theory of authentic caring in clinical relationships. *Patient Educ Couns.* **82**(3): 448–54.

Salmon P, Peters S, Clifford R, Iredale W, Gask L, Rogers A, Dowrick C, Hughes J and Morriss R (2007) Why do general practitioners decline training to improve management of medically unexplained symptoms? *J Gen Intern Med.* **22**(5): 565–71.

Salmon P, Ring A, Humphris GM, Davies JC and Dowrick CF (2009) Primary care consultations about medically unexplained symptoms: how do patients indicate what they want? *J Gen Intern Med.* **24**(4): 450–6.

Salmon P and Young B (2011) Creativity in clinical communication: from communication skills to skilled communication. *Med Educ.* **45**(3): 217–26.

Sandler G (1980) The importance of the history in the medical clinic and the cost of unnecessary tests. *Am Heart J.* **100**(6Pt1): 928–31.

Sanson-Fisher RW (1981) Personal communication. Faculty of Medicine, University of Newcastle, NSW, Australia.

Sanson-Fisher RW (1992) *How to Break Bad News to Cancer Patients: an interactional skills manual for interns.* The Professional Education and Training Committee of the New South Wales Cancer Council and the Postgraduate Medical Counicl of NSW Australia, Kings Cross, NSW, Australia.

Sanson-Fisher RW, Redman S, Walsh R, Mitchell K, Reid ALA and Perkins JJ (1991) Training medical practitioners in information transfer skills: the new challenge. *Med Educ.* **25**(4): 322–33.

Santrock JW (1998) *Child Development* (8th ed). McGraw-Hill, Boston, MA.

Schibbye A (1993) The role of 'recognition' in the resolution of a specific interpersonal dilemma. *J Phenomenol Psychol.* **24**(2): 175–89.

Schildmann J, Cushing A, Doyal L and Vollmann J (2005) Breaking bad news: experiences, views and difficulties of pre-registration house officers. *Palliat Med.* **19**(2): 93–8.

Schmidt HG, Norman GR and Boshuizen HP (1990) A cognitive perspective on medical expertise: theory and implication. *Acad Med.* **65**(10): 611–21.

Schofield T, Elwyn G, Edwards A and Visser A (2003) Shared decision making. *Patient Educ Couns.* **50**(3): 229–30.

Schulman BA (1979) Active patient orientation and outcomes in hypertensive treatment. *Med Care.* **17**: 267–81.

Scott JT, Entwistle VA, Sowden AJ and Watt I (2001) Giving tape recordings or written summaries of consultations to people with cancer: a systematic review. *Health Expect.* **4**(3): 162–9.

Seale C, Chaplin R, Lelliott P and Quirk A (2006) Sharing decisions in consultations involving anti-psychotic medication: a qualitative study of psychiatrists' experiences. *Soc Sci Med.* **62**(11): 2861–73.

Seidel HM (2003) *Mosby's Guide to Physical Examination* (5th ed). Mosby, St. Louis, MO.

Sepucha KR and Mulley AG (2003) Extending decision support: preparation and implementation. *Patient Educ Couns.* **50**(3): 269–71.

Seymour CA and Siklos P (1994) *Clinical Clerking: a short introduction to clinical skills.* Cambridge University PRess, Cambridge.

Shachak A, Hadas-Dayagi M, Ziv A and Reis S (2009) Primary care physicians' use of an electronic medical record system: a cognitive task analysis. *J Gen Intern Med.* **24**(3): 341–8.

Shachak A and Reis S (2009) The impact of electronic medical records on patient-doctor communication during consultation: a narrative literature review. *J Eval Clin Pract.* **15**(4): 641–9.

Shaw A, Ibrahim S, Reid F, Ussher M and Rowlands G (2009) Patients' perspectives of the doctor-patient relationship and information giving across a range of literacy levels. *Patient Educ Couns.* **75**(1): 114–20.

Shaw J, Dunn S and Heinrich P (2012) Managing the delivery of bad news: an in-depth analysis of doctors' delivery style. *Patient Educ Couns.* **87**(2): 186–92.

Shepherd HL, Barratt A, Trevena LJ, McGeechan K, Carey K, Epstein RM, Butow PN, Del Mar CB, Entwistle V and Tattersall MHN (2011) Three questions that patients can ask to improve the quality of information physicians give about treatment options: a cross-over trial. *Patient Educ Couns.* **84**(3): 379–85.

Sibley A, Latter S, Richard C, Lussier MT, Roberge D, Skinner TC, Cradock S and Zinken KM (2011) Medication discussion between nurse prescribers and people with diabetes: an analysis of content and participation using MEDICODE. *J Adv Nurs.* **67**(11): 2323–36.

Silverman J (2007) The Calgary–Cambridge Guides: the 'teenage years'. *Clin Teach.* **4**(2): 87–93.

Silverman J (2009) Teaching clinical communication: a mainstream activity or just a minority sport? *Patient Educ Couns.* **76**(3): 361–7.

Silverman J, Deveugele M, de Haes H and Rosenbaum M (2011) Unskilled creativity is counterproductive. *Med Educ.* **45**(9): 959–60; author reply 961–2.

Silverman J and Kinnersley P (2010) Doctors' non-verbal behaviour in consultations: look at the patient before you look at the computer. *Br J Gen Pract.* **60**(571): 76–8.

Silverman J, Kurtz S and Draper J (1998) *Skills for Communicating with Patients* (1e). Radcliffe Medical Press, Oxford.

Simpson M, Buckman R, Stewart M, Maguire P, Lipkin M, Novack D and Till J (1991) Doctor–patient communication: the Toronto consensus statement. *BMJ.* **303**(6814): 1385–7.

Skelton J (2011) Clinical communication as a creative art: an alternative way forward. *Med Educ.* **45**(3): 212–13.

Skelton JR (2005) Everything you were afraid to ask about communication skills. *Br J Gen Pract.* **55**(510): 40–6.

Slack WV (1977) The patient's right to decide. *Lancet.* **2**(8031): 240.

Slade D, Scheeres H, Manidis M, Iedema R, Dunston R, Stein-Parbury J, Matthiessen C, Herke M and McGregor J (2008) Emergency communication: the discursive challenges facing emergency clinicians and patients in hospital emergency departments. *Discourse Commun.* 2(3): 271–98.

Smith A, Juraskova I, Butow P, Miguel C, Lopez AL, Chang S, Brown R and Bernhard J (2011) Sharing vs. caring: the relative impact of sharing decisions versus managing emotions on patient outcomes. *Patient Educ Couns.* 82(2): 233–9.

Smith RC and Hoppe RB (1991) The patient's story: integrating the patient and physician-centred approaches to interviewing. *Ann Intern Med.* 115(6): 471–7.

Sommer R (1971) Social parameters in naturalistic health research. In: A Esser (ed) *Behaviour and Environment: the use of space by animals and men.* Plenum Press, New York, NY.

Sonntag U, Wiesner J, Fahrenkrog S, Renneberg B, Braun V and Heintze C (2012) Motivational interviewing and shared decision making in primary care. *Patient Educ Couns.* 87(1): 62–6.

Sowden AJ, Forbes C, Entwistle V and Watt I (2001) Informing, communicating and sharing decisions with people who have cancer. *Qual Health Care.* 10(3): 193–6.

Spiegel D, Bloom JR, Kraemer HC and Gottheil E (1989) Effect of psychosocial treatment on survival of patients with metastatic breast cancer. *Lancet.* 2(8668): 888–91.

Spiro H (1992) What is empathy and can it be taught? *Ann Intern Med.* 116(10): 843–6.

Spitzer J (2003) *Caring for Jewish Patients.* Radcliffe Medical Press, Oxford.

Starfield B, Wray C, Hess K, Gross R, Birk PS and D'Lugoff BC (1981) The influence of patient–practitioner agreement on outcome of care. *Am J Public Health.* 71(2): 127–31.

Steele DJ (2002) Overcoming cultural and language barriers. In: S Cole and J Bird (eds) *The Medical Interview: the three function approach* (2nd ed). Mosby, Philadelphia, PA.

Steele DJ and Hulsman RL (2008) Empathy, authenticity, assessment and simulation: a conundrum in search of a solution. *Patient Educ Couns.* 71(2): 143–4.

Steihaug S, Gulbrandsen P and Werner A (2012) Recognition can leave room for disagreement in the doctor–patient consultation. *Patient Educ Couns.* 86(3): 316–21.

Stepien KA and Baernstein A (2006) Educating for empathy: a review. *J Gen Intern Med.* 21(5): 524–30.

Steptoe A, Sutcliffe I, Allen B and Coombes C (1991) Satisfacton with communication, medical knowledge and coping style in patients with metastatic cancer. *Soc Sci Med.* 32(6): 627–32.

Stevenson FA, Barry CA, Britten N, Barber N and Bradley CP (2000) Doctor–patient communication about drugs: the evidence for shared decision making. *Soc Sci Med.* 50(6): 829–40.

Stevenson F and Scambler G (2005) The relationship between medicine and the public: the challenge of concordance. *Health (London).* 9(1): 5–21.

Stewart M (2001) Towards a global definition of patient centred care. *BMJ.* 322(7284): 444–5.

Stewart M, Belle Brown J, Donner A, McWhinney IR, Oates J and Weston W (1997) The impact of patient-centred care on patient outcomes in family practice. Thames Valley Family Practice Research Unit, London, ON.

Stewart M, Brown JB, Boon H, Galajda J, Meredith L and Sangster M (1999) Evidence on patient–doctor communication. *Cancer Prev Control.* 3(1): 25–30.

Stewart M, Brown JB, Donner A, McWhinney IR, Oates J, Weston WW and Jordan J (2000a) The impact of patient-centered care on outcomes. *J Fam Pract.* 49(9): 796–804.

Stewart M, Meredith L, Belle Brown J and Galajda J (2000b) The influence of older patient–physician communication on health and health-related outcomes. *Clin Geriatr Med.* 16(1): 25–36.

Stewart M and Roter D (eds) (1989) *Communicating with Medical Patients.* Sage Publications, Newbury Park, CA.

Stewart MA (1984) What is a successful doctor–patient interview? A study of interactions and outcomes. *Soc Sci Med.* 19(2): 167–75.

Stewart MA (1985) *Comparison of two methods of analysisng doctor patient communication.* Paper presented at the North American Primary Care Research Group Conference, Seattle, 14–17 April 1985.

Stewart MA (1995) Effective physician–patient communication and health outcomes: a review. *CMAJ.* 152(9): 1423–33.

Stewart MA, Belle Brown J, Wayne Weston W, McWhinney I, McWilliam C and Freeman T (1995) *Patient-Centred Medicine: transforming the clinical method*. Sage, Thousand Oaks, CA.

Stewart MA, Brown JB, Weston WW, McWhinney IR, McWilliam CL and Freeman TR (2003) *Patient-Centered Medicine: transforming the clinical method* (2nd ed). Radcliffe Medical Press, Oxford.

Stewart MA, McWhinney IR and Buck CW (1979) The doctor/patient relationship and its effect upon outcome. *J R Coll Gen Pract*. 29(199): 77–82.

Stiles WB, Putnam SM, James SA and Wolf MH (1979) Dimensions of patient and physician roles in medical screening interviews. *Soc Sci Med*. 13A(3): 335–41.

Stillman PL, Sabers DL and Redfield DL (1976) Use of paraprofessionals to teach interviewing skills. *Pediatrics*. 57(5): 769–74.

Stimson GV and Webb B (1975) *Going to See the Doctor*. Routledge and Kegan Paul, London.

Stivers T (2012) Physician–child interaction: when children answer physicians' questions in routine medical encounters. *Patient Educ Couns*. 87(1): 3–9.

Storstein A (2011) Communication and neurology: bad news and how to break them. *Acta Neurol Scand Suppl*. (191): 5–11.

Street RL Jr, Makoul G, Arora NK and Epstein RM (2009) How does communication heal? Pathways linking clinician–patient communication to health outcomes. *Patient Educ Couns*. 74(3): 295–301.

Strull WM, Lo B and Charles G (1984) Do patients want to be participate in medical decision making? *JAMA*. 252: 2990–4.

Suchman A, Deci E, McDaniel S and Beckman H (2002) Relationship centered administration. In: R Frankel, T Quill and S McDaniel (eds) *Biopsychosocial Care*. University of Rochester Press, Rochester, NY.

Suchman A, Sluyter DM and Williamson PR (2011) *Leading Change in Healthcare: transforming organizations using complexity, positive psychology and relationship-centered care*. Radcliffe Publishing, Oxford.

Suchman AL (2001) The influence of health care organizations on well-being. *West J Med*. 174(1): 43–7.

Suchman AL (2003) Research on patient–clinician relationships: celebrating success and identifying the next scope of work. *J Gen Intern Med*. 18(8): 677–8.

Suchman AL, Markakis K, Beckman HB and Frankel R (1997) A model of empathic communication in the medical interview. *JAMA*. 277(8): 678–82.

Sudore RL and Schillinger D (2009) Interventions to improve care for patients with limited health literacy. *J Clin Outcomes Manag*. 16(1): 20–9.

Sultan ASS (2007) Medicine in the 21st century: the situation in a rural Iraqi community. *Patient Educ Couns*. 68(1): 66–9.

Sutherland HJ, Llewellyn-Thomas HA, Lockwood GA, Tritchler DL and Till JE (1989) Cancer patients: their desire for information and participation in treatment decisions. *J R Soc Med*. 82(5): 260–3.

Svarstad BL (1974) *The Doctor–Patient Encounter: an observational study of communication and outcome*. Doctoral dissertation, University of Wisconsin, Madison.

Swayden KJ, Anderson KK, Connelly LM, Moran JS, McMahon JK and Arnold PM (2012) Effect of sitting vs. standing on perception of provider time at bedside: a pilot study. *Patient Educ Couns*. 86(2): 166–71.

Tai-Seale M, Bramson R and Bao X (2007) Decision or no decision: how do patient–physician interactions end and what matters? *J Gen Intern Med*. 22(3): 297–302.

Tait I (1979) *The history and function of clinical records*. Unpublished MD dissertation thesis, University of Cambridge.

Takemura Y, Atsumi R and Tsuda T (2007) Identifying medical interview behaviors that best elicit information from patients in clinical practice. *Tohoku J Exp Med*. 213(2): 121–7.

Tamblyn R, Abrahamowicz M, Dauphinee D, Wenghofer E, Jacques A, Klass D, Smee S, Blackmore D, Winslade N, Girard N, Du Berger R, Bartman I, Buckeridge DL and Hanley JA (2007) Physician scores on a national clinical skills examination as predictors of complaints to medical regulatory authorities. *JAMA*. 298(9): 993–1001.

Tarn DM, Heritage J, Paterniti DA, Hays RD, Kravitz RL and Wenger NS (2006) Physician communication when prescribing new medications. *Arch Intern Med.* **166**(17): 1855–62.

Tate P (2010) *The Doctor's Communication Handbook* (6th ed). Radcliffe Publishing, Oxford.

Tates K and Meeuwesen L (2000) 'Let mum have her say': turntaking in doctor–parent–child communication. *Patient Educ Couns.* **40**(2): 151–62.

Tates K and Meeuwesen L (2001) Doctor–parent–child communication: a (re)view of the literature. *Soc Sci Med.* **52**(6): 839–51.

Tattersall MH, Butow PN and Ellis PM (1997) Meeting patients' information needs beyond the year 2000. *Support Care Cancer.* **5**(2): 85–9.

Tattersall MH, Butow PN, Griffin AM and Dunn SM (1994) The take-home message: patients prefer consultation audiotapes to summary letters. *J Clin Oncol.* **12**(6): 1305–11.

Teal CR and Street RL (2009) Critical elements of culturally competent communication in the medical encounter: a review and model. *Soc Sci Med.* **68**(3): 533–43.

Teherani A, Hauer KE and O'Sullivan P (2008) Can simulations measure empathy? Considerations on how to assess behavioral empathy via simulations. *Patient Educ Couns.* **71**(2): 148–52.

Thorne SE, Hislop TG, Stajduhar K and Oglov V (2009) Time-related communication skills from the cancer patient perspective. *Psychooncology.* **18**(5): 500–7.

Thornton H (2009) Statistical illiteracy is damaging our health: doctors and patients need to understand numbers if meaningful dialogues are to occur. *Int J Surg.* **7**(4): 279–84.

Thornton H, Edwards A and Baum M (2003) Women need better information about routine mammography. *BMJ.* **327**(7406): 101–3.

Toon PD (2002) Using telephones in primary care. *BMJ.* **324**(7348): 1230–1.

Towle A and Godolphin W (1999) Framework for teaching and learning informed shared decision making. *BMJ.* **319**(7212): 766–71.

Tresolini CP and the Pew-Fetzer Task Force (1994) Health professions education and relationship-centred care. Pew-Fetzer Task Force on Advancing Psychosocial Health Education, Pew Health Professions Commission and the Fetzer Institute, San Francisco, CA.

Trevena L and Barratt A (2003) Integrated decision making: definitions for a new discipline. *Patient Educ Couns.* **50**(3): 265–8.

Truax CB and Carkhuff RR (1967) *Towards Effective Counselling and Psychotherapy*. Aldine, Chicago, IL.

Tse CY, Chong A and Fok SY (2003) Breaking bad news: a Chinese perspective. *Palliat Med.* **17**(4): 339–43.

Tuckett D, Boulton M, Olson C and Williams A (1985) *Meetings between Experts: an approach to sharing ideas in medical consultations*. Tavistock, London.

UK Royal College of Psychiatrists (2013) *Cognitive Behavioural Therapy*. Available at: www.rcpsych.ac.uk/expertadvice/treatments/cbt.aspx (Accessed 11 June 2013).

Vail L, Sandhu H, Fisher J, Cooke H, Dale J and Barnett M (2011) Hospital consultants breaking bad news with simulated patients: an analysis of communication using the Roter Interaction Analysis System. *Patient Educ Couns.* **83**(2): 185–94.

Van Bilsen HP and Van Emst AJ (1989) Motivating heroin users for change. In: GA Bennett (ed) *Treating Drug Abusers*. Routledge, London.

Van den Brink-Muinen A, Spreeuwenberg P and Rijken M (2011) Preferences and experiences of chronically ill and disabled patients regarding shared decision-making: does the type of care to be decided upon matter? *Patient Educ Couns.* **84**(1): 111–17.

Van der Meulen N, Jansen J, van Dulmen S, Bensing J and van Weert J (2008) Interventions to improve recall of medical information in cancer patients: a systematic review of the literature. *Psychooncology.* **17**(9): 857–68.

Van Thiel J, Kraan HF and Van der Vleuten CPM (1991) Reliability and feasibility of measuring medical interviewing skills: the revised Maastricht History-Taking and Advice Checklist. *Med Educ.* **25**(3): 224–9.

Van Thiel J and van Dalen J (1995) *MAAS-Globaal criterialijst. versie voor de vaardigheidstoets Medisch Basiscurriculum*. Maastricht University, Netherlands.

Ventres W, Kooienga S and Marlin R (2006) EHRs in the exam room: tips on patient-centered care. *Fam Pract Manag.* **13**(3): 45–7.

Verderber RF and Verderber KS (1980) *Inter-Act: Using Interpersonal Communication Skills.* Wadsworth, Belmont, CA.

Vetto JT, Elder NC, Toffler WL and Fields SA (1999) Teaching medical students to give bad news: does formal instruction help? *J Cancer Educ.* **14**(1): 13–17.

Von Fragstein M, Silverman J, Cushing A, Quilligan S, Salisbury H and Wiskin C (2008) UK consensus statement on the content of communication curricula in undergraduate medical education. *Med Educ.* **42**(11): 1100–7.

Waitzkin H (1984) Doctor–patient communication: clinical implications of social scientific research. *JAMA.* **252**(17): 2441–6.

Waitzkin H (1985) Information giving in medical care. *J Health Soc Behav.* **26**(2): 81–101.

Wasserman RC, Inui TS, Barriatua RD, Carter WB and Lippincott P (1984) Pediatric clinicians' support for parents makes a difference: an outcome based analysis of clinician–parent interaction. *Pediatrics.* **74**(6): 1047–53.

Watzlawick P, Beavin J and Jackson D (1967) *Pragmatics of Human Communication.* WW Norton, New York.

Wear D and Varley JD (2008) Rituals of verification: the role of simulation in developing and evaluating empathic communication. *Patient Educ Couns.* **71**(2): 153–6.

Weiner JS and Roth J (2006) Avoiding iatrogenic harm to patient and family while discussing goals of care near the end of life. *J Palliat Med.* **9**(2): 451–63.

Weinberger M, Greene JY and Mamlin JJ (1981) The impact of clinical encounter events on patient and physician satisfaction. *Soc Sci Med.* **15E**(3): 239–44.

White J, Levinson W and Roter D (1994) 'Oh, by the Way': the closing moments of the medical interview. *J Gen Int Med.* **9**: 24–8.

White JC, Rosson C, Christensen J, Hart R and Levinson W (1997) Wrapping things up: a qualitative analysis of the closing moments of the medical visit. *Patient Educ Couns.* **30**(2): 155–65.

White SJ, Stubbe MH, Macdonald LM, Dowell AC, Dew KP and Gardner R (2013) Framing the consultation: the role of the referral in surgeon–patient consultations. *Health Commun.* Epub Feb 12.

Whitfield G and Williams C (2003) The evidence base for cognitive–behavioural therapy in depression: delivery in busy clinical settings. *Adv Psychiatr Treat.* **9**(1): 21–30.

Williamson PR (2011) Appendix 1: a 4–step model of relationship-centered communication. In: A Suchman, DM Sluyter and PR Williamson (eds) *Leading Change in Healthcare: transforming organizations using complexity positive psychology and relationship-centered care.* Radcliffe Publishing, Oxford.

Windish DM, Price EG, Clever SL, Magaziner JL and Thomas PA (2005) Teaching medical students the important connection between communication and clinical reasoning. *J Gen Intern Med.* **20**(12): 1108–13.

Wissow LS, Roter DL and Wilson MEH (1994) Pediatrician interview style and mothers' disclosure of psychosocial issues. *Pediatrics.* **93**(2): 289–95.

Wolff JL and Roter DL (2012) Older adults' mental health function and patient-centered care: does the presence of a family companion help or hinder communication? *J Gen Intern Med.* **27**(6): 661–8.

Wolfolk R and Allen L (2006) *Treating Somatization: a cognitive-behavioral approach.* Guilford Press, New York, NY.

Woolley H, Stein A, Forrest GC and Baum JD (1989) Imparting the diagnosis of life-threatening illness in children. *BMJ.* **41**: 1623–6.

World Health Organization (1985) *Targets for Health for All.* WHO Regional Office for Europe, Copenhagen.

Wright LM, Watson WL and Bell JM (1996) *Beliefs: the heart of healing in families and illness.* Basic Books, New York, NY.

Young HN, Bell RA, Epstein RM, Feldman MD and Kravitz RL (2008) Physicians' shared decision-making behaviors in depression care. *Arch Intern Med.* **168**(13): 1404–8.

Young B, Dixon-Woods M, Windridge KC and Heney D (2003) Managing communication with young people who have a potentially life threatening chronic illness: qualitative study of patients and parents. *BMJ.* **326**(7384): 305.

Zaleta AK and Carpenter BD (2010) Patient-centered communication during the disclosure of a dementia diagnosis. *Am J Alzheimers Dis Other Demen.* **25**(6): 513–20.

Zandbelt LC, Smets EM, Oort FJ, Godfried MH and de Haes HC (2007) Patient participation in the medical specialist encounter: does physicians' patient-centred communication matter? *Patient Educ Couns.* **65**(3): 396–406.

Ziebland S, Evans J and McPherson A (2006) The choice is yours? How women with ovarian cancer make sense of treatment choices. *Patient Educ Couns.* **62**(3): 361–7.

Zimmermann C, Del Piccolo L, Bensing J, Bergvik S, De Haes H, Eide H, Fletcher I, Goss C, Heaven C, Humphris G, Kim YM, Langewitz W, Meeuwesen L, Nuebling M, Rimondini M, Salmon P, van Dulmen S, Wissow L, Zandbelt L and Finset A (2011) Coding patient emotional cues and concerns in medical consultations: the Verona coding definitions of emotional sequences (VR-CoDES). *Patient Educ Couns.* **82**(2): 141–8.

Zimmermann C, Del Piccolo L and Finset A (2007) Cues and concerns by patients in medical consultations: a literature review. *Psychol Bull.* **133**(3): 438–63.

Zolnierek KBH and Dimatteo MR (2009) Physician communication and patient adherence to treatment: a meta-analysis. *Med Care.* **47**(8): 826–34.

Index

References to figures, tables and boxes are in **bold**; references to footnotes are followed by n.

Author index

References to footnotes are followed by n.

CPD with Radcliffe

You can now use a selection of our books to achieve CPD (Continuing Professional Development) points through directed reading.

We provide a free online form and downloadable certificate for your appraisal portfolio. Look for the CPD logo and register with us at: www.radcliffehealth.com/cpd

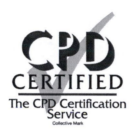